*PROTECTING CHILDREN
FROM ABUSE AND NEGLECT*

Protecting Children from Abuse and Neglect

Foundations for a New National Strategy

Edited by
Gary B. Melton
Frank D. Barry

Foreword by Richard D. Krugman

The Guilford Press
New York   London

© 1994 The Guilford Press
A Division of Guilford Publications, Inc.
72 Spring Street, New York, NY 10012

Printed in the United States of America

This book is printed on acid-free paper.

Last digit is print number: 9 8 7 6 5 4 3 2 1

Library of Congress Cataloging-in-Publication Data

Protecting children from abuse and neglect : foundations for a new
   national strategy / edited by Gary B. Melton, Frank D. Barry.
      p.   cm.
   Includes bibliographical references and index.
   ISBN 0-89862-265-4
    1. Child abuse—United States.   2. Child abuse—United States—
Prevention.   3. Social networks—United States.   I. Melton, Gary B.
II. Barry, Frank D.
HV6626.52.P76   1994
362.7'6'0973—dc20   94-18298
                                                            CIP

Contributors

Frank D. Barry, MS, Senior Extension Associate, Family Life Development Center, College of Human Ecology, Cornell University, Ithaca, New York

James Garbarino, PhD, Director, Family Life Development Center, College of Human Ecology, Cornell University, Ithaca, New York

Jill E. Korbin, PhD, Professor, Department of Anthropology, Case Western Reserve University, Cleveland, Ohio

Kathleen Kostelny, PhD, Senior Research Associate, Erikson Institute for Advanced Study in Child Development, Chicago, Illinois; Assistant Professor, Loyola University, Chicago Illinois

Paul Lerman, DSW, Professor Emeritus, School of Social Work, Rutgers University–State University of New Jersey, New Brunswick

Gary B. Melton, PhD, Director, Institute for Families in Society, University of South Carolina, Columbia

Leroy H. Pelton, PhD, Professor, School of Social Work, Salem State College, Salem, Massachusetts

Ross A. Thompson, PhD, Professor, Department of Psychology, University of Nebraska, Lincoln

David A. Wolfe, PhD, ABPP, Professor, Department of Psychology, University of Western Ontario, and Institute for Prevention of Child Abuse, London, Ontario

Foreword

The last three decades have seen remarkable growth in the recognition of the extent and significance of child abuse and neglect in the United States and around the world. What was thought in 1960 to be a problem that affected fewer than 1,000 children annually is now known to affect more than 1,000 times that number. Society's response, as measured through its organized child protection system and state and federal statutes, recently has been studied by the U.S. Advisory Board on Child Abuse and Neglect (hereafter "the Board"), and found to be in an "emergency" state. In its landmark 1990 report, the Board called attention to the emergency and suggested that a new, comprehensive, neighborhood-based, child-centered, family-focused system should replace the existing one in the United States.

The chapters in this volume form part of the intellectual matrix for the new system the Board envisioned. Following the issuance of the 1991 report that set forth the changes that would be necessary in the federal government in order to allow the development of a new child protection system, the Board commissioned the chapters in this volume to inform its discussions. All those interested in children and their protection will find valuable conceptual and practical lessons here.

Any major redirection in an enterprise as large, complex, and costly as a nation's child protection system surely is difficult. Such change inevitably will be fought by those who believe that with a little more money and a little more time, the existing problems with the system can be solved and children can be served and protected. After several years of deliberation and review of the existing data, the Board felt that such an approach would fail. There is neither the time nor the space here to enumerate all the reasons for this position—the reports of the Board are comprehensive in scope and documentation—but the readers of this volume would be advised to understand the context in which these chapters were developed. There is no quick fix to rebuilding a system that is beyond repair. Accomplishment of society's goal of protecting children from all forms of maltreatment will require the new system suggested by the Board and built on the framework put forth in these papers.

Anyone who *cares* for children, in every sense of that word, will find this volume useful. Anyone who is involved in policy development or implementation in the field of child welfare and child abuse and neglect should heed the messages that are clearly stated here.

RICHARD D. KRUGMAN
Dean, School of Medicine
University of Colorado, Denver

Contents

*PROTECTING CHILDREN
FROM ABUSE AND NEGLECT*

Neighbors Helping Neighbors: The Vision of the U.S. Advisory Board on Child Abuse and Neglect

Gary B. Melton
Frank D. Barry

The U.S. Advisory Board on Child Abuse and Neglect has concluded that child abuse and neglect in the United States now represents a national emergency. (U.S. Advisory Board on Child Abuse and Neglect, 1990, p. 2)

With this terse but dramatic proclamation, a new federal advisory board grabbed headlines across the nation one day in August 1990. For a day or two, the threat of catastrophe—perhaps more aptly, the *description* of a catastrophe occurring daily—in the nation's child protection system was the focus of attention on most of the network news talk shows and in many of the nation's major newspapers.

Initially appointed in the transition between the Reagan and Bush administrations, the U.S. Advisory Board on Child Abuse and Neglect (the Board) may have been an improbable source of activism—particularly of activism that anyone noticed. Created by the 1988 amendments to the Child Abuse Prevention and Treatment Act of 1974 (CAPTA), the Board consists of 15 members appointed to represent various constituencies in the child protection system (in our cases, adolescent services and psychology). Few among the original appointees knew each other prior to their appointment, and few were widely known in the child protection field. Although few of the members had obvious ties to the Republican Party,[1] there is little question that midlevel officials in the Department of Health and Human Services expected that this board, like scores of other federal advisory bodies, would confine its activity to attendance at occasional meetings and preparation of reports offering advice about narrow questions of agency administration.[2]

Coming from their diverse backgrounds, the Board members shared a concern with the state of the field of child protection and, in particular, the lack of leadership in responding to the problems within it, at least within recent years. Collectively, the Board decided to use its broad, vague statutory charge to review progress in fulfilling the purposes of CAPTA—an act without express purposes—as the authority to consider the state of the field as a whole. In essence, the Board conceptualized its primary mission as the evaluation of the nation's progress in ensuring the safety of its children and the development of a vision for more effective protection of children. This inquiry and the resulting reports provided the first comprehensive look at the effectiveness of the child protection system.

THE NATURE OF THE PROBLEM

As the Board struggled to understand what needed to be done to protect the nation's children, we developed what became a typical practice of sometimes exhilarating, often frustrating meetings that ran late into the night and were followed by countless hours of writing and conference calls. The exhilaration came at those peak moments when our conceptualization of a particular aspect of the problem or its solution "clicked" among ourselves or the audience with whom we were communicating. The frustration came as we recognized the scale and severity of the problem and the lack of a coherent prevailing understanding of it, and confronted the lack of official care and responsiveness in dealing with it.

The Board began its work by developing and attempting to respond to a list of hundreds of issues in the prevention, investigation, adjudication, and treatment of child abuse and neglect. It was at that point that the Board reached the collective conclusion that the problems in the child protection system were of such enormity and pervasiveness that a declaration of a national emergency was appropriate.[3] That conclusion was based on three broad factual findings and a value perspective.

The Board found first that the declaration of a national emergency was justified by the sheer scope of the problem: "In spite of the nation's avowed aim of protecting its children, each year *hundreds of thousands* of them are still being starved and abandoned, burned and severely beaten, raped and sodomized, berated and belittled" (U.S. Advisory Board on Child Abuse and Neglect [U.S. ABCAN], 1990, p. 2, emphasis in the original).

When Kempe and his colleagues identified the battered child syndrome in the early 1960s (Kempe, Silverman, Steele, Droegemueller, & Silver, 1962), their revelation was sufficiently startling to lead within a few years to a mandatory reporting system in all 50 states, but they estimated that the phenomenon applied to only about 300 children in the United States. By the time that the Board released its 1990 report, the number of officially recorded reports of suspected maltreatment had reached 2.4 million; by the time of the release of the 1993 report, the number had climbed to almost 3 million (McCurdy & Daro, 1993).

The Board's second major finding was that: "the *system* the nation has devised to respond to child abuse and neglect is *failing*. It is not a question of acute failure of a single element of the system; there is chronic and critical multiple organ failure" (U.S. ABCAN, 1990, p. 2, emphasis in the original).

Stated differently, the enormous problem of child maltreatment is mirrored in the enormous failure of the child protection system. This mismatch between the nature and scope of the problem and the nature and scope of the response is not limited to Child Protective Services, although the Board gave special attention to the short-term need to bolster that critical element of the child protection system as it now exists. Rather, the failure in child protection extends to education, health, mental health, justice, housing, and other service and research systems that should be involved in a comprehensive child protection strategy.

Third, the Board found that the declaration of a national emergency was warranted by the huge direct and indirect costs of a failed system:

> The Board estimates that the United States spends *billions* of dollars on programs that deal with the *results* of the nation's failure to prevent and treat child abuse and neglect. Billions are spent on law enforcement, juvenile and criminal courts, foster care and residential facilities, and the treatment of adults who themselves were maltreated in a prior generation. Billions more are spent on efforts to prevent substance abuse, eating disorders, adolescent pregnancy, suicide, juvenile delinquency, prostitution, pornography, and violent crime—all of which have substantial roots in childhood abuse and neglect. (U.S. ABCAN, 1990, p. 3, emphasis in the original)

The Board made clear, however, that urgent attention to the problem of child maltreatment would be warranted even if it did not exact such a heavy cost:

> *Child abuse is wrong. Not only is child abuse wrong, but the nation's lack of an effective response to it is also wrong. Neither can be tolerated. Together they constitute a moral disaster....* Tolerating child abuse denies the worth of children as human beings and makes a mockery of the American principle of respect for the rights and needs of each individual.
> *Child neglect is also wrong.*
> Children must be given the basic necessities of life—food, shelter, clothing, health care, education, emotional nurturance—so that they do not suffer needless pain. If children are to become full participants in the community, then they must be given basic sustenance so that they will then be in a position to develop their own personality and point of view. When those who have as-

sumed responsibility for providing the necessary resources for children (usually parents) fail to do so, it is wrong. When parents and other caretakers have the psychological capacity to care for their children adequately but lack the economic resources to do so, *society itself is derelict* when it fails to provide such assistance. (U.S. ABCAN, 1990, pp. 3–4, emphasis in the original)

People at all points on the continuum of political ideology acknowledge that government has a responsibility to ensure the safety of dependent persons, especially children. Faced with this moral imperative and the failure of the existing child protection system, the Board argued that the time had come to develop a new national child protection strategy that would be *comprehensive, child centered, neighborhood based*, and *family focused*. Although the Board recognized that there was an immediate need to repair the gaping holes in the existing child protection system, we also concluded that ultimately a new approach was needed, and we promised to develop it across the following decade.

THE INHERENT PROBLEMS
IN THE CHILD PROTECTION SYSTEM

The Board identified the current system as fundamentally flawed in its primary emphasis on reporting and investigation. When the problem was thought to exist for only a few hundred children, the greatest need appeared to be identification of the children and families involved—hence, the enactment of mandatory reporting laws:

> At the time, this strategy seemed reasonable. Child maltreatment was thought to be an uncommon, though egregious problem, and the major obstacle to an effective solution was uncovering the cases. It is unlikely that anyone foresaw either the complexity of the cases that would ultimately emerge or the stunning and continuing increase that would occur in their numbers. (U.S. ABCAN, 1993, p. 10, footnote omitted)

Not only did the states focus their attention on reporting laws, but the federal government later stimulated a broadening of these laws by requiring certain provisions as a condition for funding under CAPTA. From the beginning, the requirements for reporting and investigation were far more explicit than those for prevention or treatment. It should not be surprising, therefore, that the response to the reporting hot lines has far outstripped workers' ability to help the families reported. Even more fundamentally, it is questionable whether a system so focused on ferreting out abusers and subjecting them to coercive interventions could be effective even if the resources were dramatically increased. As the system currently exists, nearly half the families in which maltreatment is substantiated do not receive even the pretense of any "service" other than investigation (McCurdy & Daro, 1993).

It is difficult to discern now whether the focus on investigation caused or resulted from a mistaken formulation of the policy questions underlying development of the child protection system. What is clear, though, is that far more attention is given in discussions about child protection to the question of the threshold and limits for justifiable coercive intervention in family life than to the broader, more fundamental question of the steps that society can take to prevent harm to children.

Analogously, at the level of individual families, practice tends to focus on determination of what happened, not what can be done to help. The system responds to allegations, not needs. This investigative focus—what the Board termed "checking off boxes" (U.S. ABCAN, 1993, p. 10)—detracts from development of effective plans to prevent initial or further harm and, ironically and tragically, often results even in ignoring children's own experience in the system.

THE BOARD'S APPROACH

The Policy

Although the Board found many grave problems in the child protection system, none was more troubling than the lack of a coherent sense of mission. Too often investigation seems to occur for its own sake. Put succinctly, the system is not child centered. Children are the parties least likely to be represented in the child protection system, and they themselves rarely receive therapeutic services. Most fundamentally, their interests are lost in the focus on what their parents did or did not do.

The Board made clear that its espousal of a child-centered child protection system did not mean a lack of an emphasis on strengthening families. Concern for children as people will be reflected in due respect for the relationships important to them:

> The Board believes that the time has come for a Federal policy *based on respect for the inherent dignity and inalienable rights of children as members of the human community.* That policy should be rooted in the companion ideas that *the family* (whether biological, adoptive, or foster) is the unit in society *most likely to secure children's safe and healthy development* and that *children have a meaningful right to live safely in a family environment.* (U.S. ABCAN, 1991, p. 35, emphasis in the original)

Recognizing that respect for children's dignity "requires protection of their integrity as persons," the Board argued for adoption of an explicit policy acknowledging that "the several Governments of the United States share a profound responsibility to ensure that children enjoy, at a minimum . . . protection of their physical, sexual, and psychological security" (U.S. ABCAN, 1991, p. 43). Such a fundamental duty implies the need for care: a system that is *planned*. To promote such care, the Board (U.S. ABCAN, 1991) advocated adoption of a national child protection policy that would articulate the principles that should guide government action and that would establish a duty of federal officials to act with due urgency in fulfilling them.

In that regard, the Board argued that "the principal goal of governmental involvement in child protection should be to facilitate comprehensive community efforts to ensure the safe and healthy development of children" (U.S. ABCAN, 1991, p. 46). This focus on facilitation of help by neighbors for each other was based on the premises that child protection should be part of everyday life, that services that are highly integrated into neighborhood settings have been shown to be the most effective means of prevention and treatment of child abuse and neglect, and that neighborhood quality is an important factor in rates of child maltreatment.

The Vision

The Board's vision is one of a "neighborly" society—a society in which "all American adults . . . resolve to be good neighbors—to know, watch, and support their neighbors' children and to offer help when needed to their neighbors' families" (U.S. ABCAN, 1993, p. 82). Although such a view has seldom been related to the protection of children, it is consonant with the American tradition of volunteerism and mutual assistance. The Board recognized, though, that achievement of such a vision of "natural" helping no longer can be assumed to occur without diligent planning and action:

> Although the Board's strategy builds on such historic values of our society, it does so with recognition of the need to accommodate to trends in the post-industrial age that have weakened the expectation of voluntary help by neighbors for each other and that have reshaped not only neighborhoods but also the families within them. (U.S. ABCAN, 1993, p. 81)

The Board noted further that fulfillment of its vision would not be easy:

> It will require reversal of powerful social trends, within neighborhoods at highest risk (those that have been "drained") and the nation as a whole. . . .
> [If American children are to have a society in which they need not live in fear, then we must create not] utopia but . . . instead a society that cares enough about children as people to permit childhood. . . .
> To that end, the Nation must strive diligently to overcome the isolation created by the demands of modern life and exacerbated by the ravages of poverty. We must tear down the walls that divide us by race, class, and age, and

we must create caring communities that support the families and shelter the children within them. We must take the time to see the need and lend a hand. (U.S. ABCAN, 1993, pp. 81–82)

The Strategy

The Federal Role

After the release of the 1990 report declaring a national emergency, the Board began its work in the pursuit of such a vision by examining the role of the federal government. In part, this starting point was driven by institutional concerns; after all, the Board is a federal body. There also were substantive considerations:

> Although the Board concurs that Federal action alone is insufficient for the social transformation that is necessary for the protection of children, it is also clear that such fundamental change cannot occur on a national scale without a reformation of Federal policy. Indeed, it is clear that community change— even more basically, comprehensive services for individual maltreated children and their families—will remain difficult to accomplish without Federal reform. (U.S. ABCAN, 1991, p. 147)

The Board described its report on the federal role in child protection as "but a way-station (albeit an important one) on the road to a new national strategy for child protection" (U.S. ABCAN, 1991, p. 148). In that regard, the Board indicated its intent to stimulate federal programs that are as follows:

> • Sufficiently intensive and diverse to provide communities with the support that they need to develop a comprehensive neighborhood-based, child-centered, and family-focused approach to child protection; and,
> • Sufficiently flexible that they can adapt to both (1) the needs and strengths of particular States, Tribes, and communities, and (2) changes in the state of the art as the neighborhood-based strategy is tested and evolves. Attention to the Federal role is necessary now for development of structures and programs to facilitate communities' efforts to protect their children and strengthen their families. (U.S. ABCAN, 1991, p. 148)

Building on the federal government's historic roles, the Board recommended establishment of a national child protection policy (as already discussed), development of programmatic emphases on child abuse and neglect in many agencies (with the intent of fostering involvement by the relevant professional constituencies), establishment of a major research initiative bolstered by state and regional resource centers, and blended funding for neighborhood-based child protection programs (with funding obtained through a single state interagency plan).

Ironically, most of the response to the report on the federal role came from the private sector.[4] The Board highlighted a recommendation to move toward universal voluntary neonatal home visitation (see Melton, 1993):

> The Federal Government should begin planning for the sequential implementation of a universal voluntary neonatal home visitation system. The first step in the planning process should be the funding of a large series of coordinated pilot projects. Instead of reaffirming the efficacy of home visiting as a preventive measure—already well-established—these projects should aim at providing the Federal Government with the information needed to establish and administer a national home visitation system. (U.S. ABCAN, 1991, Recommendation G-1)

Conceived as a well-validated way of building neighborhood-level support for families at a time of developmental transition, the Board's proposed federal initiative for home visitation was taken up instead by the National Committee to Prevent Child Abuse (NCPCA), with funding by the Ronald McDonald Charities. Although no state is yet close to *universal* infant home visitation, the NCPCA has succeeded in building initiatives in most states, usually through partnerships between state government and private groups (Mitchel & Donnelly, 1993). Other foundations also have expressed interest in promoting home visitation (see, e.g., Behrman, 1993).

The National Strategy

As the example of infant home visitation illustrates, it is our impression that the Board's reports have had substantially more impact outside Washington than within it. In keeping with the idea that the real action in child protection is necessarily at the neighborhood level, the primary audience for the ultimate report on the new national strategy (released in 1993) was the field as whole. The report describes ways in which people in every sector, including local officials and civic, religious, and business organizations, can carve a niche in a neighborhood-based child protection system.

The strategy consists of five elements (see U.S. ABCAN, 1993, for specific recommendations and their justification):

1. *Strengthening urban, suburban, and rural neighborhoods as environments for children and families.* The Board noted that it is time to start paying as much attention to the environment for our own species as we do for the environment for fish and wildlife. That shift requires "strengthen[ing] neighborhoods, both physically and socially, so that people care about, watch, and support each other's families" and so that child protection becomes "a part of everyday life, a function of all sectors of the community" (U.S. ABCAN, 1993, p. 3, emphasis removed). The Board's top-priority recommendation was for "*the creation of Prevention Zones—*model neighborhoods in which intensive efforts are made to facilitate neighbors helping neighbors and to pro-

mote economic and social development for the purpose of preventing child abuse and neglect" (U.S. ABCAN, 1993, p. 3, emphasis in the original).

2. *Reorienting the delivery of human services "so that it becomes as easy to provide services to prevent child maltreatment and other forms of family disintegration as it is to place a child in foster care after the fact"* (U.S. ABCAN, 1993, p. 4). Help should be easily available to families before a crisis occurs; services provided afterward are in some respects already too late. Prevention and treatment should be integrated into neighborhood settings so that giving and receiving help are part of everyday life.

Foster care itself should be reconceptualized as part of a neighborhood-based system in which foster families often serve as partners to—rather than substitutes for—biological or adoptive families. In such a circumstance, children may have additional caretakers but still maintain strong ties with their biological or adoptive parents.

3. *Improving the role of government in child protection.* Government fiscal incentives should be reoriented to emphasize prevention and treatment rather than investigation and foster care. Fiscal policies should promote blending of funding streams in order to facilitate integration of services.

Child protection efforts should be carefully planned, whether at the federal or the neighborhood level. They should be consistent with a national child protection policy (as proposed by the Board).

4. *Reorienting societal values that may contribute to child maltreatment.* Due respect should be given to children's rights and needs; an important starting point would be ratification of the U.N. Convention on the Rights of the Child. Steps must also be taken to reduce the acceptance of violence as a means of resolving conflict, change attitudes that may contribute to the exploitation and sexualization of children, and promote appreciation of cultural differences as a source of strength in our society.

5. *Strengthening and broadening the knowledge base about child maltreatment.* A problem as serious as child maltreatment demands care in developing and applying policies and practices. Unfortunately, however, the nation's research capacity in this regard is woefully underdeveloped. Funding has been abysmal, and federal research management in this area has been little better. Program evaluation has been given little attention; the proposed program of prevention zones would offer a natural laboratory in that regard. Research programs should be reshaped so that more is learned about the experiences of children themselves as well as other actors in the child protection system.

THE SIGNIFICANCE OF THIS VOLUME

The process by which the new national strategy was devised was methodical. Besides holding hearings and symposia and conducting site visits, the

Board commissioned the papers collected as chapters in this book in order to provide background for its work. The papers themselves and discussions with their authors helped the Board to define its vision and to articulate what is needed to move toward its realization; accordingly, ideas drawn from all the papers were incorporated into the Board's 1993 report. Each paper is provocative and scholarly—apart from the immediate significance to the Board, an important contribution to the field. This book resulted from the conviction that the papers ought to be widely available to scholars and practitioners in the field.

Two of the papers were especially influential in helping the Board to develop the general framework for its work: Barry (Chapter 2) turns the focus to the need to create safe *environments* for children, and he clarifies the meaning of neighborhoods in the lives of children and families. Garbarino and Kostelny's paper (Chapter 7)—as well as their research (reviewed in the paper) on the link between neighborhood quality and the prevalence of child maltreatment—led the Board to make the establishment of prevention zones the number one recommendation in its 1993 report and identified elements that must be present in a neighborhood-based strategy.

The Board's questions about the usefulness of material, informal social, formal social supports in protecting children resulted in the papers by Pelton (Chapter 4), Thompson (Chapter 3), and Wolfe (Chapter 6), respectively. In combination with several of the other papers in this volume, Pelton's work encouraged the Board to emphasize the importance of an economic base for neighborhood development, provision of direct material supports to strengthen troubled families,[5] and development of strong housing programs as critical elements in a child protection strategy. These points were given further emphasis by Thompson's thorough review of the complexity of effective social support—a review that concludes that social support by itself is not enough—and by Wolfe's exhaustive review of the treatment outcome research, which also pointed out the limitations of a post hoc therapeutic approach in having a significant effect on the problem of child maltreatment.

Thompson and Wolfe also reinforce the Board's view that a *comprehensive*, multifactor approach is needed to address the complex problems typically experienced by families in which child abuse or neglect occurs. Thompson's paper also stimulates a focus on *reciprocity* of helping and, therefore, the Board's emphasis on community service and development of settings (e.g., neighborhood centers) that promote "natural" helping, including an expectation that families will give as well as receive help.

These papers—along with those by the other authors—also point out the sparseness of research useful in building a comprehensive child protection strategy. The contributors' observations in that regard not only served as the foundation for the Board's recommendations (included in its 1993 report) on research specifically related to a child-centered, neighborhood-based child protection strategy, but also lent support to the Board's evolving views about the serious defects in the nation's capacity for research on child maltreatment (Melton & Flood, 1994).

Korbin's paper (Chapter 5) confirms the view that race or ethnicity, apart from social class, is not an important factor in rates of child maltreatment, but she also emphasizes the signficance of persistent, concentrated poverty. In addition, her chapter underscores the need to understand, appreciate, and incorporate different cultures in our approach to reduce child maltreatment— a view that is reflected in the Board's recommendations in regard to the need to change societal attitudes.

Lerman's paper (Chapter 8) derived from the Board's concern with building settings that "demand" safety for children. Noting that placement does not guarantee safety from child maltreatment, Lerman proposes a number of federal actions that could reduce the number of children placed out of their homes. His conclusions also bolster the Board's view that while more must be done to protect children in foster care and institutional placement, much more must be done to reduce the necessity for such placements in the first place. Lerman's paper resulted in recommendations for federal leadership in development of research-based standards for children's care.

Taken together, the chapters in this volume advance the conclusion that simply adding more child protection workers will not solve the problem of child abuse and neglect. What is needed is no less than a rebuilding of our society, with a particular focus on strengthening neighborhoods. We need to build a new safety net that confirms the worth of children as persons and includes both economic and social supports and that provides help to people when they need it wherever they are.

Weaving a new social fabric is undoubtedly an ambitious task, but doing so is critical if we are to address poverty, social isolation, and other problems that, especially when in pernicious combination, threaten the safety of many of our children. In an era in which life has become so complex that people have less and less time for each other, we need new policies, programs, and grass-roots action that build or rebuild connections among and within families. The chapters in this book go far toward the development of the knowledge base necessary to plan and implement such change.

ACKNOWLEDGMENT

The authors were members of the U.S. Advisory Board on Child Abuse and Neglect from its inception in 1989 until 1993. The authors wish to acknowledge their colleagues on the Board for their contributions to the deliberations that led to the proposal for a new national strategy for child protection, but the opinions expressed do not necessarily reflect those of the Board as a whole. All royalties from the sale of this volume have been donated to Parents Anonymous, Inc.

NOTES

1. In making this point, we wish also to make clear that the Board has regarded child protection as a matter that should be of concern to everyone, regardless of party. We do not know the party identification of most of our former colleagues. When members apparently had been appointed at least in part for political reasons, nonetheless they generally transcended partisan or political–ideological concerns in their approach to the Board's work. The Board was as vociferous in criticizing the Democrat-controlled Congress for its inaction as it was in cajoling the Republican administrations to develop a strategy commensurate with the enormity and seriousness of the problem of child maltreatment.

2. Beyond the fortuitous mix of unanimous commitment, diverse expertise, and an executive director and several members with more than ordinary *chutzpah*, the Board's ability to take a broad view has been facilitated by its statutory dual reporting line (to Congress as well as the secretary of the Department of Health and Human Services and the director of the National Center on Child Abuse and Neglect). This placement between the executive and legislative branches has enabled the Board and its staff to communicate directly with Congress and the public without the usual administrative clearance.

3. The Board conceptualized the *child protection system* as encompassing the range of sectors that are or should be involved in prevention, investigation, adjudication, or treatment of child abuse and neglect. As such, it is far broader than Child Protective Services (CPS), the social services agency with responsibility for civil (family court) investigation of child protection cases. Although the failings of CPS agencies are well known, the Board was as concerned about the lack of effective prevention, treatment, and research programs, including programs addressing schools and other settings important in children's lives.

4. Although most of the action took place outside the D.C. area, the 1991 report did stimulate a vociferous debate in Washington. Perhaps for the first time, representatives of relevant interest groups (e.g., psychology, social work, and child advocacy organizations) engaged in protracted and sometimes heated debate about the strategies that should be adopted to protect children. The House also insisted on a 1-year rather than 3-year reauthorization of CAPTA in order to have extra time to develop the legislation needed to effect the Board's far-reaching view of the federal role in child protection. In the end, though, the changes to CAPTA in the 1992 reauthorization were largely cosmetic.

5. On its site visit to programs in Hennepin County, Minnesota, the Board also was impressed by an experimental voucher program that enabled troubled families to purchase services that they would find helpful.

REFERENCES

Behrman, R. E. (Ed.). (1993). Home visiting [Special issue]. *Future of Children*, 3(3).
Child Abuse Prevention and Treatment Act of 1974, Pub. L. No. 93-247, 88 Stat. 4.
Kempe, C. H., Silverman, F., Steele, B., Droegemueller, W., & Silver, H. (1962). The battered child syndrome. *Journal of the American Medical Association*, 181, 17–24.

McCurdy, K., & Daro, D. (1993). Child maltreatment: A national survey of reports and fatalities. *Journal of Interpersonal Violence, 9,* 75–94.

Melton, G. B. (1993, Winter). Infant home visitation: One step toward creation of caring communities. *APSAC Advisor,* pp. 5–6, 26–27.

Melton, G. B., & Flood, M. F. (1994). Research policy and child maltreatment: Developing the scientific foundation for effective protection of children. *Child Abuse and Neglect, 18*(Supp. 1), 1–28.

Mitchel, L., & Donnelly, A. C. (1993, Winter). Healthy Families America: Building a national system. *APSAC Advisor,* pp. 9–10, 27.

U.S. Advisory Board on Child Abuse and Neglect. (1990). *Child abuse and neglect: Critical first steps in response to a national emergency* (Stock No. 017-092-00104-5). Washington, DC: U.S. Government Printing Office.

U.S. Advisory Board on Child Abuse and Neglect. (1991). *Creating caring communities: Blueprint for an effective federal policy on child abuse and neglect.* Washington, DC: Author.

U.S. Advisory Board on Child Abuse and Neglect. (1993). *Neighbors helping neighbors: A new national strategy for the protection of children.* Washington, DC: U.S. Government Printing Office.

Chapter 2

A Neighborhood-Based Approach: What Is It?

Frank D. Barry

Both researchers and practitioners have written about the importance of the neighborhood and the community in relation to family and child development and about the importance of relating human service intervention to the neighborhood level (Cochran, Larner, Riley, Gunnarsson, & Henderson, 1990; National Commission on Child Welfare and Family Preservation, 1990). A neighborhood-based approach is listed as a cornerstone of the recommendations of the U.S. Advisory Board on Child Abuse and Neglect (U.S. ABCAN, 1990) in its first report. This chapter attempts to identify and analyze various factors that must be considered in understanding and developing a neighborhood-based strategy for preventing child abuse and neglect.

THE CASE FOR A NEIGHBORHOOD FOCUS

The Board's (1990) first report emphasized the importance of the neighborhood family ecology in terms of its potential to either prevent or provoke child abuse and neglect. The report specifically mentions the effect of "dysfunctional communities":

> [Such communities are] unable to provide even the basic necessities of food, clothing, shelter and employment for large numbers of their residents, let alone amenities most take for granted, such as adequate health care, adequate education, and opportunities for social networking, recreation and personal development in legitimate and constructive activities. (p. 45)

Schorr (1988), in *Within Our Reach*, says:

> Both common sense and research tell us that as family stress, regardless of its source, increases, the capacity for nurturing decreases, and the likelihood of

14

abuse and neglect increases. Whether the stress stems from insufficient income, a difficult child, an impaired adult, family violence and discord, *inadequate housing, chronic hunger and poor health, or surroundings of brutality, hopelessness and despair*, these are circumstances in which affection withers into hostility, *discipline turns into abuse*, stability dissolves into chaos, and *love becomes neglect*. (p. 151, emphasis added)

The National Commission on Children (1991) concurs. The Commission's final report states that "rebuilding a sense of community and reinvigorating informal systems of support for families and children should be a primary goal of social policies" (pp. 70–71).

Kromkowski (1976) writes, "A neighborhood's character is determined by a host of factors, but most significantly by the kinds of relationships that neighbors have with each other" (p. 228). Cochran and Brassard (1979) argued that the relationships parents have with other adults play a major role in helping (or hindering) them in their task of raising their children successfully. Cochran (1988) later found that expansion of the personal network of single mothers positively affected the performance of their children in school.

According to Garbarino and Sherman (1980), an impoverished neighborhood environment can make it very difficult to develop and maintain social support relationships:

The high risk neighborhood is not a good place to bring up children. A family's own problems seem to be compounded rather than ameliorated by the neighborhood context, dominated as it is by other needy families. Under such circumstances strong support systems are most needed, but least likely to operate. (p. 195)

In a more recent paper, Garbarino and Kostelny (1992) compared neighborhood characteristics, attitudes, and child abuse reporting rates in several Chicago neighborhoods. They concluded that "child maltreatment is a symptom of not just individual or family trouble, but neighborhood and community trouble as well" (p. 463).

In short, if we are to prevent child abuse and neglect, we cannot ignore environments that, by their nature, predispose families to abuse or neglect their children. Yet, the child protective system in place today focuses largely on individual families rather than on neighborhood or environmental factors. It is based on the assumption that most families function reasonably well and that direct individual attention will be effective for the occasional family that does not. While a system emphasizing an individual approach might be adequate in a healthy community, it cannot work well when the environment in which families live is itself so dysfunctional that even strong families must exert strenuous efforts just to survive. It cannot work well in conditions which Garbarino and Kostelny (1992) refer to as "an ecological conspiracy against children" (p. 463).

HISTORICAL PERSPECTIVE

There is nothing really new about the neighborhood-based approach. In a *Social History of Helping Services*, Levine and Levine (1970) describe the beginnings of mental health and helping services in response to social disorganization resulting from rapid industrialization, immigration, and urbanization after the Civil War. They note that the settlement houses, which began in the 1880s, the first psychological clinic (1896), and other service innovations of the time were heavily community oriented.

> Those early services were embedded in the community, were concerned with the educational process, and were oriented toward prevention. In short . . . our predecessors began with the types of services the community mental health movement seems to be struggling toward today. (p. 1)

What happened in the mental health field was happening in other fields as well. Levine and Levine's (1970) description of the early settlement houses, visiting teachers, and the first probation workers portrays a strong ecological approach in which considerable attention was devoted to environmental problems as a means of meeting individual needs.

During the 1920s and 1930s, according to the Levines, the settlement houses, social workers, mental health clinics, and courts became more bureaucratic and professionalized. In addition, the political climate became more conservative. Collaboration between clinics and schools grew more tenuous; confidentiality became a barrier to interagency communication (Levine & Levine, 1970). Professions developed more rigid identities, and mental health professionals in particular began to suffer what Sarason refers to as professional preciousness—an attitude that holds that "they are the only ones who truly understand . . . individuals beset with problems in living and adjustment" (Sarason, Levine, Goldenberg, Cherlin, & Bennett, 1966, p. 34). This attitude began to overshadow the holistic approach of the early days when settlement house workers, clinicians, and probation officers were feeling their way and working closely with each other and with other elements in the community. By the end of the 1930s, psychoanalysis—perhaps the antithesis of the neighborhood-based approach—had become very popular, especially among upper-class clients. Psychiatric clinics responded by shifting their attention away from their initial constituency, low-income children with behavior problems in school (Levine & Levine, 1970). The neighborhood-based approach was out.

But something deeper was at work as well. The Levines (1970) describe two competing approaches to social work and helping services, "situational" and "intrapsychic," which stem from two fundamentally different assumptions about the nature of people in need of help.

The situational mode assumes a person who is basically "good" but who has been exposed to poor conditions, and therefore has not developed to his fullest potential. Improving his situation (making adjustments to his environment) will result in far-reaching improvement in his psychological state. . . . The intrapsychic mode assumes "goodness" of the environment . . . a person is in difficulty, not because of his situation, but because of his inner weaknesses and failings . . . what has to be changed is not the circumstance but the person. (p. 8)

The Levines (1970) hypothesize that the situational, or community, approach has historically been popular in times of change and reform; the intrapsychic approach has tended to be popular in more conservative eras.

In retrospect, it seems clear that neither approach alone is sufficient; in fact, both are needed. Certainly child abuse and neglect result from serious human deficiencies. Not all, or even most, parents maltreat their children, no matter how poor they are. Yet, if we ignore ecological factors that force many families to live under extremely stressful conditions—conditions that aggravate and may even cause the personal deficiencies that push some of them over the edge—we are unlikely ever to solve the problem. As the Board (1990) has made clear, there is simply no capacity to address all these deficiencies on an individual basis. The present individually based system has become overwhelmed by sheer numbers, and as long as we think chiefly in individualistic terms, it probably always will be.

ECOLOGICAL EFFECTS: BASIC PRINCIPLES

In order to address the prevention of child maltreatment from a community or neighborhood perspective, I propose a set of assumptions that incorporate elements of both approaches described by the Levines:

1. *Child abuse and neglect result in part from stress and social isolation.* The degree of stress and social isolation or integration one experiences depends on both internal (psychological) and external (environmental) factors.

2. *The quality of neighborhoods can either encourage or impede parenting and social integration of the families who live in them.* Because neighborhoods constitute the family environment, some child abuse and neglect can be prevented by improving neighborhoods to reduce stress and facilitate social integration.

3. *The quality of life in neighborhoods is influenced by both external and internal forces.* The quality of life in neighborhoods is influenced both by the nature and the abilities of the people who live in them (internal) and by external forces such as economic conditions, political relationships, and

availability of services and other resources (external). Some of these forces (internal and external) can be easily influenced; others cannot.

4. *Any strategy for preventing child maltreatment should address both internal and external dimensions and should focus on both strengthening at-risk families and improving at-risk neighborhoods.* No comprehensive strategy can afford to ignore either the internal or external (personal vs. environmental) dimensions. Focusing only on helping high-risk families to overcome the effects of an inadequate environment is clearly less effective than attacking the environment itself, but concentrating only on improving the neighborhood environment (providing additional housing, employment, parks, etc.) is not enough when many of the residents have major deficits (such as lack of work experience, inadequate social skills, and an inability to relate well to other people). Schorr (1988) stresses that it is not one factor alone that causes adverse outcomes in childrearing; the "interplay between constitution and environment is far more decisive in shaping an individual than either alone" (p. 25). Schorr says further that "putting together what is known about childhood risk factors shows clearly that the plight of children bearing these risks is not just individual and personal, and therefore requires a societal response" (p. 30).

Schorr (1988) is concerned with far more than child maltreatment, but maltreatment is one of many factors she describes that lead to a series of "rotten outcomes" for children. For Schorr, child maltreatment is also one of a number of negative results of environmental pressures on at-risk families.

SIGNIFICANCE OF NEIGHBORHOOD ACCORDING TO INCOME

Fitchen (1981), Garbarino and Sherman (1980), and Cochran et al. (1990) have written on the importance of the neighborhood environment for the families that reside in it. However, in our highly mobile society many functions once performed in geographical neighborhoods are now accomplished through diverse and extended networks that include contacts at one's job, civic, religious, social, and other organizations that extend far beyond one's geographical area of residence. The automobile, the telephone, and television have greatly reduced the extent to which vital socialization functions are performed on a face-to-face basis among family members and acquaintances living in the same immediate area. For many in middle- and upper-income families, the concept of a close-knit neighborhood as the basis for socialization has been relegated to nostalgia.

However, this is not the case for everyone. While automobile-owning middle-class families can move freely beyond their residential area, low-income families tend to have less ability to move about beyond their neighborhood and fewer connections beyond their immediate environment. Consequently, they are much more vulnerable to conditions within the limited geographic area in which they live (Chavis & Wandersman, 1990). By the same token, the quality of the neighborhood may have much more impact on children than on their parents, because again, children cannot so readily escape it.

For this reason, improving or maintaining the neighborhood becomes critically important for low-income and other low-mobility families. Unfortunately, the neighborhoods that most need help often have the fewest resources available for improvement (Garbarino & Sherman, 1980). Cutbacks in federal and state revenue sharing and other local assistance programs within the last 10 years have aggravated this reality (Hinds & Eckholm, 1990). So has the "brain drain," which has occurred as the more upwardly mobile minority families have left inner-city neighborhoods for less stressful suburban environments, as discriminatory housing practices have broken down (Schorr, 1988).

COMMUNITY VERSUS NEIGHBORHOOD

The terms *community* and *neighborhood* are used frequently, and at times seemingly interchangeably, to denote a grass-roots approach. However, there are real differences in the meanings and they are important for this discussion. *Webster's New Collegiate Dictionary* (1980) makes it clear that the term *community* is the more general of the two. It may refer either to a place or to a class of people having something in common. The community may be small or as large as a "state or commonwealth" or a "community of nations." Chavis and Wandersman (1990) suggest that the idea of a broader sense of community that transcends place is a relatively recent theoretical concept, resulting from the advances in communication and mobility mentioned above.

The term *neighborhood* has not taken such a leap, however. All *Webster's* (1980) definitions still involve the concept of nearness, proximity, or "neighborliness," which presumably requires geographic proximity. As a result, people may belong to a number of communities, depending on their interests, affiliations, and the way community is defined. But most will presumably belong only to one neighborhood, based on the location of their primary residence.

The term *neighborhood* is often used in an urban context, whereas the word *community* may be heard more frequently with respect to rural settings. The term *community* is also more likely to refer to an entire town, city, or county than to a "neighborhood." An urban neighborhood may consist of one or several blocks, whereas a rural neighborhood might consist of several square miles or even more in very sparsely settled areas. For our purposes, a neighborhood constitutes a geographic area within which people feel physically (if not always socially) close to each other. We are especially concerned with neighborhoods whose residents have limited ability to belong to larger communities on the outside because these residents are most profoundly affected by the quality of life in their neighborhoods.

THE NEIGHBORHOOD-BASED APPROACH

A neighborhood-based approach will presumably focus both on improving the viability of the neighborhood itself and on organizing services to individual families in the neighborhood in ways that respond effectively and holistically to their needs. These two facets are intertwined, as some of the individual needs will result from shortcomings of the neighborhood environment and, conversely, the quality of the neighborhood environment will be influenced by the abilities and limitations of the families that live in it. "Families both shape their surroundings and are shaped by them. This interactive process can enhance or undermine family functioning" (Garbarino & Sherman, 1980, p. 189).

For our purposes it may be useful to discuss services to individuals separately from services to the neighborhood; although the two are intertwined, they evolve from different starting points.

Providing Neighborhood-Based Services to Individuals

Perhaps it will be most helpful to view the various aspects of a neighborhood-based service on a continuum, beginning with the most basic characteristics and gradually evolving toward a more complex version of the concept. The neighborhood-based service concept, as presented here, begins with an almost exclusive focus on individual needs within the neighborhood. But as we move across the continuum, the concept takes on characteristics that respond to neighborhood needs in addition to those of the individual. Following is a discussion of five criteria for assessing neighborhood-based services, beginning with the most basic (geographic accessibility), and moving toward the most demanding (neighborhood controlled). The purpose is not to imply that a service is only neighborhood based if it meets all five criteria, but that some services are more neighborhood based than others. The criteria proposed here are offered as a measure for assessing the extent to which different services are neighborhood based.

Geographic Accessibility

The neighborhood-based service concept implies that at least some service should be physically located in the area to be served. This is more important for poor neighborhoods than for middle- and upper-class areas because of the superior mobility of middle- and upper-class residents, yet it is the latter rather than the former who tend to have the most access to facilities. Accessibility may be provided through outposts, shared facilities, or circuit riders if necessary.

Accessibility will always be limited. Obviously it is not practical to have a highly specialized professional such as a surgeon or psychiatrist in every census tract or neighborhood; in fact, the more specialized the service, the more difficult it is to get it out of a centralized location. But accessibility to specialized services can be strengthened when local neighborhood-based services, which are more general in nature, perform outreach, intake, referral, coordinating, and follow-up functions. All this can greatly facilitate access to specialized services located elsewhere. For example, a neighborhood center can improve access to medical care simply by providing a worker to accompany a non-English-speaking immigrant on her first visit to a surgeon located outside the neighborhood.

The important thing is to have at least some services physically present in the neighborhood itself; this can vary from a traveling van that stops regularly to visit rural trailer parks to a full-scale family resource center, settlement house, community center, community school, clinic, outpost, or "one-stop" center.

The locally based center can invite social workers, counselors, doctors, or other specialists into the neighborhood, perhaps on a regular basis, or it can assist local residents in making contacts and arranging transportation to services outside the neighborhood. Such a center might also arrange preventive services such as well-baby clinics, child development classes, play groups, support groups, and home visits that in the long run may reduce the need for more specialized treatment. The key is to have a nonthreatening place where local people can go for help and support without the stigma implied by extensive eligibility requirements.

Accessibility also has a cultural dimension. In neighborhoods with high numbers of ethnic or minority populations, it is important to ensure that program staff reflect the cultural composition of the neighborhood; for members of some cultural groups, an all-white staff who speak English only can be just as much of a barrier to participation as transportation problems or a high fee.

Comprehensiveness

Schorr (1988) has concluded that services that succeed with multiproblem families are comprehensive and flexible. They "typically offer a broad spectrum of services" (p. 256) that may include housing, medical care, food, income, employment, or anything else that seems to the family to be an insurmountable barrier before they can make use of other interventions such as advice on parenting. "No one says, 'this may be what you need, but helping you get it is not part of my job'" (p. 258).

This is not always easy to achieve. According to Schorr (1988):

> What is perhaps most striking about programs that work for the children and families in the shadows is that all of them find ways to adapt or circumvent traditional professional and bureaucratic limitations when necessary to meet the needs of those they serve. (p. 258)

Local Networking and Coordination

"Neighborhood based" implies a connection with all aspects of the neighborhood, including other service agencies and systems, both formal and informal. Local task forces, planning councils, and interdisciplinary teams, supplemented by encouragement of agency staff to form their own interpersonal interagency networks, can make services more effective (Barry, 1989). Coordination at all levels is an important aspect of accessibility; if agencies responding to different problems do not work together, families may get caught up with several agencies at once, some of which may be working in different directions.

Coordination must be measured primarily from the perspective of the recipient of services, which may differ from that of the provider. Consolidated intake procedures, interdisciplinary case management teams, one-stop service locations, ease of referral, and follow-up, all directly benefit those receiving the services.

Neighborhood Involvement in Decision Making

The neighborhood-based service concept presumably implies some involvement of neighborhood residents and organizations in planning and decision making. Rudolph Sutton, of the Philadelphia Health Department, says it well: "Ask them what should be done about the problem: that's how you build trust—by sharing power" (in Cohen & Lang, 1990, p. 13). At the most basic level, involvement can be achieved through consultation with organizations and opinion leaders within the community. A more sophisticated level is reached when community residents serve on advisory or governing boards and hold line and/or administrative positions. Involving people in dysfunctional neighborhoods in planning and service development is somewhat paradoxical because sometimes it can be extremely difficult to find effective, positive leaders in such communities. But this fact simply underscores the urgency of the task. Highly dysfunctional neighborhoods desperately need positive leadership, and planning activities can provide an opportunity for potential leaders to develop their skills. For 25 years, Head Start and other antipoverty agencies have required recipient participation in program planning and governance, and their success has demonstrated that it is possible, if not always easy, to do. The nonprofit Citizens Committee for New York City, which provides assistance and training in leadership development for neighborhood and block associations, now communicates directly with 16,000 such groups, over 5,000 of which it has helped to organize. Many are in low-income, minority neighborhoods (Kaye, 1990).

Neighborhood input and involvement are especially important when the neighborhood is made up of minority cultural groups, particularly when different languages are involved. It can be important also in rural areas, where low-income people's needs and lifestyles may be poorly understood by service administrators and planners. Neighborhood involvement is a means of ensuring that services are relevant to neighborhood needs, gaining acceptance in the neighborhood, and empowering otherwise disenfranchised people to influence their environment and the conditions that affect their lives.

Often neighborhoods with large minority or ethnic populations have more leadership than may be apparent to an outsider. It is important to acknowledge and involve local leadership in any effort to develop neighborhood-based services. Involving local neighborhood leadership permits building the program in such a way as to respect and take advantage of cultural customs and traditions. All cultures have their own mechanisms for responding to human problems, and some practices may be more acceptable and more effective for their members than are standard practices such as counseling and psychotherapy. To the extent possible, neighborhood-based services should be consistent with the cultural values and traditions of neighborhood residents.

Finally, leadership development in dysfunctional neighborhoods is also important, not only to mobilize internal resources but also to utilize external assistance effectively. Such neighborhoods are unlikely to be able to "turn around" with internal resources alone, but neither can they do so solely with external resources. Internal leadership is essential for bringing both together.

Neighborhood Control

Neighborhood services may be developed and provided by community-based organizations that are controlled within the neighborhood. Such organizations may provide local services under contract to state or local public agencies. This is perhaps the most sophisticated example of the neighborhood-based service concept, and neighborhood-based agencies can provide unique opportunities to develop the leadership and skills essential for major neighborhood improvement.

Some neighborhood-based organizations have evolved far beyond the realm of human services, to provide housing, employment, transportation, medical, and even financial services. Such organizations can provide both advocacy on the outside and success stories and role models for those growing up inside the neighborhood. Their success can serve as a source of hope and pride, which are essential for neighborhood improvement.

Strengthening the Neighborhood

Although the previous section focuses on providing services to families, it must be clear by now that such services may have a decidedly positive effect on the neighborhood as well. This section focuses on interventions that start out to strengthen the neighborhood and in the process meet individual family needs as well.

Environmentalists have developed legal procedures and standards to preserve individual species of fish and wildlife. Standards have been established for air and water quality to ensure the survival of those who depend on it.

If a river or lake, or the air in a metropolitan area, fails to meet environmental standards, somebody is required to take action. Government agencies must identify the sources of pollution, prosecute any illegal polluters, and develop and implement plans to reduce the pollution.

Environmental impact studies are now required before any major construction project can go forward, and major projects have been stopped completely because they threatened the environment of a particular species of bird or fish.

The children who live in impoverished and dysfunctional neighborhoods are surely no less important to the survival of our civilization than the snail darter fish or spotted owls now protected under environmental law. Perhaps it is time we invested our energies and legal skills to ensure at least minimally suitable environments for our families and children. Perhaps neighborhoods should be rated on a scale of adequacy versus risk in terms of raising children. Neighborhoods at high risk would receive special attention, just as the discovery of a high level of pollution would bring special attention to a body of water.

Improving the viability of the neighborhood involves attention to physical, social, and psychological aspects. Physical aspects involve housing, jobs, stores, facilities for recreation, day care, and other needs. Social and psychological aspects include improving safety and strengthening various organizations (churches, clubs, sports leagues, civic and political organizations, youth activities) that provide a setting in which people can belong and interact positively with each other. Belonging and interacting are important not only in their own right but also because they facilitate the development and expansion of informal networks among neighborhood residents. Besides strengthening the ability of parents to parent, these networks are essential for achieving the norm of "neighbor helping neighbor" rather than dependency on outside services.

A comprehensive neighborhood improvement approach would involve strategies on several levels.

Neighborhood-Based Planning

Because neighborhoods do not necessarily coincide with political jurisdictions, it can be difficult to ensure that neighborhoods receive adequate attention in the various planning and funding processes that affect them. Planners and politicians often oversee areas that encompass many neighborhoods, and they typically respond most favorably to communities that are best organized rather than those with the greatest needs. A truly neighborhood-based approach would require that local government not only monitor the condition of the various neighborhoods within its boundaries, but also identify those neighborhoods most in need of improvement and develop and implement a plan, in cooperation with their residents, to remedy the most serious problems.

Allocation of Resources

At present, many federal and state funds are distributed to states, counties, cities, and towns without regard to neighborhoods. Because planning often takes place on a larger level there is no guarantee that plans will be responsive to the neediest neighborhoods, or even that they will have a neighborhood focus. A neighborhood-based approach would not only ensure that appropriate resources are distributed to neighborhoods but, as suggested above, also employ criteria to identify at-risk neighborhoods with special needs.

Such at-risk criteria could be based on social indicators such as rates of unemployment, high school dropouts, teen pregnancy, infant mortality, low birth weight, adequacy of prenatal care, child maltreatment reports, and drug usage—all potential indicators of a dysfunctional environment. Once high-risk neighborhoods have been identified, several actions can be taken.

Federal and state governments could establish procedures to ease or waive state restrictions that target funds to narrow problem categories such as housing, alcoholism, or unemployment. Although a typical multiproblem family may face problems in each of these categories and others as well, it is difficult for a community agency to develop a comprehensive response, since each problem category has its own funding streams, regulations, and restrictions. Consequently, addressing more than one problem often means combining and managing funds from different sources and coping with different accounting requirements and regulations, which sometimes even conflict with one another. Perhaps a waiver could be granted to allow regulations and rules from the primary funding source to take precedence over others when funding streams are combined for one family.

The American Public Welfare Association (National Commission on Child Welfare and Family Preservation, 1990) emphasizes the importance of offering some preventive services to everyone rather than following what Cochran and Woolever (1983) call the "deficit model," which requires demonstration of incompetence and dysfunction in order to receive help.

Although it may be too much to provide universal services on a preventive basis immediately, it may be a wise allocation of society's resources to begin by doing so for those individuals who live in a dysfunctional environment. Schorr points out that the most dysfunctional inner-city neighborhoods comprise only 1% of the U.S. population (Schorr, 1988). Even assuming a large undercount factor, providing key preventive services to people in these neighborhoods on a geographic eligibility basis would not unduly strain our country's financial resources, especially compared to the results of our failure to do so (Schorr, 1988). In these neighborhoods, an important objective may be simply to bolster the efforts of families that are presently functional in order to ensure that they remain so.

Finally, extra funds could be provided to help those communities most in need, perhaps through a set-aside for impoverished neighborhood development in existing community development block grant programs. This would follow precedents set by the Appalachian and model cities programs of the 1960s and could offset the vicious cycle of decline in which each level of deterioration sets off others. For example, a local bank closes, making it very difficult for would-be homeowners to buy property; as existing homeowners leave, they are replaced by absentee landlords and renters; crime rates increase, causing some businesses and services to close down, throwing people out of work, and driving some out of the area. Crime increases still more, still more businesses close down. . . .

In assessing the needs of different neighborhoods, particular attention should be paid to several key areas.

1. *Safety.* Gang wars in Chicago, Los Angeles, and elsewhere not only kill many innocent people—children and adults—but have virtually cut off basic human interaction of the type needed to develop and maintain the support networks required to successfully raise children. For parents in these neighborhoods, sheer survival for themselves and their children has become an all-consuming preoccupation (Garbarino, Kostelny, & Dubrow, 1991).

It is ironic that despite the collapse of the Soviet Union we continue to spend hundreds of billions of dollars on weapons of mass destruction and we continue to train and equip our soldiers to combat guerrilla movements in faraway places. We have done far less to end the guerrilla warfare now going on right in some of our own cities—even though the resulting violence is tragically affecting and warping our own children and families. Because of the fear and danger involved, often relatively little can be done to improve community life in neighborhoods where such violence continues. Top priority needs to go to ending the siege-like conditions faced by those who live there.

There are other neighborhoods where violence is less pervasive but still viewed as a serious problem. Here there may be a greater possibility for improvement, or at least prevention of further degradation. It is important to encourage such prevention, lest such neighborhoods fall victim to the kind of violence mentioned above. Some of these neighborhoods have largely been able to banish crack and cocaine dealing by organizing their citizens effectively.

2. *Housing.* Cochran et al. (1990) argue that housing ownership is a critical factor in the stability of neighborhoods and the ability of parents to form individual support networks. When most residents are renters, their commitment to the appearance of the buildings they live in tends to be low, and an atmosphere of disorder results. Perhaps even more important, renting tends to be associated with high residential mobility among the very poor. An illness or any other emergency can consume cash needed for rent payments with predictable results. When families are constantly moving, it is very hard to establish and maintain friendships and support networks. Other countries have found ways to give low-income residents a piece of ownership in their living quarters (Cochran et al., 1990). Whether through subsidized mortgage payments or other means, increasing home ownership would go far in improving social interaction and the quality of life in low-income neighborhoods. Some of the problems faced by dysfunctional neighborhoods have resulted from practices of "redlining" by banks. The refusal to make home improvement or purchase loans to residents of a particular neighborhood virtually guarantees the neighborhood's further decline, as those with the potential and desire to improve their homes are literally forced to move elsewhere. Fortunately, there is now some movement among banks to end this practice (Wayne, 1992).

In addition to inequitable banking practices, the sharp decline in federal investment in low-income housing in the 1980s has been followed by a severe shortage of livable housing units and single-room apartments. In many low-income neighborhoods there simply are not enough homes and apartments available for all who need them. Resolving the problem of low-income housing supply will ultimately require new fiscal priorities at the federal level. Until these priorities change, many low-income neighborhoods are likely to remain unable to provide an adequate environment for families to raise their children successfully. The scarcity of housing units will continue to seriously impede the ability of low-income families to maintain the social support networks that work to prevent child abuse and neglect.

However there are things that can be done on a local level. In Chicago, Shorebank, a community-based corporation, managed to reverse urban blight by bringing together enough investors to establish an island of rehabilitated apartments in a distressed neighborhood. Local residents then came forward to ask for help in buying neighboring buildings. These people would not have risked buying a building in isolation, but "they saw a halo effect from the ongoing project. . . . [and] the island of improved housing grew larger" (Gugliotta, 1994, p. 55). Today, these efforts have succeeded in rehabilitating about 30% of all housing in the neighborhood, and residents are now safer as a result (p. 53).

3. *Education.* Cochran et al. (1990) found that the size of the family network depends directly on the amount of education attained, and he consequently argues for more access to and better post secondary education as a means of improving parenting. Although there are exemplary schools in some low-income neighborhoods, a more flexible approach is needed in many others. Such flexibility might include direct involvement of business and industry to underscore and ensure the relevance of schooling. It might include elements of an apprenticeship program and use of more active teaching tools than reading and lecturing, as well as a more concerted effort, involving parents, to instill an interest in reading.

Clearly more attention is needed to make education more relevant for children who come in without much hope. Schools in a number of communities are finding better ways to involve parents, employers, and the children themselves to make education a more relevant neighborhood enterprise. New York State has developed a "community school" program that provides extra funding to help schools to more fully exploit their potential to involve parents and to strengthen the community.

4. *Municipal Services.* Wallace (1989) has found a high correlation between the closing of fire stations in certain low-income neighborhoods in New York City and the subsequent catastrophic decline of these neighborhoods. Wallace found that in neighborhoods without adequate fire protection, fires were more likely to destroy an entire building rather than simply the room or apartment in which they start. Such fires destabilize a neighborhood, forcing many people to move, often causing overcrowding in the remaining units, which can in turn lead to more fires. Burned-out buildings lead to abandonment by landlords and withdrawal of municipal services, and these ills force many to become "precariously housed" with other family members or friends. Many ultimately leave the neighborhood and/or become homeless. Wallace concludes that the acute housing shortages and population pressure lead to more burnouts, higher rates of substance abuse, homicides, suicides, and AIDS, coincident with the "disruption of personal, domestic and community social networks" (Wallace, 1990, p. 811).

Closing a fire station in a low-income neighborhood can have devastating consequence, as one destroyed building can make scores of people homeless. In contrast, one destroyed building in an upper-income neighborhood usually affects one or two families at most.

Although Wallace picked fires as perhaps the most dramatic consequence of reductions in municipal services, he notes similar results from the reduction in other services such as garbage pickups, health care, and police protection. Any action that weakens the neighborhood increases stress levels for parents, makes survival more difficult, and diminishes their ability to maintain friendships and the support network they need to parent their children successfully.

5. *Economic Development.* Perhaps the most important area of all is economic. Clearly none of the above needs would arise if there were not a serious economic problem in the community. Addressing social needs without addressing fundamental economic issues essentially means treating symptoms while ignoring the cause. Poverty and unemployment have been associated with high rates of child abuse, and the lack of economic opportunity works against the formation of stable families (U.S. Advisory Board on Child Abuse and Neglect, 1993).

But solving economic problems on a neighborhood scale is extremely difficult. Attracting a large manufacturing plant, a common dream for many depressed communities in past years, is unlikely to work today, as many manufacturers are downsizing or moving elsewhere. Instead, the economic solution probably lies in mobilizing both indigenous and outside investment, as Shorebank does in Chicago. And it will probably include several other elements as well, such as (1) good transportation to get at least some people out to employment elsewhere, (2) good education, to help them compete for jobs once they get there, and (3) capital and other assistance to help some local residents establish very small businesses—even businesses they can run from their apartments. Small businesses will not make many millionaires, but they will provide rewards for hard work while retaining some independence, and providing an element of hope that is too often missing. Furthermore, profits from small businesses are more likely to recirculate locally than profits earned in the neighborhood by large corporations, chain stores, banks, and insurance companies that are headquartered elsewhere (U.S. Advisory Board on Child Abuse and Neglect, 1993).

Attending to the Social Dimension

In addition to the aspects mentioned above, specific attention should be given to social structures themselves. What mechanisms are there to bring people together in a positive way? Churches, bowling leagues, clubs, and civic groups all do this. But in some settings, such as rural trailer parks, there may be few if any such activities. Could trailer parks organize their own sports leagues? High mobility would be a problem, but probably not an insurmountable one.

In this regard it is particularly important to focus on youth—not only on the mechanisms that bring them together but, equally important, the mechanisms for helping youth to make the transition from youth to adulthood. Failure in this area can lead to teen pregnancy, substance abuse, and criminal activities, all of which can result in child abuse and neglect. Neighborhoods need to pay attention to the mechanisms that exist for positive contact between youth and adults. Job situations that allow a youth to work closely with an adult help—but are often scarce in depressed neighborhoods. Sporting and recreational activities involving teamwork and contact with adults are important, as are extended family relationships involving close contact with aunts and uncles, as well as neighborhood or cultural events that involve children.

Unfortunately, in many neighborhoods there are simply too few opportunities of this type. Bronfenbrenner (1986, p. 53) sees a need for "programs that create and strengthen consensus and connections between the family, the school and the peer group, [and] programs that increase the involvement of responsible adults in challenging activities with children, adolescents and youth."

A disturbing dimension of the youth issue involves latchkey children. In a rural bedroom community in upstate New York, one of the top concerns of parents and community leaders was, "What happens with our children between the end of school and the time we get home from work?" For children too old to be in day care, there were few structured activities. The school provided a late bus only one day a week. Perhaps not coincidentally, alcoholism among teenagers was also a major concern in this community. A new committee of children and adults now organizes after-school activities for children.

As indicated previously, many human service programs designed to help individuals actually work in ways that strengthen the neighborhood as well. To some extent, the neighborhood is strengthened by their very presence. But it can be strengthened even more if the service operates to bring people together in ways that increase positive interaction and neighborliness. Actually, schools do this when they sponsor sports events, and perhaps for this reason, schools often serve as the center of the community, especially in rural areas. People may belong to different churches, but all their children go to the same school. It is the one institution that brings virtually everyone together.

Head Start centers work with individual families, but they also involve parents in the classroom as volunteers and in social and recreational activities, as well as policymaking. From my experience as a Head Start trainer years ago, it is clear that these parent involvement activities actually create networking opportunities for families that would otherwise be isolated. Family resource centers often do the same, involving neighborhood parents in recreational and educational activities and creating new groupings in the process.

A major tool of the settlement houses was the club—which provided a place for people in the neighborhood to belong (Levine & Levine, 1970). Clubs were formed for people of all ages for various purposes. They helped to ensure that people felt that they were important—that they mattered. In the process, they helped people to develop their own network of friends. To some extent, family resource centers, where they exist, have become today's equivalent of yesterday's settlement houses.

In their desire to help individuals—particularly those with few social skills—it is important for human services not to replace or take over the function of social networks. Initially, human service workers may be a person's only friend, but they cannot fill that function indefinitely if they are going to work with others too. Human service agencies that encourage people to develop their own networks contribute to the viability of the neighborhood; agencies that actively develop group activities strengthen the neighborhood still more. By establishing new settings for people to get together and interact, these agencies increase the neighborliness in the area involved. By implication, the quality of parenting will improve as people feel more comfortable with their neighbors and extend their social support networks as a result.

Human service agencies also strengthen the neighborhood when they help its residents to develop their leadership potential and participate in resolving community issues. To the extent that they can organize and empower neighborhood residents to resolve the major issues they face, they strengthen the viability of the neighborhood. Community action programs may do this by organizing a tenants' association or a day care group to address child care issues. A local police department may do it by organizing neighborhood watch groups that address crime problems. Youth programs, which provide constructive challenges and responsibilities to kids who would otherwise be on the streets, strengthen the neighborhood even more. By encouraging people to work together, all these efforts tend to increase neighborliness.

Cultural Relevance

Cultural relevance is a basic tenet of any neighborhood-based approach. In neighborhoods with large immigrant or minority populations, the most basic step is to ensure that the approach involves people able to communicate in the language(s) of the neighborhood. Those offering a service, organizing, or otherwise intervening in community life must be either part of the local culture or very familiar and comfortable with it. Otherwise community residents will not feel understood, accepted, and welcomed by those developing and offering the program. This is particularly important in neighborhoods in which education and income levels are low.

In neighborhoods with a strong ethnic culture, residents often develop their own local networks and support systems, and any neighborhood-based approach needs to be able to identify this capacity and reinforce it. It is also important to understand the significance of cultural customs and traditions, particularly regarding child rearing, so as to be able to distinguish between legitimate cultural differences and practices harmful to children. Finally, it is important to understand the local culture well enough to celebrate it—to enjoy and participate in festivals and customs and to reinforce parents in instilling a positive sense of cultural pride and identity in their children.

Many neighborhoods will incorporate several cultures, and it may not be possible to employ someone from each. But it is usually possible to find someone in the community from each culture who will be willing to advise and assist in understanding that culture and in communicating with someone in need of help. When several cultures are involved, neighborhood-based programs can play a major role in promoting intercultural understanding and appreciation, and a multicultural staff will provide a visible role model for accomplishing this. Celebration of cultural traditions may become even more important in this regard, by serving as a vehicle for instilling mutual appreciation rather than conflict. Celebrations can also provide a supportive setting for parents to develop and expand their own support networks of friends and relatives.

For neighborhoods with high immigrant populations, teaching literacy and English as a Second Language courses can be very important in helping people to become more competent in adapting to this culture, as well as in locating and keeping an adequate job.

Although cultural differences tend to be most obvious in urban inner-city neighborhoods with large immigrant populations, they can be significant in rural areas, too—even when residents look like those of the predominant culture. Differences in rural areas may have more to do with social class and neighborhood of origin than with race or ethnic background, but they should not be overlooked. To be effective, a rural program needs to involve people from the population it serves, just as in urban settings.

MINIMAL REQUIREMENTS
FOR A NEIGHBORHOOD-BASED APPROACH

Following the environmentalist model suggested earlier, perhaps there should be minimum requirements for responding to dysfunctional neighborhoods. Perhaps human ecologists can agree on several key responses that should be established in every dysfunctional neighborhood, along with more fortunate neighborhoods, where needed. These might include neonatal home visiting services for families, health clinics in middle and secondary schools, and at least one agency that offers intensive, comprehensive, individualized flexible services with, as Schorr (1988) puts it, "aggressive attention to outreach and to maintaining relationships over time—perhaps frills for fortunate families, but rock-bottom essentials for high risk populations" (pp. 285–286).

Other things to aim for—in addition to basics such as housing, health care, and adequate education—are organizations and institutions that provide an opportunity for people in the neighborhood to interact with each other. People who do not belong anywhere or have nothing to participate in will find it more difficult to develop the kind of individual support networks essential for maintaining their own families. As long ago as 1958, Maccoby, Johnson, and Church found that juvenile delinquency was inversely proportional to the "integration" of the neighborhood (the extent to which residents knew their neighbors by name, felt free to borrow something they needed, belonged to the same church, attended church, and held positive feelings about the neighborhood). Churches, settlement houses, bowling and baseball leagues, Head Start programs, school PTAs, Kiwanis clubs, and sewing clubs all provide means of integrating the community by giving its residents something to belong to and a setting in which they can interact with each other positively.

DEFINING NEIGHBORHOODS

Part of the difficulty encountered in any neighborhood-based approach is defining neighborhood boundaries. Typically neighborhood boundaries do not coincide with political or other jurisdictions, and often it may not be clear where neighborhood boundaries lie—it may depend on whom one talks to. A true neighborhood-based approach would begin with an effort to identify and map all the major neighborhoods in a jurisdiction—an effort that could consume substantial amounts of time and energy in a large city. Political wards and election districts may be somewhat useful in establishing boundaries, and they may be meaningful in terms of political connections—but the lines may shift every few years when census results are tallied. School districts are often larger than neighborhoods, and in rural areas they may cross several towns or even county lines. But they do have some legitimacy inasmuch as schools provide an important center for neighborhood activities, especially in rural areas.

Schorr (1988) refers to the census tract as the "statistical equivalent" of the neighborhood—certainly this measure has the advantage of being the most convenient breakdown in terms of demographic data.

Clearly, to serve as a meaningful unit a neighborhood needs to have some center(s) of economic or other activity around which people can come together. These centers could include factories or other places of employment, schools, churches, parks, businesses, and stores. Second, in order to develop any significant improvement effort, an entity is needed that can exert leadership and receive and disburse funds. This entity could be a neighborhood or civic association or a locally based agency. In some places (e.g., rural trailer parks), such an entity may be difficult to find, and a new association may have to be developed.

The neighborhood concept may be easier to define in urban settings than in sparsely populated rural areas. In an urban area it is presumably possible to include every home in some neighborhood or another, but in a rural area this may not be the case, as some houses may simply be too isolated. Also, in very sparsely settled rural areas, there may not be the critical mass of people necessary to get things done. Finally, while it is relatively hard to envision a major city with no economic base, rural areas can and do lose their economic basis (a mineral deposit may become exhausted; family farms may cease to be profitable; an external economic base—e.g., a military installation—may disappear; etc.). In some neighborhoods that have lost their economic base, it simply may be no longer possible to sustain a reasonable quality of life.

It may be premature to spell out how neighborhoods should be defined at this stage. Each of the above categories has advantages and disadvantages. Initially, at least, it may be enough to allow localities to use flexibility in defining their neighborhoods, provided local input is included. The point is to get planners, politicians, administrators, agency personnel, and residents to identify needy residential areas and to work together to improve them— however the boundaries are defined.

WHERE TO START

Ideally, a neighborhood-based approach would be comprehensive, beginning on several fronts at once. The problems facing our most needy neighborhoods have taken a long time to develop, and they will not go away easily. Just as comprehensive services are recommended for multiproblem families, comprehensive approaches are needed to "turn around" the neighborhoods in which many such families live.

The actual reality may be somewhat different, however. Despite the desirability of a massive, comprehensive approach, this turnaround requires a level of coordination and backing by various levels of government that rarely exists. For most people working to strengthen neighborhoods and neighborliness, the key question is not "What is ideal?" but "What can I do with what I've got?" and "Where do I start?"

In fact, many model neighborhood-based programs considered comprehensive today did not start out that way. Most started small and have gradually gained the confidence of those they set out to serve, increasing their ability to serve them and to strengthen the neighborhood over time. A model that started on all fronts at once might well be slowed by natural resistance to change, even from those who would benefit most.

Where one starts depends in part on where one sits; a county executive or a community planner will have different orientations, resources, and skills than an agency director or a grass-roots neighborhood leader. A state governor or legislator will have still other orientations and assets. The key is for every initiator to bring to bear those resources most easily available, and as the work progresses, to gradually integrate his or her efforts with those of others who have similar goals.

Methodologically, a good place to start is simply to ask people in the neighborhood what they feel is most important to make it a better place to live and raise children. Such querying can be done through interviews with key people, meetings with parents, door-to-door surveys, and so on. Such a down-to-earth approach has several advantages—it gives those developing the effort direct contact with those they will be serving, and a clearer sense of purpose and stronger convictions are likely to result. It also provides direct personal exposure as well as first-hand data—both essential to building the program and gaining support for the effort. Finally, it is likely to result in contacts with indigenous leaders who can provide support within the neighborhood as well.

The basic, simple rule is to start where the people of the neighborhood are, using those resources one has or can bring to bear.

Those developing a neighborhood-based effort may face a choice between starting with a direct service to individuals, which can be broadened to strengthen the community, or starting from the perspective of strengthening the community and expecting this to "trickle down" to affect individuals. Head Start, home visiting programs, and similar organizations use the former approach, providing tangible, concrete services in ways that strengthen the community by involving and empowering its members. Starting with a concrete service involves some risk, however, as it may become too easy for both neighborhood residents and staff to see the service in a narrow context, losing sight of the broader neighborhood-strengthening goal.

The opposite approach, community strengthening, may result in formation of a task force, coordinating council, or advocacy group. Community strengthening can help to unify the various agencies and organizations within the community, but it also involves a risk. It may be perceived as less than helpful and will lose its support if it does not fairly quickly produce some tangible outcome.

As the approach evolves, it should involve work on both internal and external levels. It should involve self-help and outside help. The outside help may come from the local, state, or even federal government. It may come from a bank or business willing to invest in some way; such investment might mean a plant or housing loan, or it might consist of a contribution of funds or in-kind assets, including buildings or personnel. Economic development is crucial to healthy neighborhoods, and outside help in training residents for employment, as well as in helping them to start their own small businesses, through training, loans, and other forms of support, is critical.

Outside help may also come from churches or civic organizations willing to mobilize their members. For many years the American Friends Service Committee (Quakers) mobilized weekend work camps to allow young suburban residents to paint and make minor repairs to inner-city apartments in downtown Philadelphia.

The effort should promote the realization that no city or county can be healthy unless all its neighborhoods are healthy; if the worst neighborhoods are ignored, sooner or later the problems there will affect not only those who live there but the larger community as well.

LIMITATIONS OF THE
NEIGHBORHOOD-BASED APPROACH

Although it is unlikely that child abuse and neglect can be effectively reduced without taking into account and strengthening the neighborhood environments within which families live, it would be a mistake to view a neighborhood-based approach alone as a panacea to reducing child abuse and neglect. Neighborhoods themselves and the families within them exist in a larger societal environment that can be either hostile or supportive.

Researchers are clear on the relationship between poverty and child maltreatment (Bronfenbrenner, 1986; Garbarino, 1990; Pelton, 1978). Federal policies that push some groups into poverty and limit their ability to escape it contribute to child maltreatment. Garbarino (1990) goes further to point out that "low income is a better predictor of deficits in the United States than in other countries because our social policies tend to exaggerate rather than minimize the impact of family income on access to preventive and rehabilitative services" (p. 86). In other words, the effects of poverty in this country are aggravated by our failure to provide maternal and infant health care, or basic child support subsidies as other countries do. Such policies presumably have the effect of weakening the ability of the neighborhood to perform the positive functions its residents desperately need.

Similarly, a national media that glorifies violence and sex and plays down individual responsibility can make it very difficult to prepare teenagers for responsible parenthood, despite admirable efforts within the neighborhood. This is especially true when many children spend more time watching television than interacting with their parents.

An effective national neighborhood-based strategy will involve not only strengthening neighborhoods by working at the local level, but also working toward a more benign national and societal environment within which neighborhoods exist.

SUMMARY

The goal of a neighborhood-based approach is to strengthen the quality of neighborliness among the people living in a geographic area by encouraging each to take greater responsibility for the other's welfare—essentially, neighbor helping neighbor. This can be accomplished by involving people with each other in positive, constructive ways. To the extent this approach succeeds, every parent will have a network of people concerned with his or her welfare, made up of people about whose welfare he or she is concerned as well. Some personal networks will be large, others small, but no one will be totally isolated. Although at first various agencies may engage isolated people, the ultimate objective will be to involve them in activities and relationships that survive without the agency that began the process.

All this will be accomplished through direct services and through improving the physical and social environment where people live. This approach involves and empowers the residents of the neighborhood. It places a high value on decentralization, closeness, and personal relationships as opposed to centralization, specialization, and depersonalization. It encourages development and expansion of local institutions. It requires involvement and support of traditional human services agencies in organizing and providing services at the neighborhood level, but it requires involvement of local networks, organizations, and institutions—formal and informal—as well. It requires both self-help and external help from other levels of government and the private sector.

The big issue, of course, is how to achieve all this. I have attempted to spell out ways to start—which may vary somewhat according to who takes the initiative. I have recommended an incremental approach, which identifies and builds on strengths and accomplishments, while keeping long-term goals and objectives clearly in focus.

The above is far from exhaustive. Much more has been written on neighborhood-based approach issues than could be absorbed in preparation for this chapter. A more comprehensive review of the literature is required.

Attention should be given to definition of neighborhoods and their boundaries. Particular attention should be given to defining the viability of neighborhoods—what is minimally required for a neighborhood to survive?

More attention needs to be paid to the relationship between neighborhood interventions and improvements and child abuse and neglect. While Garbarino (1990) has demonstrated that child maltreatment is related to the neighborhood environment, it is not entirely clear what the most cost-effective neighborhood improvements or interventions will be in terms of reducing child maltreatment. More sorting out needs to be done in terms of the proper role of agencies and the types of services that can best be provided on a neighborhood level.

Over the years, there have been a number of success stories involving neighborhood and community intervention as a means of improving parenting and presumably reducing child abuse and neglect. There is a need to chronicle these stories and to draw conclusions regarding the most effective ways to stimulate neighborhood improvement.

Finally, there is a need for information and a framework that could be used to help in establishing "minimum environmental standards" for neighborhoods, along the lines suggested in this chapter.

REFERENCES

Barry, F. (1989). *Coordinating services for abused adolescents: How to do it.* Ithaca, NY: Family Life Development Center, Cornell University.

Bronfenbrenner, U. (1986, Fall) A generation in jeopardy: America's hidden family policy. *Developmental Psychology Newsletter,* pp. 47–54.

Chavis, D., & Wandersman, A. (1990). Sense of community in the urban environment: A catalyst for participation and community development. *American Journal of Community Psychology, 18,* 55–81.

Checkoway, B. (1985). Neighborhood planning organizations: Perspectives and choices. *Journal of Applied Behavioral Sciences, 21,* 471–486.

Cochran, M. (1988). *Parental empowerment in family matters: Lessons learned from a research program.* In D. Powell (Ed.), *Parent education and support programs: Consequences for children and families* (pp. 33–34). New York: Ablex.

Cochran, M., & Brassard, J. (1979). Child development and personal social networks. *Child Development, 50,* 601–615.

Cochran, M., Larner, M., Riley, D., Gunnarsson, L., & Henderson, C. (1990). *Extending families: The social networks of parents and the children.* Cambridge, England: Cambridge University Press.

Cochran, M., & Woolever, F. (1983). Beyond the deficit model: the empowerment of parents with information and informal supports. In I. Siegel & L. Laosa (Eds.), *Changing families* (pp. 225–246). New York: Plenum.

Cohen, S., & Lang, C. (1990). *Application of principles of community based programs.* Atlanta: Education Development Center.

Fitchen, J. (1981). *Poverty in rural America, a case study.* Boulder, CO: Westview Press.

Garbarino, J. (1990). The human ecology of early risk. In S. Meisels & J. Shonkoff (Eds.), *Handbook of early childhood intervention* (pp. 78–96). Cambridge, England: Cambridge University Press.

Garbarino, J., & Kostelny, K. (1992). Child maltreatment as a community problem. *Child Abuse and Neglect, 16,* 455–464.

Garbarino, J., Kostelny, K., & Dubrow, N. (1991). *Growing up in a war zone.* Lexington, MA: Lexington Books.

Garbarino, J., & Sherman, D. (1980). High-risk neighborhoods and high-risk families: The human ecology of child maltreatment. *Child Development*, *51*, 188–198.

Gugliotta, G. (1994, Spring). Banking for the Community. *Responsive Community*, *4* (2), 51–59.

Hinds, M. de C., & Eckholm, E. (1990, December 30). 80's leave states and cities in need. *New York Times*, p. 17.

Kaye, G. (1990). A community organizer's perspective on citizen participation research and the researcher–practitioner partnership. *American Journal of Community Psychology*, *18*, 151–157.

Kromkowski, J. (1976). *Neighborhood deterioration and juvenile crime*. South Bend, IN: South Bend Urban Observatory.

Levine, M., & Levine, A. (1970). *A social history of helping services: Clinic, court, school and community*. New York: Appleton-Century-Crofts.

Maccoby, E., Johnson, J., & Church, R. (1958). Community integration and the social control of juvenile delinquency. *Journal of Social Issues*, *14*, 38–51.

National Commission on Children. (1991). *Beyond rhetoric: A new American agenda for children and families*. Washington, DC: U.S. Government Printing Office.

National Commission on Child Welfare and Family Preservation. (1990). *A commitment to change*. Washington, DC: American Public Welfare Association.

Pelton, L., (1978). Child abuse and neglect: The myth of classlessness. *American Journal of Orthopsychiatry*, *48*, 608–617.

Sarason, S. B., Levine, M., Goldenberg, I., Cherlin, D., & Bennett, E. (1966). *Psychology in community settings: Clinical, educational, vocational and social aspects*. New York: Wiley.

Schorr, L. (1988). *Within our reach: Breaking the cycle of disadvantage*. New York: Doubleday.

U.S. Advisory Board on Child Abuse and Neglect. (1990). *Child abuse and neglect: Critical first steps in response to a national emergency* (Stock No. 017-092-00104-5). Washington, DC: U.S. Government Printing Office.

U.S. Advisory Board on Child Abuse and Neglect. (1993). *Neighbors helping neighbors: A new national strategy for the protection of children*. Washington, DC: U.S. Government Printing Office.

Wallace, R. (1989). Homelessness, contagious destruction of housing and municipal service cuts in New York City: 1. Demographics of a housing deficit. *Environment and Planning*, *21*, 1585–1603.

Wallace, R. (1990). Urban desertification, public health and public order: "Planned shrinkage," violent death, substance abuse and AIDS in the Bronx. *Social Science Medicine*, *31*, 801–813.

Wayne, L. (1992, March 14). New hope in inner cities: Banks offering mortgages. *New York Times*, p. 1.

Webster's new collegiate dictionary. (1980). Springfield, MA: Merriam.

Chapter 3

Social Support and the Prevention of Child Maltreatment

Ross A. Thompson

Parents who abuse or neglect their offspring are distinguished from non-abusive parents in many ways (e.g., by their socioeconomic status, their life stress and difficulty, their capacities to cope with anger and frustration, and/or their recognition of the boundaries of appropriate sexual conduct with children). One of the commonly noted features of maltreating families is their social isolation: Parents who abuse offspring are believed to lack significant social connections to others in the extended family, the neighborhood, the broader community, and to the social agencies that can provide assistance. As a consequence, their maltreatment of offspring is likely to remain undetected, and their social connections with support agents who can buffer the effects of stress, promote healthy behavior, and socialize parenting are less influential.

Because of the often-cited association between social isolation and child maltreatment, social support interventions are commonly identified as potential means of preventing child abuse and neglect. By integrating a variety of formal and informal support agents into the lives of high-risk families, program planners hope that the affirmative, informational, socializing, and instrumental functions that social support commonly assumes in nonabusive families can help reduce the likelihood of child maltreatment in high-risk families. Such a view has guided the development of a wide variety of preventive intervention programs that are targeted either to nonabusive families at considerable risk for child maltreatment or to abusive families at risk for the reabuse of children.

Social support interventions have become the *cause célèbre* of scholars and practitioners concerned not only with child maltreatment but also with the broader effects of stress on physical and mental health. They argue that social supports buffer the effects of disease pathology and psychological distress on stressed individuals and, thus, contribute to less severe symptomatology, quicker recovery, enhanced coping, and diminished long-term effects of stress. Social supports also foster healthy functioning, they argue, by encouraging and reinforcing healthy behavior in at-risk individuals. Current enthusiasm for social support as a stress buffer and stress prevention dates from Cassel (1976; see also Cassel, 1974a, 1974b) and Cobb (1976), both of whom focused on social support as a buffer of life stress (House, Umberson, & Landis, 1988). Social support quickly became "the latest mental health fad" (Heller & Swindle, 1983, p. 89), as scholars and practitioners eagerly embraced the value of social support interventions for a broad variety of challenges to physical and psychological functioning. The President's Commission on Mental Health (1978), for example, enthusiastically endorsed strengthening natural support systems that exist in families, neighborhoods, and communities in the treatment and prevention of mental health problems.

No doubt, the appeal of social support interventions has been enhanced more recently by the growing need and diminished funding, during the past 15 years, for formal mental health services. Reliance on informal social support in the family and neighborhood provides a less costly means of providing needed assistance to stressed individuals. As a consequence, even in the absence of a firm research foundation for such conclusions, the arguments of Meyer (1985) are representative of emerging professional views:

> The research evidence is in: There is a strong relationship between individual physical-social-psychological health and social supports and between social isolation and the breakdown in these areas of functioning. In view of the importance of natural support networks, social workers can do no less than explore the linkages between them and professional intervention. (p. 91)

By 1985, however, other scholars had concluded that "the era of unrestrained enthusiasm that has dominated social support research and interventions for over ten years is coming to a close" (Shumaker & Brownell, 1984, p. 11). Although the links between social support and diminished stress remain viable, scholarly enthusiasm for preventive interventions based on this association is currently more restrained for several reasons (Vaux, 1988). First, the nature of social support itself, and the components of social support that assume stress-buffering and stress-preventive functions, has been vaguely and inconsistently portrayed in both conceptual and empirical analyses (Barrera, 1986). As a result, it is more difficult than expected to move from research to applications of social support concepts because social support is a complex, multidimensional phenomenon with different components that have different consequences for physical and mental well-being (Rook & Dooley, 1985). Second, the strength of the effects of social support on stress, symptomatology, and coping has often been unimpressive (Heller & Swindle, 1983). This may derive, for example, from (1) the fact that social networks can be supportive but also demanding and stressful, (2) the realization that the impact of social support may be moderated by the personal skills and characteristics of the recipient (e.g., social competence and reactance to aid), and (3) the awareness that social support must assume different functions for different problems (Brownell & Shumaker, 1984; Cohen & Wills, 1985; Heller & Swindle, 1983; Shinn, Lehmann, & Wong, 1984). Third, because of the multidimensional nature of social support and the diverse avenues and agents through which it is available, devising social support interventions requires a detailed understanding of the needs and conditions of recipient populations that is seldom available (Shinn et al., 1984). Moreover, the effects of specific supportive agents in the social networks of stressed individuals are often specific to the needs and characteristics of the population requiring aid (e.g., older adults or single parents), making generalization of social support effects much more difficult.

These considerations—and others—are pertinent to evaluating the potential role of social support in the prevention of child maltreatment. This chapter is devoted to a critical review and analysis of the literature in relation to our understanding of child maltreatment and its causes. Instead of examining the documented outcomes of intervention programs that include a social support component (which is the task of Garbarino and Kostelny's Chapter 7, this volume), this analysis draws on basic research literatures to better understand what social support *is* and *does* in the lives of children and their families. More specifically, the goal is to "unpack" the broad concept of social support to identify more precisely the following: (1) its potential functions in child development and family life, (2) the multidimensional features of social support that may—independently and in concert—affect child and family functioning, and (3) the diverse considerations entailed in predicting the effects (both positive and negative) of social support on the incidence of child maltreatment. Moreover, this analysis applies these formulations to a reconsideration of the nature of the social isolation experienced by maltreating families to better understand what aspects of social support are lacking in these families and, consequently, what kinds of interventions are most likely to prove helpful. It is important to note that there is little good research on the nature of the social isolation of maltreating families, the dimensions of social support that are likely to prove most beneficial to them, the interpersonal resources they can draw on, or the efficacy of social support interventions. Consequently, allied research concerning stress and social support in other family conditions (e.g., socioeconomically stressed families, single mothers, or children experiencing divorce) is surveyed to identify potentially valuable heuristics to apply to maltreating families, and important new avenues for future research are identified.

At a minimum, this chapter underscores the facts that social support and its effects are considerably more complex than is usually assumed and the design of interventions that entail social support must be carefully crafted to take these complexities into account. Adding social support agents to a family's social ecology is not a panacea for problems in abuse prevention, but there is evidence that thoughtfully designed supportive interventions can strengthen children and families against the risk of maltreatment. Issues such as the potential recipient's construals of social support agents, the multiple (and sometimes conflicting) purposes of social support interventions, and the manner in which natural social support networks in the neighborhoods of high-risk families may influence the risk of child maltreatment can alert program planners to the necessity of thoughtfulness in conceptualizing the supportive needs of maltreating families and to how these needs can best be addressed in the context of social support interventions. This chapter identifies (1) problems to be avoided, (2) potentially helpful strategies, and (3) needs for future research in the design of social support programs for these families.

SETTING THE STAGE

A preliminary step to such an analysis is to define more clearly the scope and nature of the problem of child maltreatment that social support is intended to address. Doing so reveals that social support can potentially serve many different goals in diverse contexts, and that distinguishing between these is an essential prerequisite to properly conceptualizing how social support can be enlisted on behalf of maltreated children and their families.

Primary, Secondary, and Tertiary Prevention

Prevention efforts can occur at three levels of intervention. *Primary prevention* concerns services provided to the general population to reduce or prevent the occurrence of maltreatment. *Secondary prevention* concerns services targeted to specially identified high-risk groups to reduce or prevent maltreatment. *Tertiary prevention* concerns targeting services to perpetrators and/ or victims of maltreatment either to prevent its recurrence or to minimize its detrimental consequences. Primary prevention programs might include, for example, high school parenting classes that foster caregiving skills, secondary prevention would focus on developing these skills in teenage parents and other identified groups that are at high risk for child maltreatment, and tertiary prevention programs would emphasize the development of parenting skills in adults who have already been identified as abusive or neglectful.

Social support interventions can be part of primary, secondary, or tertiary prevention efforts to prevent maltreatment (Helfer, 1982). Primary prevention programs emphasizing social support might seek to strengthen the capacity of neighborhoods and communities to provide social resources that parents can enlist in coping with the demands of caregiving (e.g., family resource centers or respite child care services). Secondary prevention programs with a social support component might target specific neighborhoods where the risk of maltreatment is high for such services, as well as providing other targeted interventions such as school-based programs for teenage parents or "welcome baby" perinatal visitation programs for new parents who are especially likely to be stressed by child care. Tertiary prevention programs emphasizing social support might intervene with families who have already experienced an abusive episode either to strengthen parental and family functioning (e.g., by providing crisis-intervention "hot line" or stress management "warm line" services or offering supervised visitation between parents and children who have been removed from the home) or to reduce the detrimental outcomes to children who have been maltreated (e.g., through developmental day care and after-school programs). Thus, the scope of potential preventive efforts entailing social support is necessarily broad, and this analysis (consistent with the mandate from the U.S. Advisory Board on Child Abuse and Neglect, 1990) focuses primarily—although not exclusively—on secondary and tertiary prevention.

It is important to note that the role of social support is not the same in these alternative prevention contexts, even though the consistent goal is the prevention of child maltreatment. One obvious difference is in the nature of the population targeted for prevention efforts and their receptivity to social support interventions. Social support can be enlisted in the family ecology much more easily for untroubled families (in the context of primary prevention) than for high-risk families (in secondary prevention efforts), and may be most difficult for families who have already experienced child abuse or neglect (tertiary prevention). This is not only because of the greater number and severity of life stresses experienced by troubled and abusive families, and how stress may affect the range and nature of their potential supportive agents, but also because the same psychological and familial dysfunction that contributes to high-risk status may also reduce their receptivity to supportive interventions. Moreover, if tertiary prevention efforts are guided by the growing number of studies identifying the correlates of reabuse in maltreating families (e.g., Ferleger, Glenwick, Gaines, & Green, 1988; Herrenkohl, Herrenkohl, Egolf, & Seech, 1979), services will be targeted to families typified by a constellation of serious personal, familial, and ecological problems, which does not bode well for the efficacy of social support programs.

Another important difference between primary, secondary, and tertiary prevention efforts is how, from the family's perspective, social support is enlisted in the context of other interventions that are either coercive or volitional. Although most social support interventions are more effective when they are voluntarily enlisted by their beneficiaries, legal authorities and public and private social service personnel have multiple goals for their involvement with families in secondary and tertiary prevention contexts. When tertiary prevention is involved, for example, the state also has a responsibility to ensure child protection and to adjudicate child abuse allegations in ways that necessarily enhance the state's coercive role in family life. Consequently, social support interventions in the context of tertiary prevention are more likely to have the goal of quickly effecting and documenting behavioral change, may entail significant privacy intrusions, and will likely be regarded by their recipients as obligatory and coercive, which may undermine some of the potential benefits. By contrast, when secondary prevention is involved, society's respect for the integrity of family functioning and parental autonomy limits the state's coercive role and changes the state's function to an empowering or "provisioning" one, and in this context social support interventions are likely to be perceived as voluntary, self-regulated, and individually determined, with the goals of emotional support, access to services, and counseling, as well as skills acquisition. The same is true of primary prevention efforts. This suggests that apart from the nature of the families who are targeted, it may be more difficult to design effective social support interventions in the context of tertiary than secondary prevention efforts, and that with tertiary prevention, issues concerning the avenues and agencies of support may be a more paramount consideration.

Subpopulations of Maltreatment

Although researchers and policymakers commonly refer to child abuse and neglect as if it is a homogeneous phenomenon, child maltreatment assumes diverse forms. Recognizing the different—but overlapping—subpopulations of maltreatment is essential to understanding the potential effects of social support interventions because different goals and strategies are likely to be effective with different subpopulations.

Researchers have recently sought to distinguish at least four subpopulations of maltreating parents: those who are physically abusive, those who are physically neglectful, those who engage in emotional maltreatment, and those who engage in sexual abuse (e.g., Daro, 1988, 1993; Herrenkohl, Herrenkohl, & Egolf, 1983). The limited evidence suggests that these parents differ in a number of important ways: in the extent to which socioeconomic stresses (such as poverty and unemployment) figure prominently in maltreatment; in the degree to which abuse derives from the perpetrator's personal problems with impulse control and/or sexual dysfunction; in the nature of the broader family problems that are associated with maltreatment; and in the characteristics of the children who are victimized. Findings from a recent study of 19 federally funded clinical demonstration programs suggest, not surprisingly, that different intervention strategies work best with different maltreatment subpopulations. For example, individual and family therapy was most successful with sexual abuse perpetrators, programs involving family counseling and community service referrals served best those families characterized by neglect, and parenting and child development classes were most successful with emotionally maltreating families (Daro, 1988, 1993). There were also differences in the effectiveness of services offered to the child victims of various maltreatment subpopulations.

Although it is premature to identify distinct typologies of different maltreatment subpopulations—especially given the considerable number of families characterized by multiple forms of abuse—it is important to delineate different maltreatment subpopulations in order to understand how social support interventions can benefit different kinds of abusive families. More specifically, subpopulation considerations are germane to clarifying the goals, agents, and design of social support interventions.

- *Goals*. Social support could be enlisted to provide appropriate models of parenting behavior, to provide a buffer against the effects of socioeconomic or other life stresses, or to enhance access to skills, services, or information, depending on the subpopulation of concern. As noted earlier, devising social support interventions in light of the recipient population's unique needs and characteristics is essential to program success. If maltreatment is reactive to poverty and limited resources, social support to enhance access to skills and services might be paramount. If maltreatment instead derives primarily from problems in impulse control, social support to provide counseling or appropriate role models may be most important.
- *Agents*. Prevalent community standards of appropriate parental conduct (e.g., with respect to physically punishing, berating, or threatening offspring or with respect to sexual misconduct with children) may help to determine the extent to which neighborhood-based social support interventions are likely to be effective in remediating certain parenting problems and the kinds of interventions that will prove most useful (cf. Garbarino & Crouter, 1978). Neighbors or extended family members may be helpful in providing material support or referrals to formal support systems even when they may not reliably provide good role models for appropriate parenting practices. By contrast, self-help groups may strengthen parenting skills but provide fewer community-based social supports for individuals at risk of child maltreatment.
- *Design*. With some subpopulations, social support interventions may need to be integrated with social skills training and access to community services; with other subpopulations interventions can be integrated with individual and family therapy or alternative counseling strategies. Recognizing that social support alone is unlikely to address the full range of difficulties encountered by maltreating parents or children, program planners' understanding of maltreatment subpopulations assists them with integrating supportive interventions into a constellation of supplementary services that addresses other needs of these families.

In sum, the consideration of social support interventions is informed by Daro's (1988) admonition that "if practitioners and policy makers have learned only one thing over the past two decades, it should be that allowing one type of maltreatment to dominate our thinking leaves us with a response system and practice standards inappropriate for the full range of concerns represented by this serious welfare dilemma" (p. 204).

However, the influence of other perpetrator characteristics contributes complexity to these considerations. The presence of a substance abuse problem makes the remediation of child maltreatment considerably more challenging, for example, because the problem of drug dependency is the paramount concern. Consequently, conventional social support programs targeted to these subpopulations may have to be considerably modified and integrated with drug detoxification programs, and the enlistment of natural social support networks must take into account the extent to which these networks foster the target individual's substance abuse problem. When child neglect or other forms of maltreatment are associated with the socioeconomic stresses of single parenting, on the other hand, social support programs in the context of guided access to material resources (e.g., affordable child care) may be advisable (cf. Belle, 1982). Adolescent parents present another challenge to the design of social support programs because of the unique constellation of their needs and interests vis-à-vis parenting as well as the demands and supports that are potentially available from their families of origin.

Therefore, the design of carefully crafted social support programs for maltreating families must take into consideration not only the characteristics of abuse that require remediation but also other features of perpetrators and victims that help to define the goals, agents, and design of an appropriate supportive strategy.

Victims as Well as Perpetrators

Tertiary prevention efforts involving social support should target the children who are victimized by child maltreatment as well as the perpetrators. (To an important extent, moreover, secondary prevention efforts providing social support to children also merit attention.) However, there are diverse considerations in designing supportive interventions in a developmentally appropriate manner that recognizes the interrelationships between the social networks of children and their parents.

Developmental concerns are important not only as they pertain to the age of the child of concern but also with respect to the consequences of maltreatment. A number of studies (see Aber & Cicchetti, 1984; Cicchetti, 1990; Egeland & Sroufe, 1981; Egeland, Sroufe, & Erickson, 1983; Erickson, Egeland, & Pianta, 1989; Pianta, Egeland, & Erickson, 1989; see also Garbarino, 1989; Toro, 1982) found that maltreated children show predictable and cumulative developmental losses that are associated with the experience of abuse or neglect. (They also noted that different forms of maltreatment have predictably different consequences for offspring.) For infants and toddlers, these losses involve the development of insecure attachments to caregivers and early deficits in the management of emotional arousal in challenging situations. By the preschool years, maltreated children show less self-control and greater distractibility in problem-solving situations and significant problems in social relationships with peers. Maltreated children are often cognitively delayed by the time of their entry into school and also show psychological problems (e.g., anxiety and/or aggression) that are sometimes indicators of emerging psychopathology. During the school years, these children show impairments in social skills (with adults as well as peers) and in self-esteem: They are more aggressive, depressed, withdrawn, and impulsive than are nonmaltreated children. These problems are also apparent in adolescence and are coupled with greater social deviance and acting-out behavior.

To the extent that tertiary preventive programs involving social support are designed in a developmentally sensitive manner to address the detrimental consequences of abuse or neglect, they will address the age-salient problems experienced by maltreated children at different periods of their growth. Social support to promote the development of secure attachments to alternative caregivers might be emphasized in programs for maltreated infants, for example, supportive programs fostering competent social skills with peers might be employed during the preschool and grade-school years, and social support to enhance self-esteem and buttress perceptions of personal competence in maltreated children and adolescents might be emphasized in later years. Moreover, given that the deficits of maltreated children are not only developmentally variable but also cumulative, intervention programs must be flexibly responsive to the changing constellation of challenges experienced by these children over time. In other words, the consequences of maltreatment of children must be considered not only at the time of occurrence, but also later, as these deficits have potentially long-term effects. Intervening with social support at the time that maltreatment is detected requires considering the history of developmental consequences of abuse and their future implications.

Developmental concerns are pertinent not just to the goals of social support interventions but to the actors and agencies by which they are provided. As they mature, children enter into and emerge from different ecological networks that provide different opportunities for enlisting social support. In infancy and during the toddler and preschool years, for example, social networks are largely home and family based, with parents mediating interaction with outsiders and with extended kin by arranging contact and transporting children (Cochran & Brassard, 1979; Feiring & Lewis, 1988, 1989; Lewis, Feiring, & Kotsonis, 1984; Parke & Bhavnagri, 1989). At the same time, child care during parental working hours is a prominent concern both for parents (especially in balancing the availability, quality, and affordability of accessible care) and for children (because of reliable links between the quality of care and their development). In these contexts, developmental child care services are an important avenue for social support both for maltreated children and for their parents (and may assume secondary preventive value with high-risk families). In middle childhood the schools become an important means for providing social support for children and secondarily for parents (Asp & Garbarino, 1983; Hirsch & DuBois, 1989). Not only school-based supports but after-school activities may be potential intervention avenues, especially given the need for after-school programs for the offspring of working parents.

As they get older, children become involved in other extrafamilial social ecologies that also present potential social supports, ranging from youth groups to athletic teams to neighborhood gangs (cf. Bryant, 1985; Medrich, Roizen, Rubin, & Buckley, 1982). In adolescence, social support can involve more complex peer networks that are largely independent of the family system, especially given the greater mobility and independence that most adolescents enjoy, and that provide many significant benefits, as well as risks, to teenagers (Berndt, 1989; Blyth, Hill, & Thiel, 1982; Blyth & Traeger, 1988; Garbarino, Burston, Raber, Russell, & Crouter, 1978). In short, the changing developmental capabilities and needs of children result in changing social ecologies that present different social support opportunities for maltreated children. This issue is explored later in greater depth when alternative avenues for the social support of maltreated children are reconsidered.

Another feature of the ecology of maltreated children that merits consideration is out-of-home placement. Any program of social support that seeks to prevent severe psychopathological outcomes in maltreated children must consider the nature of the foster care system in which many abused and neglected children are placed and its relevance to the natural, informal support systems on which children previously relied. Although extended consideration of the nature and quality of foster care is beyond the scope of this analysis (and is also the subject of Lerman's Chapter 8, this volume), it is important to note that foster care arrangements that can maintain the benefits of the child's informal support systems developed around the family of origin are likely to assist the child's adjustment to out-of-home placement and enhance the child's emotional well-being. Such arrangements might involve kin-based care placements that can preserve the child's ties with extended family members as well as neighborhood supports. Alternatively, they might involve foster care placements in the same neighborhood in which the child has grown up if foster parents are available. Such arrangements might require identifying important members of the child's social network within that neighborhood and maintaining those relationships while the child is in foster care; alternatively, they might involve creating "specific" foster care placements involving limited licensing of foster families to care for a particular child in need, with foster parents drawn from the "natural helpers" in the child's neighborhood or community (Lewis & Fraser, 1987). Although there are problems inherent in all these kinds of arrangements (including limited accountability and diminished professionalism of foster parents), they offer one avenue to maintaining natural support networks for children at risk.

A final concern related to the provision of social support to the victims of child maltreatment is the intersection of the social networks of children and parents within the family. Various avenues of social support have different consequences for children and parents, and predicting these outcomes requires considering how parents and offspring are jointly influenced by the social networks of each. As noted earlier, parents are often arrangers, facilitators, and monitors of their children's contacts with community resources, which means that extended family and neighborhood-based supports are usually mediated by parents (O'Donnell & Steuve, 1983; Parke & Bhavnagri, 1989). Parents also mediate children's contact with extended family members based on the relationships they share with extended kin and because of the kinds of relationships they want offspring to have with kin (Robertson, 1975; Thompson, Scalora, Castrianno, & Limber, 1992). Parental social networks are likely to have important consequences for offspring as they influence parents' access to material and emotional assistance, provide models and other stimulation for children, and help regulate parents' child-rearing behavior (Cochran, 1990a, 1990b; Cochran & Brassard, 1979).

The intersection of parental and offspring social networks means, however, that interventions intended to benefit one family member may have unpredictable consequences for other family members or provoke undesirable consequences for the intervention target. For example, if tertiary prevention efforts involve social support for children through extrafamilial activities and groups (such as a Big Brother or Big Sister program), parents or siblings may respond aversely to the new experiences, attitudes, and values children are acquiring in ways that increase stress for children at home. Also, at times, kin or neighborhood contacts can provide emotional support for parents while reinforcing authoritarian or punitive childrearing practices that heighten stress (and the risk of maltreatment) for children. These issues are also reconsidered later in the context of predicting the effects of alternative social support interventions on maltreating families.

Taken together, efforts to enlist social support to benefit maltreated children as well as their parents in the context of secondary or tertiary prevention efforts seriously complicate the design of support interventions because social support programs require considering the intersection of parental and child social networks as well as the developmental needs of offspring. In the end, program planners must strive to implement social supports that have complementary benefits for parents and children rather than targeting interventions for only one family member. However, doing so requires anticipating the effects of interventions on different family members in ways that stretch existing research and theoretical knowledge.

Conclusion

Indeed, virtually all these "stage-setting" considerations take us quickly beyond the boundaries of existing knowledge concerning the potential efficacy of social support interventions for maltreating families. Beyond researchers' awareness of the social isolation of abusive and neglectful families (about which, as we shall see, more knowledge is needed), little is known about the range of social supports that can assist maltreated children and their families or their effectiveness in either preventing maltreatment or remediating its consequences. As a result, this analysis remains, at times, uncomfortably speculative: Generalizing beyond existing research and theory to the special needs, demands, and circumstances of high-risk families is risky but necessary to provide useful heuristics for program design. The considerations discussed here with respect to the distinctions between primary, secondary, and tertiary prevention; the subpopulations of maltreatment; and the distinct but complementary needs of victims and perpetrators underscore, however, the need for careful thought concerning the complexity of the scope and the nature of the problem of child maltreatment that social support is intended to address.

WHAT IS SOCIAL SUPPORT?
UNPACKING AN ELUSIVE CONCEPT

There are a variety of definitions of social support used by community psychologists, family sociologists, developmental psychologists, and others who are concerned about child and family functioning. For purposes of this analysis, I will define social support as *social relationships that provide (or can potentially provide) material and interpersonal resources that are of value to the recipient, such as counseling, access to information and services, sharing of tasks and responsibilities, and skill acquisition.* Such a definition provides a beginning to understanding what social support is and does in child development and family life. However, much more is needed to elucidate its potential functions and the relationships in which it is embedded. An analysis of what social support entails underscores not only the multifaceted nature of social support but also its variable purposes in preventing and remediating maltreatment. Such an analysis also points to the importance of careful thinking in efforts to design interventions to strengthen supportive ties in the lives of children and families.

Social Networks and Social Support

Except when it is provided in the context of formal social services, social support is typically provided by members of one's social network. This network can include members of the immediate and extended family, local or distant friends, colleagues at the workplace or school, neighbors, employees at businesses and services in the community (e.g., barbers, grocers, and post office personnel), clergy, community and neighborhood leaders, and, for children, peers at school and in the neighborhood, siblings, older children, teachers, and other adult personnel associated with school, recreational programs, or other activities. One's personal social network is potentially diverse, and given that individuals are also influenced by the social networks of other family members, diversity is especially characteristic of the family social network, which may be defined as the aggregate of the social networks of its members.

Characteristics of Personal and Familial Social Networks

A considerable amount of recent research has been devoted to mapping and understanding the influence of personal and familial social networks (see especially Cochran, Larner, Riley, Gunnarsson, & Henderson, 1990; Fischer, 1982; Litwak & Szelenyi, 1969), and at least four conclusions from this research are noteworthy.

First, as suggested above, personal and familial social networks include neighborhood and nonneighborhood membership. However, the majority of network members are not neighborhood based and, instead, can be found in the broader metropolitan area and/or in outlying regions (Belle, 1982; Cochran & Henderson, 1990). This is generally true of children as well (Larner, 1990b), although school-based network members usually enhance children's neighborhood contacts (Cochran & Riley, 1990). This is not very surprising given that members of the extended family, friends and associates who have moved from the neighborhood, and colleagues in the workplace or school often live outside one's neighborhood. For many children, in addition, school-based social contacts are not neighborhood based (e.g., when children are bused to school or go to a "magnet" school outside their neighborhood).

However, because most social network members are not neighborhood based, a program of strengthening neighborhood social supports for high-risk families will enlist only some of the social networks on which individuals commonly rely. Moreover, given the importance of kin support and reliance on supportive agents outside the neighborhood (Cochran, Gunnarsson, Grabe, & Lewis, 1990; Gunnarsson & Cochran, 1990; Litwak & Szelenyi, 1969) and the heightened rates of turnover in neighborhood-based social networks (Larner, 1990a, 1990b, and below)—trends that are as apparent in high-risk subpopulations as in other subpopulations—a neighborhood-based program may not even enlist the supportive figures who are the most salient and potentially most valuable resources in individual and family social networks. In her study of socioeconomically stressed single mothers, Belle (1982) confirms this conclusion in arguing that the reason women interacted with neighborhood members was simply because they had nowhere else to go, and those who were in frequent contact with community members did not differ on measures of perceived support, tangible assistance, or emotional well-being compared with those who infrequently saw their neighbors— perhaps because of the importance of nonneighborhood supports.

Second, there is considerable turnover in personal social networks. In a 3-year follow-up study of the personal and familial social networks of a sample of 240 parents in Syracuse, New York, nearly one quarter (22%) of the network members on average were dropped from adults' social networks between the first and follow-up interviews (Larner, 1990a). When Larner examined the nature of the social relationships that were dropped or retained, she found highest turnover among nonkin ties (34% turnover), neighbors (32% turnover), and friends, acquaintances, and former workmates (31% turnover). The lowest turnover rate was, not surprisingly, among kin (only 9% turnover). More surprisingly, neighbors did not figure prominently in the social networks of most people in this study and were readily dropped or added to personal networks with little influence on an individual's or family's primary support systems (Larner, 1990b). This is not surprising given the rather high rates of mobility, job change, educational completion, marital change, and other factors that can alter social networks and social support systems. But these findings from one of the few longitudinal studies of social networks suggest that certain features of the network—those that are neighborhood based and non-kin-related—are especially susceptible to turnover.

Third, there are distinctive characteristics of the social networks of certain subpopulations that are of the greatest interest to students of child maltreatment (Vaux, 1985). In particular, social network attributes have been examined for lower-socioeconomic-status (SES) group members and for single mothers, which are two groups at heightened risk for child abuse and neglect (Daro, 1988; Pelton, 1978). In general, the personal and familial social networks of lower-SES families tend to be smaller and more kin based than those of middle- and upper-SES families (Cochran, Gunnarsson, et al., 1990; Fischer, 1982; Vaux, 1988). In the Cochran study, SES differences were apparent for kin, neighbors, and "others": For each component of the social network, higher-SES families had a larger number of social ties than did lower-SES families. In addition, a higher proportion of higher-SES mothers worked compared to their lower-SES counterparts, which enhanced their occupation-related social network ties. To Cochran (1990c), Fischer (1982), and other commentators, these differences derive also from the resources, skills, and opportunities that education and income provide individuals in constructing and maintaining social networks, as well as from the constraints imposed by neighborhoods that are sometimes dangerous and unpredictable and which, thus, engender suspicion and wariness in contacts with neighbors.

Single mothers also have smaller personal social networks with higher rates of turnover (Larner, 1990a; Leslie & Grady, 1985; Weinraub & Wolf, 1983). Single mothers have more frequent contact with network members than do married mothers and rely on them for tangible childrearing and child care assistance as well as emotional support (Belle, 1982; Gunnarsson & Cochran, 1990). However, the networks of white single mothers are more focused on nonkin friends and neighbors, while black single mothers place greater emphasis on kin (Cochran & Henderson, 1990; Cross, 1990; Fischer, 1982; Gunnarsson & Cochran, 1990; but see Colletta, 1979; Leslie & Grady, 1985). These differences may derive from neighborhood and cultural processes: the importance of kin supports in black families (McAdoo, 1980; Stack, 1974) and the greater ease of access to same-race neighborhood social networks and supports by white mothers (Cochran, 1990c). However, kin supports are also important to white single mothers, who may especially benefit from a strengthening of kin ties immediately following a divorce (Colletta, 1979; Leslie & Grady, 1985).

Fourth, the foregoing discussion strongly implies that the differences between kin and nonkin ties figure prominently in any analysis of social networks and social support. There are many reasons for this. Relationships with members of the immediate and extended family (even when one includes relations with a former spouse and the spouse's family) have a history of interaction and support that provides a foundation for continuity in the future (Litwak & Szelenyi, 1969; Tinsley & Parke, 1984). Family members have greater opportunities for maintaining sociability through various formal events (e.g., holidays, birthdays, and anniversaries) and informal occasions that enable them to continue contact even when geographically separated. Nonkin ties do not benefit from these opportunities, especially when they are geographically distant. Kinship is also built on strong cultural foundations of respect for family and family integrity that provide added incentives (sometimes obligations) to maintain and strengthen these ties. Consequently, family members figure more prominently in the primary social networks of most individuals than do other partners in the neighborhood, workplace, or broader community. To be sure, individuals usually form intimate relations with only a selected subset of kinship ties (based on age, gender, frequency of contact, and the nature of support required) (see Hoyt & Babchuk, 1983), but kin nevertheless remain preferred sources of primary support among most individuals.

Description of Social Networks

In light of the importance of social networks to social support, the next step is to understand the dimensions of a social network that are most critical to the support individuals experience from those around them (e.g., Barrera,

1986; Ladd, Hart, Wadsworth, & Golter, 1988; Mitchell & Trickett, 1980; Vaux, 1988). Do people benefit most from a large social network, from the intimacy of relationships, or from the stability in the network, or from some combination of these and other factors? Answering this question is crucial to understanding what features of personal and familial social networks should be the targets of social support interventions, as well as to predicting the likely consequences of such intervention efforts.

Unfortunately, most assessments of social networks focus largely on network size, which is the number of persons with whom the individual has contact. Network size is a rather insensitive measure of the supportive features of social networks because many members of the social network may not assume a supportive role. There is evidence that a large social network may aid mental and physical well-being by providing a supportive community (Cohen & Wills, 1985), but large social networks are clearly not necessary to social support. Research indicates, for example, that only one or a few confidantes may be sufficient to assume a stress-buffering role for distressed individuals (Cohen & Wills, 1985; Gottlieb, 1985). Measures of sheer network size may not, therefore, sensitively index the features of social networks that are relevant to coping with stress. There are, however, other dimensions of personal and familial social networks that likewise index their *structural* characteristics:

* *Social embeddedness* is the frequency of contact with network members. By distinguishing individuals who have regular interaction with others from those who have relatively infrequent contact—even though the size of their social networks may be comparable—it is possible to identify individuals who are socially isolated in terms of their social embeddedness.

* *Dispersion* is the ease with which individuals can contact social network members. This is typically indexed in terms of geographical proximity and, thus, distinguishes neighborhood-based from non-neighborhood-based social supports. It is partly because of differences in dispersion, for example, that theorists like Litwak and Szelenyi (1969) argue that neighbors can best help with immediate emergencies and everyday assistance whereas kin are most helpful in the context of long-term commitments (e.g., childrearing support) and nonkin friends can provide reference group and emotional support. Dispersion can account for these important functional differences in network relationships. Moreover, for socioeconomically impoverished individuals, dispersion may be the most important dimension of social networks because of the difficulties impoverished individuals encounter in obtaining transportation, telephone service, and other means of access to nonneighborhood network members.

* *Stability* is the consistency of network features over time. As indicated earlier, there is surprising turnover in social network membership, but different components of the network evidence different rates of stability over time (e.g., kin vs. nonkin network components). It is not clear from research

how the stability of network membership affects social support, but one would expect greater support from those with whom one shares the most stable relationships over time.

• *Extensivity* is the degree to which social interaction within the network occurs in small groups (including dyads) rather than large groups. Extensivity is thus a structural feature of social networks that may have important implications for intimacy and perceived support, although it is not clear that intimacy/support and extensivity are directly linked.

Unfortunately, although structural dimensions of social networks are easiest to measure and have been the focus of most assessments of network functioning (including studies of the social isolation of maltreating families, which are reviewed later), they may be the least informative dimensions of the supportive qualities of social networks. Consistent, perhaps, with an intuitive view that intimate relationships with a few confidantes may be more valuable than a large number of connections to a broad social network, researchers such as Barrera (1986) have noted that measures of social embeddedness are only moderately associated with measures of perceived social support and/or enacted (or realized) social support from network members. Similarly, Cohen and Wills (1985) concluded, from an extensive literature review, that the stress-buffering aspects of social support (i.e., how support protects individuals from the potentially adverse effects of stressful events) are revealed only by measures of perceived support from network members, not from structural measures of sheer network size or embeddedness (although the latter showed other benefits to individuals). Thus, other, nonstructural dimensions of social networks must be considered and assessed in order to evaluate their social supportive features.

These alternative dimensions—like perceived support—often focus on the *affiliational* characteristics of social networks:

• *Valence* is the emotional quality of relationships with network members. Recognizing that these relationships may be stressful as well as supportive, this dimension focuses on the individual's perceptions of the affective quality of network relationships and whether they are experienced as emotionally positive or negative.

• *Reciprocity* concerns the extent to which social support in relationships is mutual or unidirectional. Thus, reciprocity has broad implications not only for how relationships are defined but for the interactional processes underlying giving and receiving assistance within them (e.g., perceptions of dependency and/or indebtedness in the context of one-way help). Reciprocity may be a central feature, for example, to the ease with which relationships with network members provide support to stressed individuals because of the extent to which unidirectional assistance may be stigmatizing to adults (Fisher, Nadler, & Witcher-Alagna, 1982) and unpleasant for help providers (cf. Polansky, Ammons, & Gaudin, 1985). On the other hand, reciprocity is typically not expected of children, who are commonly recipients of one-way assistance without stigma or expectations of reciprocal aid. These issues are reexamined later in this chapter.

• *Homogeneity* is the extent to which network members share common attributes, such as their socioeconomic status, occupational goals, religious values, and other features. Homogeneity may heighten supportiveness within social networks when congruence of values and norms fosters emotional and instrumental aid. However, this congruence may, at the same time, blunt other goals of social support: Homogeneous social networks may be less effective in altering an individual's childrearing beliefs and practices, for example, when these practices are consistent with neighborhood or subgroup norms.

• *Multidimensionality (multiplexity)* concerns the number of different supportive functions assumed by individuals within one's social network. Married mothers tend to enjoy relationships with network members that are characterized by one primary function (e.g., emotional support, childrearing assistance, and recreational activities), while single mothers have multifunctional or multidimensional relationships within their smaller social networks (Cochran, Gunnarsson, et al., 1990; Gunnarsson & Cochran, 1990). Understanding these differences aids not only in appreciating the difference between network size and support but also in understanding how existing social supports can be enlisted to benefit targeted individuals within neighborhoods and communities. Multifunctional relationships may provide stressed individuals with important social supports, but the capacity of network members to provide support is affected also by their complex roles in the target's life (e.g., providing child care assistance, being a neighbor, and providing counseling at the same time). At times, multifunctional relationships may be valuable sources of social support, but at other times the complexity of these relationships may undermine their potential as change agents in a parent's or family's life.

• *Density* or *complexity* is the extent to which network members are themselves associated with each other. Individuals with dense (or complex) social networks have members who are in mutual contact and can thus share information concerning the target individual. Those with less complex social networks experience relationships with network members who do not know each other. Although it is easy to assume that greater network density is desirable (especially in the intercoordination of social support to the target individual among diverse members of a social network), it is important not to underestimate the "strength of weak ties" (Granovetter, 1973) that can contribute diverse opportunities for obtaining information, ideas, and support from many different associates, each with different perspectives on the target individual. In particular, when a person is engaged in life transitions (e.g., to a new identity or way of behaving), less dense social networks may be most advantageous because the person is not wedded to a dense social network governed by past expectations for behavior among interconnected network members (Mitchell & Trickett, 1980).

• *Perceived support* is the extent to which individuals subjectively experience or expect support in the context of their relationships with network members. Although this is not the same as actual (or enacted) support, perceived support may be an even more significant predictor of the extent to which contact with social network members assumes a stress-buffering function in the lives of stressed people (Barrera, 1986; Cohen & Wills, 1985). In other words, coping with physical or social stress may depend more on one's perceptions that support is available and accessible than on the instrumental actions of social network members or the target's utilization of network resources. However, perceived support may not always be an appropriate index of social support or its potential efficacy. When social network members urge an individual to quit smoking or drinking—or to stop abusing or neglecting offspring—it is quite likely that the target individual will perceive such actions as unsupportive. In such cases, the individual's perceptions of social support may not be a valuable gauge of the extent to which network members are acting in a supportive manner.

• *Enacted support* is the frequency of specific supportive or helpful actions provided by network members. Although it is reasonable to expect congruence between measures of perceived and enacted support, research findings are consistent with the illustration in the preceding paragraph showing that there is actually a surprisingly low concordance between measures of enacted support and perceived support in research on this topic (Barrera, 1986). The helpful actions of social network members may not always be perceived as supportive by the target, in other words, and one's perceptions of support within the network may not agree with the extent to which members are truly acting helpfully.

It is clear that there are many different ways to describe personal and familial social networks. In this light, it is unfortunate that few research studies have included more than one or two dimensions in their assessments of social networks. In fact, most studies have relied largely on measures of network size or social embeddedness, and no research has comprehensively evaluated the interrelationships among these multiple dimensions of social networks for the extent to which they are mutually correlated and, perhaps, interdependent.

However, it is important to be aware of the multiple dimensions of social networks, not only for descriptive purposes, but for clear thinking about the design of social support interventions for families at risk for child maltreatment. Clearly, interventions that increase network size or enhance social embeddedness will not necessarily accomplish the same goals as interventions that are designed to enhance the density of social networks or foster perceptions of support from network members. Given the degree of independence between measures of various dimensions of social networks in current research, one cannot assume that interventions that target one dimension of social networks will necessarily influence other dimensions; thus, carefully crafted interventions designed to accomplish thoughtfully considered, specific goals are necessary. This requires careful consideration of the specific purposes of social support interventions (e.g., to enhance the amount of contact with others? to coordinate support among members of the network? to foster intimacy among a few associates? to heighten perceptions of support from network members?) and then consideration of which features of the social network to target.

Moreover, the multiple dimensions of social networks imply multiple processes by which social networks can act supportively for stressed individuals. Perceived support from network members may be valuable, for example, because it combats feelings of loneliness and isolation and aids coping. Dispersion may be an important aspect of social networks for emergency assistance but not for long-term emotional support and counseling, especially if access to geographically distant network members is problematic because of financial or transportational limitations. Density and complexity may be important factors in social networks of sufficient size that the intercoordination of the supportive efforts of network members is valuable but unimportant in networks of smaller size. Homogeneity may be valuable, as noted earlier, for some support functions (e.g., affirmation and emotional sustenance) but not for others (e.g., changing behavior that may nevertheless be normative for the neighborhood or community). House et al. (1988) offer a similar observation:

> Networks of small size, strong ties, high density, high homogeneity, and low dispersion appear to be helpful in maintaining social identity and hence health and well-being outcomes when these are promoted by identity maintenance. However, *change* in social roles and identities, and hence health and well-being during such change, is facilitated by larger networks with weaker ties, lower density, and greater social and cultural heterogeneity. (p. 304; emphasis in original; references omitted)

In short, another important reason why attention to the multiple dimensions of social networks is important is that different network dimensions are relevant to different functions of social support in the lives of stressed individuals. Consequently, we turn next to the alternative—and overlapping—functions of social support.

Functions of Social Support

One reason why clear thinking concerning the intended purposes of social support interventions is necessary is that social support can assume diverse

functions in the lives of the child and the family, many of which are not necessarily complementary and some of which may be mutually inconsistent.
Thus, a preliminary step to inquiring about the potential role of social support in preventing and remediating child maltreatment is defining the intended
functions that social support is expected to have. Defining the functions of
social support also has the added benefit, for this analysis, of identifying the
potential weaknesses of each supportive function in terms of the reasons for
enlisting support to prevent maltreatment.

Most commonly, social networks are regarded as supportive when they
provide *emotional sustenance*, such as esteem-enhancing affirmation, com-
passion and empathy, and a sense that others share one's dilemmas and
stresses. Certainly, one of the important benefits of supportive network
members is the sense that one is not alone and that, furthermore, others are
emotionally "on your side" in coping with stress (what Gottlieb, 1985, has
called "milieu reliability"). However, one potential disadvantage to the
emotional sustenance entailed in social support is that it may foster dependency in the recipient and heighten the need to reciprocate or otherwise remedy the indebtedness that sometimes results from such supportive interactions (Fisher et al., 1982). Emotional sustenance can also foster conformity
pressures in the recipient, especially if emotional support is contingent (explicitly or implicitly) upon the recipient's participation in or compliance with
group norms (such as those in adolescent peer groups). Finally, when emotional sustenance is the perceived primary function of supportive social exchanges, it is difficult for supportive agents to critically challenge the
recipient's behavior and remain supportive (at least in the view of the recipient). Exhortations to reduce smoking or drinking, end substance abuse, or
eliminate abusive or neglectful behavior toward offspring may be an essential component of social support interventions but may be regarded by recipients as emotionally unsupportive behavior.

Another function of social support is *counseling, advice, or guidance.*
Although such action may also be emotionally supportive, its primary purpose is to provide the recipient with guided direction in how to cope with
stressful demands. This direction may consist of peer counseling, including
instruction in parenting skills and coping with life stress, modeling influences
deriving from shared experiences with friends or neighbors, or advice from
members of the extended family (e.g., Cochran & Brassard, 1979). One
important purpose of such counseling is to influence the recipient's "secondary appraisal" of stressful circumstances: that is, to strengthen the individual's
awareness of the resources that exist for coping successfully with demanding conditions (Lazarus & Folkman, 1984). This influence may include but-
tressing the recipient's sense of personal competence and self-efficacy or re-
minding the recipient of interpersonal resources on which he or she can rely.
Another important purpose of counseling, however, is the transmission of
consensual social values and norms concerning behavior. Counselors often

affirm or challenge the recipient's actions when they provide advice concerning the expression of anger to others, the use of controlled substances, or the treatment of offspring. In this sense, counseling has a socializing function. However, it is important to recognize that the values and norms underlying a counselor's advice reflect not just community norms but also personal and parochial values, and insofar as social support interventions rely on neighborhood and community members, recipients may receive unhelpful as well as beneficial advice from their natural counselors. If an everyday counselor sees no harm in physical punitive behavior or berating offspring (cf. Garbarino & Crouter, 1978), for example, recipients may feel justified in their treatment of children. In such circumstances, counseling may be perceived as emotionally supportive but may accomplish little else for the recipient, and may sometimes actually be misleading and unhelpful.

A third function of social support is *access to information, services, and material resources and assistance*. In this respect, support agents act as brokers between the recipient and others who can provide tangible assistance. This mode of social support is commonly found in communities where neighbors and friends are consulted for advice about child care settings, provide referrals to community agencies where information or material resources can be obtained, or lend money or other items that are needed by the recipient. This function of social support can be especially valuable, therefore, when stress derives from inadequate access to needed information or resources (such as in low-SES settings), but it can also engender feelings of dependency, vulnerability, and, sometimes, stigma in the recipient. At times, stress owing to financial concerns (e.g., indebtedness to others) might also be enhanced.

A fourth, and related, function of social support is *skills acquisition*, for example, when social network members provide training in job-related skills, foster more competent parenting, or aid in personal skills related to household management, financial planning, or coping with stress. These functions are commonly assumed informally by workplace colleagues or friends and neighbors and are especially valuable for stressed individuals whose coping with life demands is undermined by limited personal or salable skills (which may be true of certain maltreatment subpopulations) (see Polansky, Chalmers, Buttenwieser, & Williams, 1981; Seagull, 1987, and below). When this kind of assistance can be reciprocated by the recipient, moreover, the exchange of skills can be empowering; when assistance is one way, however, perceptions of vulnerability and dependency may ensue.

These four primary functions of social support are those most commonly conceived in research on social support and the design of supportive intervention programs. However, two additional functions of social support must also be considered in the effort to enlist support in the prevention of child maltreatment.

One concerns the use of social support for *social monitoring and social control*. In other words, one important function of social support for preventing maltreatment is the regulation provided by social network members, who, uniquely, can observe the target's behavior in everyday circumstances and can impose unique sanctions on disapproved parental conduct (cf. Garbarino, 1977a). To the extent to which friends, neighbors, and extended family members are deliberately enlisted into social support networks for preventing maltreatment, it is, in fact, hard to deny that social monitoring and control are the important goals of doing so. Local members of the social network are capable of observing and regulating the target's behavior far more effectively than can formal social service or law enforcement agencies, and, to the extent to which the target is enfranchised into the social network, their sanctions may be uniquely salient in regulating maltreating behavior. Local network members can also be effective in enlisting professional helpers by reporting suspected child maltreatment to local authorities. Social control may be, on the whole, the most important function of social networks in the prevention of child maltreatment.

But this is a much different function of social support from those conceived above: Whereas conventional portrayals of social support underscore the *provision* of needed resources that are valued by the recipient (consistent with the definition of social support provided at the beginning of this discussion), this function emphasizes the *constraints* imposed on the recipient's actions by network agents (House et al., 1988). To be sure, social monitoring is a more benign form of social control than are active efforts to regulate the target's actions, but all are intended to constrain the recipient's behavior. Although this may nevertheless be a valuable goal for the prevention of child maltreatment, its integration with other functions of social support (e.g., emotional sustenance) may be problematic. In other words, it may be difficult to enlist social network members for the dual purposes of providing emotional support and monitoring and controlling the target's parental behavior—especially if the target is aware of these roles.

Moreover, it is once again important to note that characteristics of the agents of social control deserve thoughtful consideration. Even though friends, neighbors, and extended family members can assume unique roles in monitoring and regulating the parental conduct of target individuals, they may not share the values and perspectives of social service and law enforcement personnel concerning the parameters of appropriate parental conduct. Certain behavior that is viewed as physically abusive or neglectful in the eyes of child protection caseworkers (e.g., harsh physical punishment and leaving young children unsupervised) may be regarded somewhat more benignly by informal neighborhood and community agents (cf. Garbarino & Crouter, 1978).

An additional function of social support highlighted by maltreatment prevention goals is the role of supportive agents in the *developmental remediation* of the victims of child abuse and neglect. Consistent with the victim-oriented tertiary prevention concern of this analysis, social support must be conceived also for its potential contributions to remediating the developmental consequences of child maltreatment, especially those contributing to psychopathological outcomes in children. As indicated earlier, systematic research on the victims of child maltreatment has revealed many different consequences of abuse and neglect for children's capacities to master the age-relevant challenges of psychological growth, and these developmental losses constitute an agenda for the goals of social support interventions. Thus, for infants and toddlers, social support might be enlisted to provide alternative attachment figures (perhaps in the context of therapeutic day care programs) with whom children can develop secure emotional bonds. For preschoolers and grade-school children, social support might be oriented toward strengthening peer social skills and integrating children into the social networks of age-mates in day care, school, and after-school (e.g., youth sports) programs. For grade-school children, social support to strengthen academic and intellectual competence should also be considered, as well as using supportive interventions to enhance self-esteem and reduce anxiety and depression. In adolescence, when social deviance is a potential consequence of maltreatment, a broader concern for the nature of extra-familial peer and adult social support systems is warranted to channel and redirect these impulses (i.e., social support for purposes of social control).

An example of how social support can function in these ways is found in a large study of social networks by Cochran and Riley (1990). By linking their mapping of children's social networks to family structure and children's academic competence, these researchers found that children with more adult relatives who involved them in task-oriented activities (car washing, shopping, etc.) had higher contemporaneous report-card scores and higher teacher reports of the child's cognitive motivation in the classroom. This was especially true of female-headed single-parent homes, in which boys especially benefited from activities with their male kin. These findings underscore not only that network size alone is relatively insensitive to the influences of particular network members but also that social support can enhance children's developmental achievements when viewed within the context of family structure and family processes. Yet, it is important to note that when child victims of maltreatment are concerned, social support influences should be regarded from the perspective of developmental remediation but with concern for the full range of benefits children might receive from supportive social agents: instrumental assistance, emotional sustenance, counseling and advice, companionship, and other functions described earlier (Peterson, 1990). Enlisting these agents in the context of tertiary prevention efforts within the context of a troubled family or an out-of-home placement, however, is especially challenging.

It is clear that there are multiple potential purposes for enlisting social support agents in the networks of maltreating families and that these functions are not necessarily mutually consistent. Therefore, it is wise to consider carefully the specific goal for social support interventions for the prevention of child abuse and neglect. Is it to give the recipient the feeling that someone cares? Is it to provide counseling concerning the problems and stresses that may contribute to child maltreatment? Is it to enhance access and referrals to others who might provide material or instrumental assistance to the recipient? Is it to enhance society's capacity to regulate and control the parental practices of high-risk adults? Is it to provide a forum in which the target's behavior can be critically self-examined, perhaps with the assistance of intervention agents in the target's social network? Not only are these goals diverse, but they entail different risks for the recipient and for the intervention. Social support may, at times, engender feelings of dependency, vulnerability, indebtedness, or stigma; it may be rejected because the recipient is unable to reciprocate; it may reinforce behavior that is undesirable but nevertheless consistent with the norms of the neighborhood or community in which the recipient's social network can be found; it may violate personal privacy; it may enhance conformity pressures.

In the end, social support interventions must be carefully crafted to ensure that specific, intended goals are advanced while some of the potential disadvantages of the intervention are compensated for. It is quite likely that different subpopulations of maltreatment will benefit differentially from different social support functions (e.g., access to services and skills acquisition for unemployed neglectful families and counseling, emotional sustenance, and social control for different members of sexually abusive families) and that different purposes for social support are relevant to the perpetrators and victims of maltreatment, as noted earlier. In short, the functions of social support are diverse and require consideration of their mutual compatibility, the agents who provide them, and trade-offs between the costs and benefits of social support from neighborhood and community sources.

Two additional comments concerning the functions of social support merit further attention. First, social support can function either as a stress buffer or as stress prevention, and many of the alternative functions of social support listed earlier can contribute to each (e.g., Barrera, 1986; Cohen & Wills, 1985; House et al., 1988; Vaux, 1988). On one hand, social support can be enlisted to aid an individual's coping with stressful events, and this *stress buffering* aids healthy functioning through the kinds of emotional, instrumental, and regulatory functions assumed by social support agents. The stress-buffering functions of social support are thus enlisted after the onset of stressful events. On the other hand, social support can aid in *stress prevention* by surrounding the recipient with people who provide emotional and instrumental assistance and advice that contributes to healthy functioning. The company of others fosters self-esteem, a sense of belonging, access to reference figures, and compliance with social norms that can be health enhancing (Vaux, 1988). In this context, stress is prevented before it exacts a cost because of the contributions of social support to physical and mental well-being. Both stress-buffering and stress-prevention aspects of social support accord well with the enlistment of social support to prevent child maltreatment but obviously function in somewhat different ways.

The distinction between the stress-buffering and stress-prevention aspects of social support is important, however, in conceptualizing the role of social support interventions in secondary and tertiary prevention. Although both stress buffering and stress prevention are likely to be relevant, in secondary prevention the enlistment of social support for purposes of stress prevention might be preeminent. In this context, social network members might be most valuable in providing emotional sustenance, counseling and advice, access to information and resources, and skills acquisition in their overall efforts to strengthen healthy functioning in high-risk individuals and families. In the context of tertiary prevention, however, enlisting social support for purposes of stress buffering might be emphasized over its stress-prevention aspects. In these circumstances, social network members might best assume monitoring (social control) roles and assist in the developmental remediation of offspring, as well as the other supportive functions outlined above. Although it is unwise to demarcate the various functions of social support solely in terms of their stress-buffering and stress-prevention aspects, this conceptual distinction can contribute to clearer thinking about the goals of social support interventions for preventing child maltreatment.

Second, the extent to which the efficacy of social support depends on the recipient's subjective experience of being supported is an issue that both clarifies this analysis and helps to clarify the relations between different social support functions. Although it is intuitively obvious that most forms of social support are subjectively perceived as helpful by recipients (emotional sustenance, advice and counseling, access to information or services, skills acquisition, etc.), it is not true that all forms of social support must be so perceived. Social network agents enlisted for purposes of social control are one example of supportive interventions that may ultimately benefit recipients without necessarily being perceived in that manner (indeed, recipients may be averse to the regulatory activities of social network members). More colloquially, when friends, neighbors, or extended family members urge individuals to stop smoking, drinking, or engaging in substance abuse, their supportive actions may instead be rejected by the individual they are intended to benefit. These considerations are important because support agents enlisted for the prevention of child maltreatment may be subjectively perceived as either supportive or nonsupportive by target individuals, and it is important to clarify the intended role of supportive agents in the design of interventions. It may be very hard for the same supportive agents to provide emotional sustenance, counseling, and other manifestly helpful interventions while critically challenging the recipient's parenting practices or trying to change his or her behavior, and intervention programs that seek to embrace such diverse functions of social support face important (although not insurmountable) challenges. Moreover, to the extent that the maintenance of social support requires the active cooperation of the intervention target, targets are more likely to maintain contact with social agents they perceive as being supportive than with other network members who they perceive as being more critical and unsupportive.

These considerations underscore the complexity of social support when it is conceptually "unpacked." Adding further complexity to this analysis are the findings of studies that examine the predictors of the success of social support in the lives of stressed individuals. Such studies seek to answer how—once we understand what social support is and does—we can best predict the impact of social support interventions. Thus, we turn to a consideration of this literature.

PREDICTING THE EFFECTS OF SOCIAL SUPPORT

One of the considerable challenges in applying current research on social support to the design of child maltreatment prevention programs is that the effects of social support are often population specific. In other words, interventions that benefit older adults in nursing homes are not necessarily the same interventions that will assist families with a developmentally delayed child or will aid an adolescent mother. This is hardly surprising because the ecological circumstances of stressed individuals and families are different, the personal and interpersonal resources on which they can usually rely vary considerably, their own skills for enlisting social support also vary, and society has different regard for the needs and characteristics of individuals who face different stresses and demands. However, this specificity makes the generalization of studies concerning social support more problematic for an analysis of child maltreatment prevention.

Nevertheless, it is possible to distill several general factors that may underlie the likely success of social support—especially naturally occurring social support—in the lives of maltreating and high-risk families. This section discusses these factors, with special attention to their relevance to enlisting neighborhood- and community-based social supports in the prevention of child abuse and neglect. The considerations that predict the efficacy of social support include the following: the effects of stress on the availability of support, the effects of the recipient's personal characteristics on access to social support, general characteristics of recipient reactions to aid, the relationship between social support agents and their social network membership, provider reactions to help giving, the challenges of providing social support in families with overlapping social networks and multiple targets of social support interventions, and finally the acknowledgement that social networks are often sources of stress as well as support. These considerations underscore the complexity in designing and supporting successful social interventions for troubled families and the need for careful thought in such efforts.

Effects of Stress on the Availability of Social Support

In many respects, the relationship between stress and social support is reciprocal: Support may reduce the incidence or impact of stressful events, but
stress may also alter the availability of social support. Important and severe
stressors such as job loss, divorce, and hospitalization have a significant
impact on the nature of the support networks on which one can rely or on
one's accessibility to those networks (Shinn et al., 1984; Vaux, 1988). On
one hand, stressors may *enhance* social support, as support agents become
mobilized to provide assistance and as the recipient may seek aid and become more receptive to the assistance that is offered (Vaux, 1988). On the
other hand, stressors may *diminish* social support because they decrease
network size or the recipient's access to support agents (Shinn et al., 1984).
Loss of a job or divorce, for example, can eliminate access to support agents
on whom one has typically relied on the past. As a consequence, support
agents may be least available and/or accessible on precisely those occasions
when they are most needed.

The impact of stress on the availability of social support is not only
apparent with respect to episodic, severe stress. Under chronic stressful conditions—especially when those stresses are widely shared among members
of the social network or neighborhood—social support may be less obtainable
because of the impact of enduring stressful conditions on potential support
sources. As already noted, for example, individuals from lower-SES circumstances typically have smaller social networks than those from middle- and
upper-SES groups (Cochran, Gunnarsson, et al., 1990; Fischer, 1982; Vaux,
1988), and single mothers likewise have smaller social networks with higher
rates of turnover compared to married mothers (Gunnarsson & Cochran,
1990; Larner, 1990a; Leslie & Grady, 1985; Weinraub & Wolf, 1983). In
each case, networks of diminished size and stability may derive not only from
characteristics of potential recipients (e.g., how divorce and single parenting
reduce the range of potential support agents) but also from how network
members themselves may share some of the same stressors experienced by
distressed individuals (e.g., socioeconomic distress).

Enlisting neighborhood-based social support in the prevention of child
maltreatment thus requires considering not only the various potential agents
of support but how the stressors experienced by high-risk families or maltreating parents may alter potential support networks. When maltreatment
derives partly from socioeconomic stress, for example, it is likely that network members themselves suffer from the same conditions as those who need
assistance. When a substance abuse problem partly accounts for abuse or
neglect, that problem may also limit the range of potential support agents in
the parent's environment and alter the quality of support the agents can
provide (especially if the agents also have problems with drug dependency).
When parents have been found guilty of sexual abuse, the social stigma attached to this finding may itself alter the nature and number of social sup-

ports that can be found to assist in preventing reabuse, especially if neighbors and community members react with outrage or anger. In short, it is important to consider not only the unique circumstances of the distressed individuals who are targets of social support interventions, but how those stressful circumstances affect the kinds of support that may be available to distressed individuals.

Effects of the Recipient's Personal Characteristics on Social Support

Social support is usually not received passively. Especially when informal social supports are concerned, support must be sought, accessed, and maintained by the recipient. Viewed in this light, a predictor of the extent to which social support can reduce stress is not only the availability of supportive agents, but the recipient's capacity to gain help from these agents. Therefore, the recipient's personal characteristics may be an important mediating variable in the relationship between social support and well-being (Heller & Swindle, 1983; Shinn et al., 1984).

At a minimum, these personal characteristics include the basic social skills needed to establish and maintain supportive relationships with social network members. Deficits in this capacity may derive from many sources, including the effects of stress itself (e.g., when stress results in depression), constituent social skills, intellectual competency, and a sufficient degree of mental health to engage in satisfying sociability with others (which may be episodically affected by a substance abuse problem as well as periodic or chronic psychological dysfunction). Personal characteristics needed to utilize social support also include the motivational bases for help seeking, such as an awareness of the relevance of support to one's coping capacities, sufficient sociability to seek assistance from others, and perceptions that support is available. These personal characteristics also include the time and energy necessary to enlist assistance from others—which may themselves be diminished by stress or by other personal characteristics of the potential recipient. Beyond these minima, other personal characteristics of the recipient may affect the extent to which social support is obtained from network members. These characteristics include the recipient's extraversion, self-disclosure, comfort in intimate relations with others, and other social dispositions.

The recipient's developmental status is also an important personal characteristic relevant to accessing and maintaining social support. Infants and young children have little control over the social networks that potentially can provide them with support, and adult support agents do not expect them to assume much responsibility for obtaining assistance because young children have few effective competencies for establishing and maintaining their own supportive social networks. As a result, the social support they receive is usually not contingent upon their personal skills and abilities. However, even during the preschool years—and certainly by grade school—certain forms of social support become contingent upon the recipient's personal characteristics. Peers and adults increasingly evaluate the personal characteristics of children when establishing and maintaining relationships with them, and during the late preschool and early grade-school years, the social competence and attractiveness of children become important predictors of their social embeddedness, especially with peers (Hartup, 1983).

This is important because, as noted earlier, maltreated children have deficiencies in social skills that can impair peer relationships, which can make it harder to enlist peers in interventions to remediate the effects of abuse and prevent more deleterious developmental outcomes. The aggressive and impulsive behavior of children who have been abused or neglected is likely to undermine the very peer relationships that can provide assistance to them. This becomes especially significant as, with increasing age, children rely more on self-constructed peer social networks, and as the nature and quality of their social experiences depend more on the personal competencies that are needed to create and maintain satisfying peer relationships. Thus, the recipient's personal characteristics for enlisting social support are developmentally graded but become important from a surprisingly early age.

To be sure, not all forms of social support are so contingent upon the recipient's personal characteristics. It does not require significant skill, for example, to receive the kinds of material or financial assistance that others can provide or to receive unsolicited advice from others (some of which may be unwanted). Some forms of social support are provided to young children regardless of their personal skills, as noted above. However, most of the important forms of social support that are the subject of this chapter are mediated by the personal characteristics of the recipient. This means that support resources may exist in an individual's neighborhood or community without the individual benefiting from them.

These considerations have provoked a lively debate among students of social support about whether the apparent buffering effects of social support on stress result primarily from the social competence of the recipient. As stated by Heller (1979):

> The often repeated finding in naturalistic studies that persons with established support networks are in better mental and physical health than are the unsupported may be due to variables other than social support. . . . It is possible that competent persons, who are more immune to the adverse effects of stress, are also more likely to have well developed social networks as a direct result of their more general social competence. (p. 361)

While most other commentators have not adopted such a strong position, especially in light of prospective research suggesting a strong causal role for social support per se (see House et al., 1988), the argument that social competence is the basis for the apparent stress-buffering effects of social support underscores its important mediating role.

With respect to enlisting social support for the prevention of child maltreatment, moreover, social competence may be a very important mediator. Seagull (1987) has argued that studies of maltreating families provide very little evidence for social isolation, but when they do, isolation derives more from their limited social skills than from deficits in the social supports of their neighborhoods and communities. Consistently with the research of Polansky and his colleagues (Gaudin & Polansky, 1986; Gaudin & Pollane, 1983; Polansky et al., 1981; Polansky, Gaudin, Ammons, & David, 1985), Seagull argues that this is especially apparent of neglectful families, whose characterological deficits in social skills and competence constrain their capacities to access and maintain supportive networks among neighbors, friends, and kin. From this perspective, therefore, social skills training is an essential component of intervention efforts to strengthen social supports for parents who neglect their offspring. Because Seagull's argument and Polansky's research are important for understanding the social isolation of neglectful families, they will be reconsidered in greater detail later in this chapter. But from their perspective and those of other students of the etiology of child maltreatment, interventions that strengthen a recipient's capacities to access and maintain support from network members—in the context of social skills training or information concerning potential sources of informal support in the neighborhood, or by strengthening the roles of natural helpers (Collins & Pancoast, 1976) who can mediate access to supportive community agents— may be an important contribution to the efficacy of social support interventions.

Recipient Reactions to Aid

The personal characteristics of the recipient help to account for individual differences in the capacity to maintain supportive social networks and to seek assistance from network members when distressed. But for most people, the experience of receiving assistance from others engenders both positive and negative reactions that can also influence the experience of being aided and being willing to receive assistance in the future. Understanding these recipient reactions to aid is especially important when considering the role of social support in the prevention of child maltreatment because social support is usually regarded as an ongoing resource for distressed individuals. Recipient reactions to aid may be unimportant, in other words, if assistance occurs on only one occasion (e.g., a financial donation), but social support typically is conceived as a continuing, incremental benefit. Because the recipient's efforts are necessary (at least in part) for the maintenance of social support, recipient reactions to aid may significantly mediate the efficacy of social support interventions.

Assistance from others can evoke diverse reactions in recipients (Fisher et al., 1982; Shumaker & Brownell, 1984). Along with the positive feelings of support and gratitude that accompany aid, recipients may also experience feelings of failure, indebtedness, vulnerability, inferiority, and dependency. These feelings may occur for several reasons. First, norms of equity in our society motivate individuals to try to reciprocate the assistance they receive from others, and if they fail (because they cannot or are prevented from doing so), they experience discomfort and anxiety (Greenberg, 1980; Greenberg & Westcott, 1983; Hatfield & Sprecher, 1983). Discomfort may arise because of feelings of indebtedness, the experience of humiliation, and/or fears of exploitation due to the unreciprocated receipt of assistance from the benefactor. These feelings are especially acute when support is costly to the one providing aid, the benefactor's motives are voluntary and altruistic, and/or the recipient receives large benefits, which in each case heightens perceptions of inequity and indebtedness.

Second, help giving also often involves implicit assessments, not only of the benefactor's motivations but also of the reasons the recipient requires help. If help is needed because of external conditions buffeting the recipient (e.g., socioeconomic stress or sudden financial or legal difficulties), help giving involves little stigma as long as those circumstances are not attributable to the recipient's personal qualities. However, if help is needed because of the recipient's personal attributes (e.g., poor skills at personal or family management or inadequate impulse control), help giving reflects the recipient's failure and inadequacy and receiving help in these circumstances may be stigmatizing. Moreover, receiving assistance in the context of perceptions of personal inadequacy may paradoxically increase the recipient's helplessness and dependency insofar as it conveys clear messages about the recipient's inability to succeed on his or her own. Third, receiving assistance may also directly threaten self-esteem because it threatens autonomy, privacy, and self-reliance (Fisher et al., 1982). Privacy violations in the context of helping may be especially threatening to self-esteem because they attack the integrity of possessional and informational self-control.

To be sure, help giving typically involves a mingling of positive and negative perceptions of the benefactor, the assistance, the recipient, and the circumstances in which help is offered and received. Although unrequited altruism often inspires mixed feelings in those who benefit, gratitude is also almost inevitable (Hatfield & Sprecher, 1983). Attention to recipient reactions is important, however, not just because of how the reactions affect the experience of receiving help, but primarily because of their effects on future access to assistance. When recipients cannot restore equity in help-giving relationships, or experience assistance as stigmatizing or humiliating, they are less likely to seek help in the future and are more likely to terminate a help-giving relationship (Fisher et al., 1982; Shumaker & Brownell, 1984). In these circumstances, moreover, recipients are more likely to reinterpret the situation to restore their self-esteem, such as by derogating the benefactor, minimizing the extent of the assistance or its costs to the benefactor, and/or perceiving the benefactor as less altruistic and more manipulative. This is especially likely when assistance is received from strangers (with whom one does not share an ongoing relationship of mutual aid) or nonprofessionals (for whom reciprocity and equity norms are more salient than with professional help givers) and when the benefactor and the recipient come from similar social circumstances (such as sharing neighborhood and community ties) in which the inequity of the helping relationship is especially salient (Fisher et al., 1982; Greenberg & Westcott, 1983; Shumaker & Brownell, 1984). These conditions make the maintenance and continuity of assistance especially difficult in informal and neighborhood-based forms of assistance and pose special challenges for social support interventions that require, at least, the recipient's tacit participation.

The literature suggests several factors that will support, rather than undermine, recipients' positive perceptions of assistance. Recipients are most likely to regard assistance positively when they (1) have opportunities to reciprocate (or are required to repay) the aid they are receiving either to the benefactor or to others who require help, especially in the context of a relationship of reciprocal assistance; (2) have the freedom to accept assistance based on their own perceptions of need; (3) perceive the benefactor's intentions as a combination of self-interest and altruism in the helping relationship (i.e., not as wholly altruistic); (4) estimate that assistance comes at little direct cost to the benefactor (with costs borne primarily, perhaps, by impersonal social institutions and agencies); (5) regard their own need for assistance as externally instigated (e.g., arising from difficult life demands at work or neighborhood) rather than from personal inadequacies; (6) perceive assistance as an entitlement rather than a bestowal of aid; and (7) receive assistance in settings and circumstances that reduce stigma, perhaps as a component of normative benefits (e.g., assistance in the context of everyday encounters, routine transactions with social or institutional agents, and/or programs whose benefits are widely shared by community members), and ensure privacy (Pettigrew, 1983). In this regard, programs to provide assistance are most likely to succeed when they provide universal benefits (i.e., recipient populations are not stigmatized by their identification with the program) or, if this is impossible, can be incorporated into programs that target a broad and heterogeneous population.

When young children are the recipients of assistance, it is less clear that these considerations apply. One reason is that social norms of equity and reciprocity are less regularly applied to children, who are, almost by definition, regular recipients of unrequited benefits from adults. Moreover, young children are likely to be less cognizant of the attributional processes involved in receiving support in conditions that may be stigmatizing or contribute to perceptions of personal inadequacy. Although preschoolers often reciprocate the benefits they receive from others (especially peers), it is not clear that this reflects their awareness of social norms of equity rather than simply acting in a manner that maintains good relations with others (Eisenberg, 1983). However, it is important to recognize that expectations of reciprocity begin to be influential during the early school years and are especially important in late school age and adolescence, when more mature appraisals of social norms, inferences concerning motives, and attributions concerning the recipient are possible (Eisenberg, 1983). Thus, from a surprisingly early age, children become vulnerable to the feelings of indebtedness, inferiority, and dependency that commonly mark adults' reactions to aid, and pertinent considerations concerning the nature of the assistance and the contexts in which it is obtained should apply to the social support they receive also.

Support Agents and Their Social Network Membership

Another important consideration in predicting the effects of social support on stress concerns the nature of the support agents and their place in the target's social network. In essence, who is offering assistance and what other roles do they have in the life of the recipient? Encompassed within this broad question are a number of more specific issues.

First, because informal support agents—such as a relative, a neighbor, a coworker, a classmate, clergy, a doctor, barber, or hairdresser, to name several—often have additional roles and responsibilities in relation to the recipient, a potential conflict exists between providing support and the provider's institutional commitments, professional responsibilities, and personal values. Neighbor(s) may be more concerned about finding a quick exit from a troubled community than with providing support to troubled individuals who live nearby. The assistance of a relative may be colored by a legacy of family conflict, or by the kin's greater concern for the niece or nephew who has been maltreated than for the brother or sister who is abusive. Community caregivers may be as concerned about maintaining a professional partnership, pleasing a customer (or employer), or advancing a program as they are with providing emotional sustenance or counseling. A doctor, school personnel, or other professionals may be affected by their knowledge of—and personal reactions to—an abusive incident, and the existence of mandatory child abuse reporting laws may also color their interactions with parents or children from high-risk families. They may limit contact, for example, with family members who demand more attention and concern than they can provide and who additionally pose uncomfortable problems for their professional roles. Coworkers may be divided between their allegiance to a troubled fellow employee and their fidelity to the employer, especially when stress affects an employee's competence or productivity. In short, many informal support agents have multiple interests and commitments that may influence the support they can offer distressed individuals. This may be especially true when the recipient is a maltreating parent or is at high risk for child abuse or neglect, when the social stigma attached to the adult's behavior is considerable in our society.

Second, because informal support agents occupy unique "niches" in the recipient's life, they can offer unique forms of social support. A neighbor can provide respite child care, emergency assistance, and sometimes material aid; a coworker can assist in managing workplace stress and, at times, offer emotional relief from family-based demands; kin can offer understanding based on long-term personal intimacy; a schoolteacher is someone apart from family and friends who knows the child and parent and can provide helpful advice; a doctor or minister can provide a likewise dispassionate perspective and, at times, professional advice or a referral. This kind of "situation specificity" of support agents (Unger & Powell, 1980) suggests that informal network members are specialized for specific kinds of social support. Intervention programs that rely on informal support systems should be designed with this kind of specificity in mind.

Third, efforts to prevent child maltreatment seldom rely exclusively on informal support systems. Concurrent with the efforts of informal network members are the activities of formal support agencies, including social service personnel in the community, welfare workers, therapists, law enforcement agents, and people associated with a variety of public–private initiatives such as food pantries, soup kitchens, and other programs. Because these personnel often provide social support along with other services, the coordination of formal and informal support efforts should be incorporated into the thoughtful design of neighborhood- and community-based maltreatment prevention programs (cf. Collins & Pancoast, 1976; Froland, Pancoast, Chapman, & Kimboko, 1981; Lewis & Fraser, 1987; Miller & Whittaker, 1988; Tracy & Whittaker, 1987; Whittaker, Schinke, & Gilchrist, 1986).

The coordination of formal and informal helpers is important because each kind of helping agent can make unique contributions to the needs of high-risk families. Whereas professional helpers have expertise, enhanced personal and material resources, and the benefits of a clear role definition in relation to recipients and professional accountability, informal support agents can provide more ongoing and multifaceted forms of assistance in the context of mutual help giving, using approaches consistent with the values of the community in which target individuals live (Collins & Pancoast, 1976; Froland et al., 1981). Gottlieb (1983) argues that a natural support network differs from professional services in other ways also, including the following:

> (a) its natural accessibility; (b) its congruence with local norms about when and how support ought to be expressed; (c) its rootedness in long-standing peer relationships; (d) its variability, ranging from the provision of tangible goods and services to simple companionship; and (e) its freedom from financial and psychological (stigmatizing) costs incurred when professional resources are used. (p. 27)

Just as informal, neighborhood-based support agents should not try to emulate the functions and skills of professionals, it may be impossible for professional helpers to assume many of the unique roles identified by Gottlieb that social network members assume in the lives of recipients of social support. Both forms of helping are unique, and each benefits by their mutual intercoordination.

In particular, program planners should strive to avoid two potential dangers. One is that informal support systems would be undermined by enlisting formal services, which can occur when formal agencies (1) contribute to labeling or stigmatizing recipient families, (2) disrupt informal support networks by assuming their functions or diminishing their perceived importance or influence, or (3) undermine informal support agents by increasing demands upon them (Froland et al., 1981). In a sense, a successful neighborhood-based prevention strategy requires that agents of formal support systems respect and assist the informal social networks that often provide tangible and meaningful aid to targeted individuals (Collins & Pancoast, 1976). This is crucial because networks of informal helping relationships help to define neighborhood coherence and integrity—both a "sense of community" and a personal attachment to it—that the recipients of professional assistance can draw on in their efforts to establish psychological and emotional well-being (cf. Unger & A. Wandersman, 1985). In a sense, professional efforts that undermine informal helping relationships also undermine one of the defining elements of "neighborhood" when this term is defined by its relational rather than locational features.

A second danger is that informal social network members will undermine the recipient's access to formal agencies, such as when extended family members conceal abuse or seek to limit access to the perpetrator or victim, or neighbors reinforce the recipient's skepticism of the benefits of contacting formal help agents. Although this is sometimes difficult to avoid in the context of tertiary prevention, the coordination of formal and informal support systems in child protection can reduce the likelihood that agents of each system will act in a mutually antagonistic fashion or with conflicting goals.

Finally, it is worthwhile questioning whether social support always comes from individuals within personal and familial social networks. Shumaker and Brownell (1984) pointed out that self-disclosure and helpful advice may occur more easily in fairly anonymous social encounters, such as in conversations with strangers on airplanes or buses or with casual acquaintances at work or school. In these cases, it is the *lack* of personal intimacy that contributes to candid communication because the risks of self-disclosure are low. In a similar manner, crisis hot lines or "warm lines" (from which even children can benefit) (see Peterson, 1990) permit the discussion of personal conflicts or stressful circumstances with total strangers, and helpful counseling can occur in these nonthreatening circumstances because anonymity can foster self-disclosure and candid advice giving. In short, social support may be obtained from individuals who are not part of one's social network—indeed, who are sometimes completely anonymous—because some forms of social support avail when the risks of self-disclosure are low. In such cases, the disadvantages of receiving support from individuals who do not know you well, and who cannot provide ongoing assistance, are outweighed by the opportunity for candid conversation with someone who will not carry this information into future encounters with the recipient. This view, too, should be considered when designing social support programs to benefit the victims and perpetrators of child maltreatment.

Therefore, identifying potential support agents in the social networks of stressed individuals requires considering their broader roles in the individual's life. The possibility of conflicts with institutional commitments and personal values, the situation specificity of the kind of help they can offer, and the need for the integration of formal and informal support services suggest that careful network mapping is an essential ingredient to the design of effective neighborhood-based social support programs oriented to the prevention of child maltreatment.

Provider Reactions to Assistance

It is important to note also that help giving can be demanding and stressful to providers of assistance. Social support, in particular, requires emotional as well as material resources that can be quickly consumed by recipients in the context of an ongoing, long-term relationship. When these relationships are enlisted for the prevention of child maltreatment, providers experience additional stresses for several reasons. First, parents and offspring who are at high risk for maltreatment often experience multiple needs—economic, personal, residential, legal—that can overwhelm potential providers, especially those found in informal support networks. Second, parents and children from high-risk families are often unable or unwilling to reciprocate the support they receive, either because of their reactions to the experience of receiving help (as described above) or because of personal characteristics or external stresses that make it difficult for them to devote attention to others' needs and concerns. As a consequence, providers are likely to experience their relationships with recipients as frustrating conduits of one-way (rather than mutual) aid (Polansky, Ammons, & Gaudin, 1985). Third, the goals for help giving are likely to be differently conceived by the providers and recipients of social support (Shumaker & Brownell, 1984). Especially when social support is enlisted for secondary or tertiary prevention, providers are likely to be most concerned with strengthening positive parenting practices and ensuring that children are not maltreated. Recipients, by contrast, may be most interested in obtaining emotional nurturance and access to material resources. Their conflicting goals may cause both providers and recipients of assistance to feel frustrated by the relationship or disappointed in the partner, to experience their relationship as being "out of sync," or to engage in open conflict.

For these reasons, well-conceived social support programs that focus on informal neighborhood assistance will devote as much attention to "supporting the supporters" as to targeting the recipients of assistance. Indeed, far more might be accomplished by addressing the needs of support agents than by focusing on recipients alone. Because of the unique features of helping relationships with needy families (different, by definition, from other social relationships) and the potential for the exhaustion of support providers, assistance to potential benefactors is an important ingredient for the success of social support programs. As suggested earlier, this might occur as formal and informal support agents coordinate and integrate their activities in relation to high-risk families, or it might require directly targeting resources to the informal support agents identified in neighborhoods and communities.

Social Support and Overlapping Social Networks within the Family

The inherent challenges of providing social support to stressed individuals are multiplied in efforts to provide support to several family members with diverse needs, characteristics, and interests. In the context of preventing child maltreatment, of course, a family-oriented approach is essential. Support should be offered not only to parents who are at risk for abusing or neglecting offspring but also to children who may suffer from the developmental losses characteristic of maltreated children, or who may show other effects of their high-risk status. Consequently, coordinating support efforts to multiple family members requires considering not only the personal social networks that each member may rely on, but also the family social network that is the aggregate of their personal networks. The family social network is important because social support provided to one family member may have indirect consequences for others.

On many occasions, for example, social support offered to parents can have beneficial consequences for offspring. It is striking, however, how early this can occur. Cutrona (1984) reported, for example, that an overall index of social support that mothers received during pregnancy and a component index of "social integration" (i.e., homogeneity) together predicted postpartum maternal depression 8 weeks after delivery. Mothers with enhanced support experienced less depressive symptomatology (see Unger & L. P. Wandersman, 1985, for similar results). After birth, support agents can indirectly benefit offspring by providing emotional sustenance to parents, offering personal and childrearing advice, enhancing the family's material resources, providing models of appropriate parenting practices, and monitoring and (at times) regulating childrearing behavior (Cochran, 1990a, 1990b; Cochran & Brassard, 1979). As a practical example, it seems that much of the success of Hawaii's perinatal home-visitation program in reducing child maltreatment derives from the manner in which social and emotional support for young mothers reduces the personal demands and isolation that can contribute to child maltreatment.

Consistent with this view, a number of investigators found that social support that reduces sources of stress for mothers has beneficial effects on offspring. When Weinraub and Wolf (1983) observed mothers interacting with their preschoolers, for example, they found that more optimal maternal behavior was associated with diminished stress and greater amounts of parenting and emotional support for mothers in two-parent families and with diminished stress, fewer working hours, and greater parenting support for single mothers (see Crnic, Greenberg, Ragozin, Robinson, & Basham, 1983; Crnic, Greenberg, Robinson, & Ragozin, 1984, for similar results with mothers and infants). As these results suggest, however, social network characteristics that heighten stress on parents (e.g., extended working hours) can have negative consequences for offspring. For example, the transition from divorce to single parenting results in diminished social support to mothers (Belle, 1982; Colletta, 1979; Larner, 1990a; Gunnarsson & Cochran, 1990; Weinraub & Wolf, 1983) and is associated with greater punitiveness and authoritarianism in childrearing beliefs (Colletta, 1979) and with diminished supervision and greater social deviance in adolescent offspring (Dornbusch et al., 1985).

Thus, social support provided to one family member (in these cases, a parent) can have indirect benefits for other family members (such as offspring). Social support provided to one family member may, on other occasions, have undesirable indirect consequences for other family members, or even for the recipient. Extended family members who provide emotional support to parents may, at the same time, reinforce harshly punitive or neglectful parenting practices that are detrimental to offspring. Conversely, extended kin may support children who are at risk for maltreatment but, at the same time, denigrate and undermine their parents. Social support provided by nonkin may also have unanticipated indirect detriments for offspring. Weinraub and Wolf (1983) found, for example, that the total number of social contacts experienced by single mothers was *negatively* associated with competent parenting because, the authors reasoned, single mothers who sought outside relationships with supportive adults had less time to devote to offspring. The potentially deleterious effects of social support on other family members may become especially acute when obtaining support casts other family members in a humiliating, vulnerable, or dependent light. For example, Robertson, Elder, Skinner, and Conger (1991) reported that husbands who were inconsistently employed were more negative toward their spouses and more punitive in their parenting when their wives sought and obtained emotional support from outside the family, presumably because doing so confirmed the husband's sense of failure and helplessness. These associations were not observed in families in which husbands were stably employed. Thus, the availability of social support for one family member is not necessarily a uniformly positive experience: It may have indirect consequences for other family members, or for the recipient, that can complement or undermine the support provided the recipient.

At times, the direct and indirect consequences of social support within family social networks can be complex. In a study of rural towns in Australia, for example, Cotterell (1986) found that childrearing attitudes and behavior were strongly predicted by an interaction of (1) the father's absence (owing to job demands), (2) the mother's "informational support" from neighborhood agents about raising children, and (3) characteristics of the community (e.g., stability of the population), with support to the mother being the most important of these predictors. These findings suggest that the treatment of offspring is indirectly affected by familial social networks that are themselves affected by employment as well as community characteristics. In another Australian study, Homel, Burns, and Goodnow (1987) reported that measures of the socioemotional adjustment and social functioning of school-age offspring were predicted by the number of "dependable friends" parents could list and parents' affiliation with voluntary organizations (e.g., community groups, religious institutions, and business/professional organizations). The family's "neighborhood risk level" (i.e., an index of socioeconomic status, delinquency, school truancy, and related variables) also influenced the child measures, suggesting that parents may provide both role models and avenues for access to social networks from which children can potentially benefit within the constraints of their neighborhoods. Finally, O'Donnell and Steuve (1983) reported that lower-income and middle-class mothers differed significantly in the access they provided offspring to community resources and services, consistent with the findings of the Australian studies. Whereas middle-class mothers reliably tended to use regularly scheduled, publicly sponsored community services and to enfranchise themselves into these programs as volunteers and aides, lower-income mothers were more reluctant to commit themselves or their children to scheduled activities and instead preferred to give their children greater (unscheduled) freedom for "just being with friends." As a consequence, their children were afforded significantly fewer opportunities to benefit from these programs and activities.

These findings indicate that there are significant and complex relations between the personal social networks of parents and offspring and that the direct and indirect effects of the familial social network on its members can vary in its impact and valence. The studies illustrate the multidimensionality of these influence processes and the importance of considering them in efforts to provide social support to maltreating families. In essence, as students of family policy have discovered in other aspects of family functioning, efforts to influence the experience of one family member can have broader implications for other family members that are often unanticipated or in conflict with intended goals (cf. Thompson et al., 1992). Because a family is such a complex social institution, all its members are likely to be affected by interventions designed to provide social support to one family member. Moreover, because social support is a resource from which all members of high-risk families can benefit, programs to enlist supportive agents for one family member should seek to ensure that either the effects of the intervention on other family members are benign or interventions provide benefits to other family members also.

It is important to recognize occasions when social support might be targeted to one family member with relatively little impact on others. Children can benefit from Big Brother or Big Sister programs, for example, in which their activities occupy after-school time that minimally affects family life. The same is true of a variety of curricular and extracurricular school activities or day care programs for younger children. However, it is important to recognize that indirect effects on the rest of the family—or the child—may nevertheless derive from such experiences. Children who are exposed to new values, perspectives, and experiences may arouse the resentment, envy, or anger of other family members when these experiences are brought home, and the child's participation in such extrafamilial activities may also become the focus of coercive or manipulative efforts by parents. In general, therefore, social support that is broadly conceived—that takes into consideration its impact on all family members even when only one is the primary target—is likely to be more successful than are more limited intervention efforts.

Social Networks as Sources of Social Stress

As many aspects of the previous discussion have implied, relationships with social network members have diverse consequences for most individuals. Friends, neighbors, relatives, coworkers, and other social agents can be potent sources of social support but may also instigate conflict, create frustration or humiliation, and impose demands on the target individual (cf. Garbarino, 1977a). In short, social networks provide benefits but also impose costs, and any effort to enlist informal support systems for preventing child maltreatment must take into account the fact that relationships with social network members can be stressful, demanding, and evaluative. Indeed, conflict with network members may influence one's experience of stress more potently than the amount of support such members provide (Shinn et al., 1984).

This is an especially important consideration with respect to the populations that are at highest risk for child maltreatment, and that are likely to experience multiple stressors of various kinds. As Belle (1982) has evocatively noted with respect to socioeconomically distressed single mothers: "One cannot receive support without also risking the costs of rejection, betrayal, burdensome dependence, and vicarious pain. This is probably especially true among the poor, whose relatives, friends, and neighbors are likely to be stressed and needy themselves" (p. 143).

Such a conclusion is aptly demonstrated in her interviews with women who experienced their extended kin as demanding and burdensome, husbands and boyfriends as unreliable (and frequently abusive), and neighborhoods as dangerous or entrapping. As noted earlier, Belle (1982) found that women with larger social networks, who lived in close proximity to network members, and who interacted frequently with network members in their communities were no less depressed, anxious, or psychologically healthy when compared with women who were more socially isolated, contrary to the findings of other research studies reported earlier. Similarly, women who were extensively involved with their neighbors were not those who experienced the greatest social support. In short, in communities in which residents experience the greatest need for social support from neighbors (and in which social support might be most helpful in reducing child maltreatment), informal support networks are most limited because potential helpers are themselves stressed and needy ("drained" in the parlance of social researchers). Identified providers of social support may themselves be exhausted because of their efforts to assist others, and neighborhoods may undermine rather than support mutual help among community members. This is perhaps one of the greatest challenges in designing neighborhood-based social support systems that rely on informal helpers in communities where families are at high risk for child maltreatment.

Overall, predicting the effects of social support is a very complex calculus of considerations related to characteristics of the recipients, the providers of assistance, their social networks, and the physicosocial ecology in which social support occurs. These considerations are important, however, because they indicate why support providers become burned out by their roles, why recipients sometimes reject the assistance they are provided, why certain informal support agents are ineffective, why support can exist in communities without being utilized, and why social network members are sometimes the best—and worst—sources of informal support. In short, these considerations indicate mistakes to be avoided, avenues to be pursued, and complexities to be encompassed in the design of neighborhood-based social support interventions.

THE SOCIAL CONTEXT OF CHILD MALTREATMENT

With these considerations in mind, it is appropriate to consider the social conditions associated with child maltreatment and examine how the nature and functions of social networks, and of the various predictors of the success of informal social support systems, can inform our understanding of the physicosocial ecology of child abuse and neglect. Among the questions meriting consideration are the following: How does the social context of child maltreatment help to define the parameters of neighborhood-based social supports for high-risk parents and their offspring? What are the potential social resources these families can draw on for obtaining support from social network members? What is the meaning of the well-documented "social isolation" of maltreating families? Does the preceding social network analysis help us to understand the constituents of social support that are lacking in the social ecology of high-risk families and, conversely, the aspects of their social support that are comparable to those of untroubled families? What features of the social networks of maltreating families require further research? To the extent to which these families are socially isolated, what are the reasons? What potential avenues exist for strengthening informal social supports within their neighborhoods and communities?

This ambitious agenda begins with a summary of research knowledge of the broader socioeconomic conditions associated with child maltreatment. It then turns to a detailed review of studies documenting the social isolation of maltreating families to understand (1) the criteria by which these families are deemed to be isolated, (2) the dimensions of their social networks that appear to be different from and similar to those of untroubled families, and (3) the potential resources for support that may exist in their social ecologies. Finally, I reconsider why these families experience social isolation in their neighborhoods and communities. This analysis also identifies a number of areas for future research.

Socioeconomic Context of Child Maltreatment

Throughout this chapter, the link between child maltreatment and socioeconomic stress has been underscored. This is not to deny that children are abused or neglected in homes that range throughout the spectrum of family income and education, or that certain forms of maltreatment are more distally linked to socioeconomic stress. However, many researchers have noted that family income and education (together with underemployment, poor and/or public housing, welfare reliance, single parenting, and more dangerous neighborhoods) are strong correlates of child maltreatment (Daro, 1988, 1993; Garbarino, 1976; Garbarino & Crouter, 1978; Garbarino & Sherman, 1980a, 1980b; Gaudin & Pollane, 1983; Gaudin, Wodarski, Arkinson, & Avery, 1990–1991; Gelles & Cornell, 1990; Gil, 1970; Giovannoni & Billingsley, 1970; Lovell & Hawkins, 1988; Newberger, Reed, Daniel, Hyde, & Kotelchuck, 1977; Pelton, 1978; Polansky, Ammons, & Gaudin, 1985; Polansky et al., 1981; Polansky, Gaudin, et al., 1985; Salzinger, Kaplan, & Artemyeff, 1983; Smith, 1975; Smith, Hanson, & Noble, 1974; Starr, 1982; Straus, 1980; Straus, Gelles, & Steinmetz, 1980; Wolock & Horowitz, 1979; Young, 1964). In short, although child maltreatment is not limited by the boundaries of socioeconomic status, it is wise to consider this problem in the context of poverty and financial stress. This means that neighborhood-based social supports must build on the resources of economically stressed communities that are typically characterized by higher levels of crime, perceptions of danger by its residents, high residential mobility, limited local business initiatives, higher unemployment and reliance on welfare benefits, heightened use of public housing, limited local community activism, and neighbors who are themselves buffeted by these social conditions.

There are other data indicating that high-risk families are multiproblem families. Daro (1988) noted in her extensive consortium of demonstration programs that maltreating families are also characterized by other forms of domestic violence, including interspousal fighting (especially apparent in physically abusive families) and physical violence between siblings (especially apparent in emotionally maltreating families). She noted that maltreatment is more likely in families with a parent who has a substance abuse problem (which was also primarily associated with emotional maltreatment in her samples) or mental illness. Other researchers reported similar results (see Gelles & Cornell, 1990; Starr, 1982; Straus et al., 1980; Wolock & Horowitz, 1979; Young, 1964). Families with maltreated children tend to have more children and are less likely to be intact compared to nonmaltreating families, underscoring that these families have enhanced childrearing demands and child care needs (Gaudin & Pollane, 1983; Gil, 1970; Giovannoni & Billingsley, 1970; Polansky, Gaudin, et al., 1985; Smith et al., 1974; Wolock & Horowitz, 1979; Young, 1964; but see Ory & Earp, 1980). These families are also characterized by heightened residential mobility, which may also undermine the strength of community relational ties and hinder their stability and consolidation over time (Elmer, 1967, 1977; Gaudin & Pollane, 1983; Gil, 1970; Newberger et al., 1977; Polansky, Gaudin, et al., 1985; Starr, 1982; Strauss et al., 1980).

It is not surprising, then, that most researchers studying maltreating families describe them as highly stressed by their living conditions as well as by their personal problems. Their capacities to cope are limited by these circumstances and are often additionally constrained by the limited resources of their neighborhoods and communities. Supportive ties within the family unit as well as with extended kin are likely to be limited because of interfamilial conflict. Workplace supports are undermined by the association of maltreatment with unemployment and with the kinds of jobs that do not foster strong supportive relationships among employees. Child care needs and childrearing demands are heightened in maltreating families in ways that are likely to make children the focus of many of the difficulties and frustrations parents must face. Neighbors—like the families themselves—are often struggling to cope with these circumstances and are thus likely to have few resources to devote to the needs of others. Communities are likely to provide few easily accessible organized recreational, social, or educational activities outside the school system that can foster neighborhood ties and a sense of community among its residents. Schools, like the neighborhoods themselves, may be perceived by children as dangerous and unpredictable settings. In short, the normative conditions experienced by families at high risk for child maltreatment seem to offer few meaningful resources for coping with life stress and enhancing informal supportive networks.

Social Isolation of Maltreating Families

In addition to the other correlates of child maltreatment, numerous investigators have also commented on their social isolation. Daro (1988), for example, found social isolation to cut across the different maltreatment subpopulations that were the focus of her intensive demonstration programs, suggesting that isolation is a pervasive rather than syndrome-specific cause of child abuse or neglect. Other researchers (e.g., Giovannoni & Billingsley, 1970; Polansky et al., 1981) perceive social isolation to be particularly characteristic of neglectful families. All researchers, however, regard the lack of connection to supportive figures as one of the consistent features of maltreating families.

What do researchers mean when they refer to the "social isolation" of maltreating families? Are they referring to personal or familial social networks of limited size or scope? Are they concerned with the infrequency with which family members are in contact with friends, relatives, and neighbors? Are they primarily describing the loneliness and lack of perceived support from others as it appears to maltreating family members themselves? Are they referring to the extent to which interactions with others are experienced as stressful rather than supportive? Are they describing their social networks as lacking density and interconnectedness among its members? Are they implying limitations in the functional roles assumed by social network members: diminished emotional sustenance, for example, or inability to obtain counseling, advice, or access to information or services from social network members? The preceding analysis of social networks and social support invites such queries in efforts to obtain a systematic analysis of the social ecology of child maltreatment. More important, however, answers to such questions provide avenues to understanding the nature of the links that exist (and do not exist) between maltreating family members and others in the surrounding community and what can be done to improve these linkages.

Unfortunately, it is often difficult to understand what researchers mean by the social isolation of maltreating families. Many studies did not include appropriate comparison or control groups, so it is impossible to determine whether the social network characteristics of maltreating families are unique to families who abuse or neglect their offspring or instead derive from broader features of these families and their social ecologies (e.g., poverty and low socioeconomic status) (e.g., Lovell & Hawkins, 1988). Many studies relied on global impressionistic or summary measures of social isolation, which do not enable us to understand more precisely the features of social networks that are lacking. For example, Ory and Earp (1980) surveyed social service case records to identify socioeconomically comparable samples of maltreating (primarily neglectful) families and nonmaltreating families and found that they differed significantly on a composite measure of "social disorganization" that included assessments of parents' personal characteristics, family stability and family discord, and a global index of "social isolation" (see also Gaudin & Pollane, 1983; Newberger et al., 1977; Polansky et al., 1981). Global indices do not offer much precision, of course, in identifying the nature of the social isolation experienced by these families or its causes. In many cases, researchers relied on highly imprecise, secondhand, and/or potentially biased reporting sources in assessing the social networks of maltreating families. Perhaps, most distressingly, the widespread perception that these families are socially isolated in their neighborhoods led most researchers to focus largely, if not exclusively, on the deficits in the families' social networks with much less interest in the potential strengths and resources the networks might possess, despite the obvious relevance of the latter to constructing supportive social networks within neighborhoods.

Despite these characteristics, however, some conclusions can be drawn about the social network characteristics of these families that led researchers to regard them as socially isolated. In most studies, judgments of social isolation derive from the fact that these families have a smaller network size compared to that of other families (Corse, Schmid, & Trickett, 1990; Elmer, 1967; Kotelchuck, 1982; Salzinger et al., 1983; Smith et al., 1974; Young, 1964), or that these families evince limited social embeddedness: that is, they see network members less frequently than do others (Bryant et al., 1963; Crittenden, 1985; Elmer, 1967; Gaudin et al., 1990–1991; Giovannoni & Billingsley, 1970; Hunter & Kilstrom, 1979; Jensen, Prandoni, Hagenau, Wisdom, & Riley, 1977; Kotelchuck, 1982; Nurse, 1964; Polansky et al., 1981; Polansky, Gaudin, et al., 1985; Salzinger et al., 1983; Smith et al., 1974; Starr, 1982; Straus et al., 1980; Wolock & Horowitz, 1979; Young, 1964). For example, in an evocative but impressionistic study based on social service case records of 300 maltreating families, Young (1964) reported that neglectful families especially lacked steady contact with friends and relatives, and 85% belonged to no organized group. However, this was also characteristic of other maltreating families: 95% of families deemed "severely abusive," for example, had no continuing relationship with others outside the family. In a more systematic comparison of physically abusive and control families who were matched on important socioeconomic, ethnic, and other variables, Starr (1982) reported that abusive mothers visited fewer people on a regular basis, made fewer total visits, met with relatives less often, and were less likely to feel that they met with relatives frequently enough (although the groups did not differ on 24 other indices of social isolation, some of which are discussed later). Salzinger et al. (1983) reported similar findings and noted that frequency of contact with extended kin was a more important predictor of maltreatment than was regularity of peer interactions among mothers in their sample. Giovannoni and Billingsley (1970) compared socioeconomically distressed neglectful mothers with nonmaltreating mothers from similar backgrounds and found that while the two groups did not differ significantly on measures of contact with friends, the neglectful mothers were significantly less likely to see extended family on a regular basis, especially if they were white. On the other hand, in a study of physically abusive mothers, Corse et al. (1990) reported that only contact and support from peers differentiated these mothers from a matched control group; in relations with nuclear family, extended family, and professionals, the two groups were comparable. In a British study, Smith et al. (1987) compared matched samples of physically abusive and nonabusive mothers and found that when social class differences were controlled, the groups differed in their frequency of contact with extended family members (but not with neighbors and friends), and a higher proportion of abusive mothers reported having no social activities and few opportunities to have a break from the child. Wolock and Horowitz (1979) compared the social service case records of welfare recipients who either maltreated their offspring (primarily through neglect) or did not and reported that maltreating families had significantly fewer contacts with friends, relatives, and organized groups outside their households.

It is important to note that these conclusions concerning limited network size and social embeddedness in maltreating families are not entirely uniform. Starr (1982), for example, found no group differences on measures of the number of personal telephone conversations, personal letters written, good friends in the neighborhood, and neighbors known by name; help with child care; or organizational membership. Giovannoni and Billingsley (1970) found no group differences in organizational ties, which included involvement in various service systems, use of recreational facilities, and related services (only church involvement distinguished these groups, with neglectful mothers less committed to religious activities) (see also Polansky, Gaudin, et al., 1985, for similar results). Corse et al. (1990) found no group differences in the size and support of nuclear family members, extended family members, and professional network members. Crittenden (1985) found that while neglectful mothers had less contact with friends than did nonneglectful mothers, they had *more* regular interaction with relatives. Lovell and Hawkins (1988) reported that mothers referred to a therapeutic program because of child maltreatment contacted more than 46% of their network members on either a daily basis or several times weekly; another 28% were seen once a week. While Smith et al. (1974) reported that physically abusive mothers felt socially isolated compared to nonabusive mothers, they found *no* differences in the husbands' reports of their social activities compared to the husbands in nonabusive families.

The diversity of these findings probably derives from several factors. First, it is clear that researchers studied samples of maltreating families that varied, sometimes strikingly, in the severity of family dysfunction and child maltreatment. In comparison with the sample studied by Young (1964), in which severe child maltreatment was accompanied by high rates of alcoholism, mental illness, and criminality, other researchers (e.g., Giovannoni & Billingsley, 1970; Ory & Earp,1980) studied samples in which child maltreatment and accompanying family dysfunction were much less severe. Second, in some studies the samples of maltreating families were rather small, threatening the generalizability of the conclusions obtained. Third, the studies surveyed here varied significantly in the nature of the reporting sources and the detail and specificity of the information obtained concerning social network features, with some studies obtaining a rich portrayal of the strengths and weaknesses of the networks of maltreating families and other researchers obtaining a much more impoverished picture. Studies also differed in whether social network support was appraised subjectively (i.e., from the viewpoint of maltreating parents) or more objectively (e.g., in a measure of the frequency of contact or overall network size), and these two approaches differ in their sensitivity and validity in complex ways (see, e.g., Polansky, Ammons, & Gaudin, 1985; Polansky, Gaudin, et al., 1985). Fourth, the samples studied also varied in the relative preponderance of physical abuse or neglect of offspring in the maltreating families under study. Insofar as abusive and neglectful families differ in the characteristics of their social networks and their reasons for limited contact with network members, this variation may affect the patterns of results yielded by these researchers (although the overlap in subpopulations of abusive and neglectful families must also be kept in mind).

Despite this variability, some conclusions seem warranted in this review of studies concerned with network size and social embeddedness. First, when group differences were noted, they usually portrayed maltreating families as having less regular contact with social network members. Impoverished contact with members of the extended family was particularly distinctive, which is important in view of the report by Salzinger et al. (1983) that relationships with extended kin were a more important predictor of child maltreatment than were relationships with peers. This is not surprising, given the importance of kin-based supports in the preceding review of social support networks. However, enhanced contact with extended kin is not an unmixed blessing, since relatives can induce stress as well as support. Perhaps for this reason, Straus and Kantor (1987) reported that child abuse was *more* likely to occur when extended family lived within an hour's drive, which they interpreted to reflect extended kin support of punitive and authoritarian childrearing practices together with the stress that extended family members can foster (see also Cazenave & Straus, 1979; Straus et al., 1980).

Second, the picture of social embeddedness yielded by these studies may be a limited one because there are various ways that family members can establish and maintain contact with others outside the home, and these diverse modes of social contact were rarely assessed by these investigators, who instead tended to focus primarily on face-to-face interactions with social network members. However, families can also become involved in community organizations, write letters, and make telephone calls, and these are different modes of social embeddedness that an exclusive emphasis on direct interactions is unlikely to reveal. Moreover, for socioeconomically distressed families who may experience transportation difficulties, involvement in neighborhood groups as well as telephone contact can ameliorate the problems they experience in traveling to the homes of friends and relatives who live far away (although some impoverished maltreating families lack even telephone service) (see Gaudin et al., 1990–1991; Parke & Collmer, 1975; Wolock & Horowitz, 1979). Thus the picture of social embeddedness yielded by these studies may be a limited one.

Third, the findings of Smith et al. (1974) are unique in suggesting that differences in the social embeddedness of spouses within a family may be an important predictor of child abuse. Theirs is, unfortunately, the only study to independently assess the social networks of mothers and fathers within the same families. It is important to do so in future research because social isolation may not necessarily be uniformly shared by all family members, especially when one parent has regular outside employment.

Finally, these findings suggest that social network members are especially important to maltreating families in their potential child care support, whether they are extended kin (Hunter & Kilstrom, 1979) or friends and neighbors (Belle, 1982; Starr, 1982). Exchanging assistance with children not only provides families with tangible assistance in one of the most demanding aspects of their daily experience but also helps to construct relational ties with network members that may also serve other mutual purposes.

Other Dimensions of Social Isolation

As noted earlier, however, measures of network size and social embeddedness are likely to be among the least sensitive indices of the social support derived from social network members. Large social networks are not necessarily supportive networks, and frequent contact with network members may induce stress rather than support (cf. Barrera, 1986). Unfortunately, few studies of the social isolation of maltreating families have moved beyond these rather global—and conveniently evaluated—aspects of their social networks. In one impressive exception, Salzinger et al. (1983) compared the social network characteristics of maltreating mothers referred to a hospital-based family crisis program with nonmaltreating mothers seeking routine pediatric care. Based on maternal reports, they found not only that maltreating mothers had smaller networks and were more insulated from contact with network members, but that their social networks also exhibited less density (i.e., network members were infrequently in contact with each other). Salzinger et al. pointed out that circumscribed contacts with a smaller number of social network members may undermine efforts at behavioral change in the treatment of offspring because maltreating mothers receive few consistent social supports for maintaining changed patterns of child rearing as network members are in little contact with each other (for supportive evidence of this view, see also Wahler, 1980; Wahler & Hann, 1984).

Crittenden (1985), on the other hand, calculated a measure of reciprocity based on mothers' reports about the amount of help given and received from significant network members and reported that maltreating mothers experienced less reciprocity in their relationships with network members than did nonmaltreating mothers. The assistance they received from their network supporters, in other words, tended to be experienced as one-way aid by the providers. Similar results were reported in a study of neglectful mothers by Polansky, Gaudin, et al. (1985), which is discussed in detail later. These findings are important in light of the evidence, reviewed earlier, that reciprocity is an important facet of natural helping and is especially pertinent to cultural norms of equity in mutual assistance. Finally, Lovell and Hawkins (1988) also reported that maltreating mothers experienced a lack of reciprocity in relationships with social network members and also concluded that their social networks were characterized by density. This is, of course, contrary to the findings of Salzinger et al. (1983) noted above.

The dimensions of greatest relevance to understanding the importance of social networks and their supportive features to maltreating families, however, are perceived support and enacted support. On the basis of these measures, in other words, we can learn about the extent to which social network members (1) are regarded by maltreating families as accessible sources of social support and are expected to provide assistance when needed, and (2) have actually engaged in instrumental acts of assistance in the past. Unfortunately, information concerning these dimensions of the social networks of maltreating families is impoverished. There are few studies concerned with enacted support from extended kin, friends, or neighbors, and most are concerned with potential support in child care (e.g., Hunter & Kilstrom, 1979; Starr, 1982). Lovell and Hawkins (1988) reported that maltreating mothers said that the large majority of their social network members rarely provided help with child care or parenting responsibilities, even though the same mothers reported considerable satisfaction with their relationships with the same network associates (e.g., they reported enjoying seeing nearly 80% of network members very much and could "share their thoughts and feelings frequently" with nearly 50% of these associates). The incongruity between these perceptions is explained, the authors argued, by the fact that most maltreating mothers regarded most of their network members as supportive in general but lacking useful or helpful advice on parenting and child care issues.

Somewhat similar findings are reported by Corse et al. (1990), who reported that physically abusive mothers experienced significantly less satisfaction with their parenting support than did mothers in a matched control group, and that they experienced especially impoverished support from peers. On other measures of perceived support, however, researchers have found surprisingly few reliable differences between maltreating families and nonmaltreating families. Starr (1982), for example, discerned no group differences on self-report measures of relatives or friends who could be counted on when needed. Elmer (1977) noted that a sample of hospital-referred mothers of maltreated infants differed from mothers of infants hospitalized for other reasons on a global measure of social support, but although they reported lower "satisfaction with a male partner" compared with nonmaltreating mothers, there were no group differences on measures of "availability of help from friends or neighbors" or "availability of another person to confide in." As noted above, Lovell and Hawkins (1988) reported that maltreating mothers experienced considerable satisfaction with many members of their social networks. When Smith et al. (1974) compared the responses of identified abusive mothers with the rest of their sample, the former group had a significantly *lower* proportion reporting loneliness. On the other hand, Polansky and his colleagues (Polansky, Ammons, & Gaudin, 1985; Polansky et al., 1981; Polansky, Gaudin, et al., 1985) have consistently found that neglectful mothers reported greater loneliness and lack of neighborhood support compared with socioeconomically comparable nonneglectful mothers, and this series of studies is discussed in greater detail later. Similar results have been obtained by Jensen et al. (1977) and by Gaudin et al. (1990–1991) concerning physically abusive and physically neglectful families, respectively.

It appears, therefore, that much of the basis for the perceived social isolation of maltreating families is their limited amount of contact with social network members, especially extended family. This is an important difference, not only because of its consequences for maltreating parents but also for their offspring. Not only do parents who avoid, escape, or simply fail to establish relationships with others outside the home fail to benefit from the kinds of informal supports that such network contacts can provide, but their parenting behavior remains unmonitored by outside agents who might provide alternative role modeling, counseling, criticism, or information to professional support agents.

For offspring, insularity not only limits their own opportunities for contact with people outside the home (given the manner in which the social networks of parents and children typically overlap) but may also bias their perceptions of appropriate social behavior and contribute to their impoverished social skills. This is especially alarming given Young's (1964) report that abusive parents actively sought to insulate their offspring against outside contact, preventing children's involvement in neighborhood recreational, educational, and other social activities; forbidding attendance at sports and parties; and in other ways limiting contact with outsiders. As Parke and Collmer (1975) noted, such actions are likely not only to inhibit the child's development of social skills and contribute to peer rejection, but also to keep the child at home, which increases the child's association with the range of other domestic experiences that are likely to heighten the risk of abuse. In other words, parental behavior that keeps offspring close to home heightens the risk of an abusive encounter. Such parental insularity also restricts the opportunities for children to benefit from informal neighborhood supports.

However, although social isolation *qua* limited social embeddedness provides an informative picture of the social ecology of child maltreatment, it is important to note that researchers have thus far failed to elucidate whether maltreating families differ from nonmaltreating families on other—potentially more informative—dimensions of their social networks. We know very little, for example, about how maltreating family members perceive the valence of the relationships they share with different social network members—that is, whether they experience their encounters with extended family, neighbors, friends, and other associates as primarily pleasant, ambivalent, stressful, unpredictable, and meaningless or in other ways (see, however, Corse et al., 1990; Lovell & Hawkins, 1988). Does their lack of social embeddedness derive, in other words, from uncertainty about their status in the eyes of network associates, perceptions that assistance will not be available when it is needed (perhaps due to an awareness that network associates are themselves similarly stressed), conflict and stress within the relationship, limited interest and/or motivation to strengthen social ties, and/or infrequency of contact (which may occur for various reasons detailed below)? These are different—and potentially nonoverlapping—reasons for a lack of social embeddedness that existing research has failed to distinguish and examine.

We also require far greater insight into other structural and affiliational features of the social networks of maltreating families that might help us to understand whether, for example, their networks of smaller size are nevertheless characterized by greater multidimensionality (as suggested by Belle's, 1982, analysis of the social networks of lower-income single mothers) or homogeneity (which would have implications for the kinds of information and counseling maltreating families are likely to obtain). High multidimensionality in the context of networks of limited size is much less a concern because network associates are probably assuming diverse roles in the lives of parents and offspring in potentially helpful ways. High homogeneity suggests that social support may not be possible from network associates who are themselves stressed and buffeted by some of the same socioeconomic circumstances that affect the target families. As Wahler and Hann (1984) noted, such network associates may exacerbate perceptions of family stress by exchanging complaints and "war stories" about the demands of childrearing rather than enhancing constructive problem solving or other forms of tangible assistance.

We know much less than we should about how maltreating family members perceive the different support functions that are assumed by their network associates, and how these functions relate to the perceived valence of or support from their relationships with friends, relatives, neighbors, and others they see regularly. Is there a small but reliable coterie of network members who provide emotional sustenance, for example, while network associates are lacking for informational or material assistance? We know relatively little about how maltreating families regard the neighborhood contexts in which many of these functions are enacted (Polansky, Gaudin, et al., 1985; but see Starr, 1982, and Wolock & Horowitz, 1979, for indications that maltreating families may perceive their neighborhoods far more benignly than might be expected in light of Belle's, 1982, findings). We must explore further both the possibility (suggested by Smith et al., 1974) that characteristics of the social networks of maltreating mothers (who have been the focus of most research) may differ from those of their spouses and its implications for understanding the ecology of child maltreatment as well as potential avenues for intervention. What does it mean for a socially isolated woman to perceive her spouse as socially embedded in a network that is meaningful and supportive of him? We also know very little about how maltreated children and their siblings construct perceptions of *their* social networks and where they regard potential sources of interpersonal support in the psychosocial ecologies in which they live. In short, our research knowledge of the social isolation of maltreating families is breathtakingly shallow given the extent to which social isolation has been assumed to be true of family members who abuse or neglect their offspring.

The emphasis for future research is on family members' subjective perceptions of their social networks because an understanding of how they conceive the social resources available to them provides the greatest potential for insight into why they experience social isolation and what avenues for changing their social insularity might exist. Indeed, as Polansky and his colleagues have suggested, perceptions of social support may be informative especially because they differ from how the same neighborhood support resources are regarded by others in the community (Polansky, Gaudin, et al., 1985). Moreover, such an analysis might reveal resources as well as deficits in the social networks of maltreating families. Exemplary of this approach is a study by Tracy (1990) that sought to provide a comprehensive assessment of the self-perceived social networks of families with children at risk for out-of-home placement, often because of child maltreatment. Tracy reported that, consistently with other research, most network members consisted of either family or friends, with neighbors and workplace associates each constituting an additional 10% of social network membership. More significantly, respondents were in contact with 42% of their network members either daily or several times a week (by telephone or in face-to-face encounters) and reported feeling close to nearly half their network members, who could be relied on to provide either concrete support, emotional sustenance, or informational assistance. Most of these supports were provided by friends, with whom respondents also reported the greatest reciprocity in their relationships (i.e., aid was perceived as mutual rather than unidirectional) (cf. Fisher et al., 1982). Consistent with other studies (Barrera, 1986), Tracy (1990) reported no significant association between total network size and perceived support. In comprehensively mapping the social networks of high-risk families in this way, researchers in the future might achieve a better understanding of the resources on which social support interventions can be built, as well as the deficits to be addressed in supporting maltreating families.

Explanations for Social Isolation

If limited social embeddedness is an important constituent of their social isolation, why do maltreating families act in this way? The pertinent data to address this question are scarce and, in the absence of information about other social network dimensions, explanations are necessarily speculative. However, several reasons can be cited.

1. Maltreating families may isolate themselves from community contacts because they recognize that their behavior is nonnormative and they seek to escape detection. Young (1964) proposed this portrayal of abusive (but not neglectful) families in characterizing 59% of the abusive families she studied as "secretive and suspicious" in avoiding contact with outsiders. Powell (1979) similarly noted that when families detect significant discrepancies between their childrearing approaches and community norms, one solution is to avoid contact with neighbors who are likely to recognize and criticize the discrepancy.

2. Maltreated families may instead be isolated by community residents for several reasons. Many of their characteristics—including poverty, domestic violence, substance abuse, mental illness, or welfare dependency—quite apart from child abuse or neglect, are likely to inspire rejection from neighbors. In the context of their poor social skills, moreover, maltreating parents present unattractive prospects for new friendships. In addition, their children are likely to be rejected by peers for their atypical behavior and may be regarded by adults in the community as asocial, unkempt, delinquent, or simply "strange." Furthermore, encounters with maltreating families may engender salient but ill-defined anxiety in others, owing to a perception that "something is very wrong," which may cause community members to avoid contact with them even in the context of suspicions of child maltreatment.

3. Maltreating families may be unmotivated to strengthen and maintain contact with community residents because they regard neighbors as having little to offer them. This perception may derive from several sources. First, if these families are, indeed, rejected and stigmatized by their neigh-

bors, their sense that social support is unavailable within local neighborhood social networks may be confirmed. Second, if these families experience aid from neighbors and community members (or, for that matter, from friends, relatives, or other associates) as humiliating, denigrating, or demeaning, they may make a rational calculation that assistance is too costly when it comes at such a high price to self-esteem and privacy. Consequently, they may not seek enhanced sociability and may actually reject offers of assistance. Third, the diverse socioeconomic, personal, and child-related stresses experienced by high-risk families may make the expenditure of time and energy to establish and strengthen local social ties sufficiently costly that doing so appears to exceed the benefits of obtaining support from new friends and neighbors. This may be especially true for adults whose depression, distress, or other personal problems cause them to underestimate the potential benefits of supportive social relationships. Fourth, maltreating families—like others in our culture—may embrace values of family privacy and noninterference in domestic affairs that cause them not only to avoid involvement in others' families but to resent others' interest in their own family situation. For all these reasons, the motivational underpinnings to enhanced sociability with network members is undermined. This is likely to be true especially if maltreating parents are basically satisfied with their existing social relationships even in the context of their limited social networks, which existing research seems to confirm (e.g., Starr, 1982).

4. Finally, maltreating families may be marginal or peripheral community members who, even in the context of the other circumstances outlined above, are likely to be largely ignored by neighbors and other community members. Rather than regarding these families as being actively rejected by others in the neighborhood, or actively avoiding contact with outsiders, their social isolation may derive simply from the fact that there are few natural challenges to a status quo of community marginality brought about by their socioeconomic and personal conditions.

Each of these possibilities is consistent with the research literature on maltreating families, but choosing among them requires far greater insight into their social ecologies—and their perceptions of those ecologies—than researchers presently possess. These explanations define an essential research agenda for future progress in our understanding. However, two additional explanations have been proposed for the social isolation of maltreating families that also merit consideration.

Polansky on Child Neglect

In a series of studies of neglectful families conducted in Appalachia, Philadelphia, and urban and rural settings in Georgia, Polansky and his colleagues (e.g., Polansky, Ammons, & Gaudin, 1985; Polansky et al., 1981; Polansky,

Gaudin, et al., 1985) have sought to describe the personal and ecological characteristics that contribute to this form of maltreatment in lower-income families. More uniquely among investigators in this field, Polansky adopts the view of a personality theorist in arguing that enduring character disorders assume a major role in the loneliness and social isolation experienced by neglectful families (Polansky et al., 1981). He does not deny the importance of the socioeconomic stresses and neighborhood dysfunction that other investigators (especially Garbarino) have emphasized in their accounts of child maltreatment. However, Polansky has argued that what distinguishes neglectful from nonneglecting families in these settings, and what biases their perceptions of their social networks, impairs their capacity to enlist others in supportive ways, and alters the responses of network members to them, are long-standing personality problems of early origin.

In particular, Polansky argues that a high proportion of neglectful mothers use psychological defenses involving detachment to cope with the demands and stresses of their life circumstances, and this defensive style has origins in the mothers' own early histories of inadequate parental care. Polansky has identified an "apathy–futility syndrome," which, he argues, often accounts for the passive, withdrawn demeanor of these mothers and which is characterized by (1) a pervasive conviction that nothing is worth doing, (2) emotional "numbness" that is sometimes mistaken for depression, (3) limited competence in many areas of living, (4) lack of commitment to positive standards, and (5) verbal "inaccessibility" to others, as well as other maladaptive features. Other neglectful mothers are instead characterized by an "impulse-ridden character," reflecting limited self-monitoring and self-control in many behavioral domains. Polansky's neglectful mothers (like Elmer's, 1967, maltreating families, but contrary to those studied by Wolock and Horowitz's, 1979, neglectful sample) were also characterized by anomie—that is, distrust of and retreat from society. Character disorders are difficult to treat in even the best of therapeutic regimes, but Polansky argues that the social worker's role is necessarily a quasi-therapeutic one while also making efforts to limit the effects of the parent's psychopathology on children (Polansky et al., 1981).

In more recent research, Polansky and his colleagues closely examined how neglectful mothers perceive their neighborhoods (defined largely in terms of people in geographic proximity) and compared their perceptions with those of their nonneglectful neighbors (i.e., individuals who share the same communities) with somewhat startling results (Polansky, Ammons, & Gaudin, 1985; Polansky, Gaudin, et al., 1985). Polansky found that neglectful mothers perceived themselves as being significantly more lonely than a comparison group of mothers matched for socioeconomic status and other variables. Neglectful mothers also perceived their neighborhoods as less friendly (contrary to what Starr, 1982, and Wolock and Horowitz, 1979, have reported) and their neighbors as less helpful, and that there was less instrumental assistance and emotional support available to them compared with the perceptions of nonneglectful comparison mothers. When the neighbors of neglectful mothers were interviewed, however, much different perceptions of the same communities were revealed: There were no differences between neighbors of neglectful mothers and neighbors of comparison mothers in their perceptions of the friendliness of the neighborhood, the helpfulness of neighbors, or the availability of emotional and instrumental support. There was, in fact, a low correlation between the perceptions of neglectful mothers of their communities and the perceptions of their nearby neighbors, whose judgments were more comparable to those of the comparison mothers and their neighbors. In short, neglectful mothers' perceptions of the unsupportiveness and unfriendliness of their neighborhoods were rather unique and were not confirmed in the judgments of their neighbors who shared the same communities. Rather than reflecting objective features of "neighborhoods at risk," they were significantly colored by neglectful mothers' own backgrounds, needs, and experiences.

When neighbors were asked about their own social networks, furthermore, informal analyses of their responses indicated that neglectful mothers were less likely than comparison mothers to be regarded as someone neighbors could turn to for assistance and were more likely to be viewed as someone who "need[s] help in raising their children" and "it would not pay to call on." Indeed, neglectful mothers themselves reported helping others who lived nearby less frequently than did comparison mothers. There was also evidence in these responses that the offspring of neglectful mothers were being ostracized in their neighborhoods. Polansky concluded that neglectful families had become identified in their communities as families requiring assistance but not offering it, and their failure to reciprocate led to the stigmatizing of parents and offspring alike.

These findings are fairly complex and require replication because of the rather informal manner in which the results are reported and because some of these findings differ from other research on neglectful families described earlier. However, these studies contribute to a portrayal of neglectful families as neighborhood members who experience a cascading series of difficulties that result in their progressive isolation within the community. The origins of their social difficulties may derive from long-standing character disorders, as Polansky argues, or instead from lack of social skills or competence (cf. Seagull, 1987), overwhelming life stress, limited coping capacities, or other reasons. In any case, the adults in these families are needy individuals who are quickly recognized as such by neighbors. However, they become distinguished from others within the community also by their inability or unwillingness to reciprocate the assistance and help offered them within the neighborhood—perhaps for the same reasons outlined above (character disorders, life stress, social incompetence, etc.). Consequently, parents and their offspring become excluded from the network of supportive relations of the community, which probably contributes to their discordant perceptions of neighborhood friendliness and helpfulness compared to the views of others who live nearby. Moreover, their motivation to enhance and strengthen social ties within the neighborhood is likely to be further diminished by stigma, as well as by the humiliation that grudging assistance from neighbors in these contexts may involve. Whether Polansky is correct that it is not neighborhood structure per se that distinguishes the social ecologies of neglectful families from nonneglectful families (see Garbarino's research in the next section), it is certainly true that their perceptions of their communities are markedly different—and more negative—than those of nonmaltreating families living in the same area.

The important and evocative features of Polansky's account of child neglect consist largely of his portrayal of an escalating series of characterological, situational, socioeconomic, and relational problems experienced by these families that leads, together with "social distancing" by neighbors (cf. Polansky & Gaudin, 1983; Gaudin & Polansky, 1986), to their progressive isolation within the community. It is important to note that Polansky's research does not assess other features of social network ties—particularly relationships with coworkers, friends outside the immediate neighborhood, and extended kin—that may be important alternative sources of social support for these families. This remains an important limitation to this work, especially in light of research reviewed earlier that the social networks of lower-income families are smaller and more kin focused—and less neighborhood based—than those of other kinds of families (cf. Cochran, Gunnarsson, et al., 1990; Fischer, 1982; Vaux, 1988). Lovell and Hawkins (1988), for example, in another study of maltreating mothers, indicated that mothers reported neighbors as constituting only about 10% of their network associates. As a consequence, important sources of non-neighborhood-based social support may exist for maltreating families that Polansky has not included in his description of their social isolation. Work associates, former neighbors who moved elsewhere in the community, and associates from community or civic groups (e.g., church and union members) all constitute nonneighborhood (and nonkin) alternative sources of social support. Nevertheless, this research provides one of the most complex characterizations of the social isolation of maltreating families that exists in the literature and should thus provide the basis for follow-up research inquiry.

Garbarino on the Social Ecology of Child Maltreatment

In contrast, the work of Garbarino and his colleagues focused on the social conditions of the neighborhoods of maltreating families, particularly abusive ones. In a series of conceptual analyses, Garbarino (1977a, 1977b, 1980; Garbarino & Gilliam, 1980) argued that child abuse requires at least three ecological conditions: (1) a cultural context that condones domestic violence in general and violence toward children in particular, (2) families who experience stress in their life circumstances combined with isolation from important support systems that might buffer or protect them, and (3) consensual values concerning family autonomy and parental "ownership" of children. Although each is a critical component of the conditions leading to abuse, Garbarino focused on the second in creative research efforts examining the neighborhood ecology of child maltreatment.

In a series of pioneering studies, for example, Garbarino and his colleagues (Garbarino, 1976; Garbarino & Crouter, 1978; Garbarino & Sherman, 1980a) used social indicators data for specific counties in New York, neighborhoods in Omaha, Nebraska, and communities in Chicago to examine the associations between reports of child maltreatment and information concerning income, education, residential patterns and housing, neighborhood development, community attitudes, and sources of social support, especially as they affected mothers in these communities. Not surprisingly, socioeconomic indices were strong predictors of reports of child maltreatment in New York, but beyond these, other important predictors were the proportion of women in the labor force with children under age 18, the median income of households headed by females, and various measures of educational attainment (Garbarino, 1976). In Omaha, economic factors together with variables reflecting maternal stress and high geographic mobility were potent predictors of child maltreatment (Garbarino & Crouter, 1978). In each study, between 36% and 81% of the variance in child maltreatment *between neighborhoods* (i.e., not necessarily between families or individuals) was accounted for by these measures. These relationships were substantively replicated in an independent study by Young and Gately (1988), although with somewhat less predictive power, and also in a study of Chicago neighborhoods by Garbarino and Kostelny (1991).

In a follow-up study, Garbarino and Sherman (1980a) used the results of the earlier research to identify socioeconomically comparable "high risk" and "low risk" neighborhoods in the Omaha area, with "neighborhood" defined primarily in geographical terms (see Garbarino & Sherman, 1980b). A high-risk neighborhood was one in which the actual rate of maltreatment was higher than expected based on socioeconomic indices; a low-risk neighborhood, conversely, had a lower rate of maltreatment than expected. "Expert informants" in these neighborhoods (e.g., public health nurses, elementary school principals, mail carriers, Girl Scout leaders, police, clergy, and staff of the city planning department), as well as randomly selected local residents were interviewed in detail to discover differences in the supportive and stressful features of daily life in each neighborhood. In a partial report of these data, Garbarino and Sherman (1980a) noted that mothers in high-risk and low-risk neighborhoods differed significantly in their perceptions of neighborhood "exchanges" (i.e., mothers in high-risk neighborhoods were more likely *not* to ask for assistance from neighbors) and in their reports of the social networks of offspring (i.e., larger networks for children in low-risk neighborhoods). Garbarino and Sherman interpreted the former difference to reflect the limited reciprocity of assistance in high-risk neighborhoods that was noted also by other researchers. Interestingly, however, there were no significant differences in maternal perceptions of sources of help in meeting life demands, which included assessments of the types of helpers they could draw on (e.g., family, coworkers, friends, and neighbors), the helpful responsiveness of these people, and mothers' overall satisfaction with the help provided. This is, of course, contrary to some other findings concerning maltreating families. Finally, on a measure of family stresses and supports, mothers from high-risk and low-risk neighborhoods differed significantly in their perceptions of child care availability (i.e., more options in low-risk neighborhoods) and the suitability of the neighborhood as a place for raising children (i.e., viewed less positively in high-risk neighborhoods), but they did not differ in perceptions of the quality of child care, the friendliness of neighbors, recreational opportunities, and assistance in childrearing provided by family, friends, and neighbors.

Taken together, therefore, this series of studies provides a vivid portrayal of the kind of "social impoverishment" (Garbarino & Kostelny, 1991) that may contribute to heightened rates of child abuse in high-risk neighborhoods. It is apparent that when seeking to explain why certain neighborhoods (rather than individuals) are more abuse prone than others, extraordinarily powerful predictive models can be created based on several socioeconomic indicators, together with demographic data that relate to the stresses experienced especially by mothers in these communities. These data underscore the links between socioeconomic status and child maltreatment but further this understanding by identifying some of the unique attributes of especially risky lower-income neighborhoods. However, it is unclear the extent to which these data are helpful in identifying why certain families are more abuse prone than others, especially in view of the rather mixed picture provided by high-risk and low-risk neighborhood residents in their perceptions of the stressful and supportive features of their communities. Furthermore, like the research of Polansky, this series of studies emphasizes social support networks that are neighborhood based and, thus, provides much less insight into extended support systems organized around coworkers, nonneighborhood friendships, and family members. In the Omaha research, Garbarino gathered data concerning citywide support services and discovered that families in high-risk neighborhoods had less awareness and made less use of these services than did families in low-risk neighborhoods (J. Garbarino, personal communication, 1992). This reflects that the intersection of local neighborhoods and broader community support structures requires exploration. As Garbarino himself has noted, neighborhoods do not create abuse, but this research provides a provocative picture of their contributions.

Conclusions

What, then, do we learn about the origins of the social isolation of maltreating families from these studies of Polansky, Garbarino, and others? Given our impoverished understanding of the nature of their social isolation itself—that is, uncertainty about what features of their social networks beyond social embeddedness distinguish maltreating families from others—it is difficult to draw more than provocative hypotheses from these interesting studies. In other words, a variety of processes could account for the lack of social embeddedness experienced by maltreating families, including their own efforts to escape detection and criticism from others in the community, their rejection and stigmatization by neighborhood members, their undermined motivation to establish and maintain neighborhood ties owing to social stigma, reactions to receiving aid, stress and/or privacy concerns, their marginality in the community, their social pathology and limited social skills, or other reasons. Existing research does not yet provide a basis for establishing which of these alternative explanations is preeminently or insignificantly influential in the social isolation of maltreating families. It is quite likely that we will be unable to answer this question until a better understanding of the nature of their social isolation is achieved.

However, these studies do permit a few tentative conclusions. First, it seems likely that a variety of interacting processes are responsible for the lack of social embeddedness experienced by maltreating families, as suggested in the review of Polansky's research. More important, it is likely that different processes account for (1) the initial patterns of isolation that early distinguish these families as different within their neighborhoods, and (2) the perpetuation of their social stigma within the community and their progressive insularity from community contacts. It is unwise to assume, in other words, that the social insularity of maltreating families is unicausal, especially when their history of neighborhood residence is considered. It will take detailed longitudinal studies—probably initially in the form of case-study accounts—to begin to unravel these changing influences over the course of neighborhood residence.

Second, it seems equally likely that single-factor accounts—attributing their social isolation either to the character disorders of maltreating families or to the social impoverishment of their neighborhoods—will prove inadequate, both because social insularity is likely to have diverse origins in the life experience of any high-risk family and because different causes run across the population of high-risk families that concerns us. In this respect, Seagull's (1987) conclusions are basically correct but are too limited: Social isolation characterizes some, but not all, maltreating families; for some, but not all, it derives from character disorders. Multicausal longitudinal process models are a conceptual as well as an empirical necessity in elucidating these diverse, interacting influences on social insularity.

Third, there is suggestive evidence that the origins of the social isolation of physically neglectful and physically abusive families may have reliably different causes. As Young (1964) suggested nearly 30 years ago, neglectful families may become isolated largely because of their limited social competence, overwhelming stresses, and diminished motivation to find rewards in contact with outsiders, which are combined with substance abuse problems and mental disorders for a major proportion of neglectful families. Abusive families, by contrast, may be more actively (rather than passively) socially insulated, with their isolation deriving from avoidance and suspicion of others, combined with conflict with potentially supportive agents in the neighborhood and extended family. This hypothesis must remain conjectural, however, in view of the limited data addressing these differences.

Beyond this, few reliable conclusions can be drawn concerning the origins of the social isolation of maltreating families. Much important research remains to be done.

REWEAVING THE STRANDS: FROM RESEARCH TO POLICY

It is tempting but foolish to try to derive from this research review a list of recommendations for sculpting intervention programs to address the social isolation of maltreating families in the context of informal neighborhood support systems. One reason is that our understanding of their social isolation is insufficiently detailed for a sensitive assessment of the deficits and resources that exist in the social ecologies of maltreating families. Another reason is that the design of social support intervention programs—targeted for *any* needy population—is still in its infancy, with few well-designed evaluation studies of these programs and even fewer that evaluate the processes underlying program effectiveness rather than just their outcomes (cf. Unger & Powell, 1990). There are few such carefully evaluated programs concerning the prevention of abuse and neglect. As a consequence, any recommendations for program design must be regarded as speculative.

However, the problem of child maltreatment does not await the completion of the kinds of systematic research efforts necessary for well-founded program proposals. Moreover, the U.S. Advisory Board on Child Abuse and Neglect has already embarked on an ambitious agenda of policy reform focused on the development of a preventive social support strategy centered around informal social networks in communities and neighborhoods, and it is essential that this agenda be developed and refined using the best available research. Thus, in the context of a strong recommendation for support of future research that will address the significant deficits that currently exist in our knowledge of child maltreatment and social support, the following generalizations and recommendations for the development of informal social support systems for preventing child maltreatment can be tentatively proposed.

Neighborhood-based social support alone is not sufficiently broadly based to strengthen supportive resources to high-risk families. Several conclusions from the research literature summarized in this chapter suggest that a program of social support interventions—even one emphasizing informal social networks—must extend significantly beyond neighborhoods to encompass extended kin; workplace social networks; friends who live outside local neighborhoods and communities; associates through churches, unions, and other community groups; school-based associates; and other potentially valuable resources to children and their parents. First, basic research on social networks indicates that neighborhood ties do not constitute the majority of the relationships with social network members on which individuals commonly rely for social support. Most social network ties are nonneighborhood based. Second, neighborhood-based relationships are characterized by greater turnover than are other relationships (e.g., with extended kin and long-term friends) and, thus, may be a less reliable and more unstable source of supportive ties than are relationships with other network members. Third, in lower-income populations (which are at greater risk for child maltreatment), social networks are smaller but are more kin based and less neighborhood focused, suggesting that neighborhood-based relationships may not be among the most salient or potent sources of potential support to them. Fourth, maltreating families may be particularly unlikely to rely on neighborhood-based support systems because of the processes of insularity, stigma, and "social distancing" (Polansky & Gaudin, 1983) that are particularly likely to occur in relationships with neighbors, who are more prone to identify maltreating families (and their offspring) as "different" owing to the lack of reciprocity in mutual help giving, social incompetence and indifference, and (quite likely) their abuse or neglect of offspring. Evidence supporting this view comes from the study by Lovell and Hawkins (1988), earlier described, in which maltreating mothers reported considerable satisfaction with social network associates, of which only about 10% were neighbors. Fifth, the lower-income neighborhoods in which high-risk families are likely to reside are themselves "needy neighborhoods" in which a lack of economic resources, high mobility in and out of the community, a lack of broader civic commitment, and the financial and personal stresses of its residents are likely to exhaust the supportive resources on which maltreating families can rely.

To be sure, there are some important advantages to developing informal supportive relationships for high-risk families that are neighborhood based. Neighborhood support networks help to create a more positive total physicosocial ecology in which various prevention goals related to child maltreatment can be advanced because high-risk parents and offspring are benefiting from supportive relationships from diverse sources within their residential milieu. This could ultimately promise greater success than more piecemeal efforts to strengthen relations with extended kin, friends, and workplace associates on a family-by-family basis. Furthermore, neighborhood-based supportive relationships do not rely on the kinds of additional resources—transportation, telephone, and the like—that frequently hamper the efforts of lower-income families to strengthen and maintain relationships with network members who live at greater distance. Besides their easy access, many of the other benefits of informal support systems—their congruence with local norms and variability of support functions, for example (Gottlieb, 1983)—are more easily accomplished within neighborhood-based support systems than in more extended supportive network ties. Finally, it is important to note that the research summarized in this chapter used a conventional, geographically based definition of neighborhood in the operationalization of neighborhood supports. When the concept of neighborhood is broadened to encompass meaningful relational ties that may extend beyond families who live immediately nearby, some (but not all) of these problems with interventions based on neighborhood-based social supports evaporate.

However, the benefits of neighborhood supports (regardless of the breadth of definition) are likely to be constrained by the inherent neediness and structural problems of the neighborhoods themselves. Furthermore, social support efforts that focus primarily on neighborhood relationships risk missing some of the more important, and potentially more powerful, social network relationships that high-risk families may experience as more meaningful sources of social support. Although relationships with extended kin can be characterized by conflict and intergenerational animosity, for example, they are also consolidated by cultural support and formal ties that provide greater stability—and potentially, reliability—to the supportive functions they can assume. Furthermore, several studies suggest that the lack of supportive ties with extended kin distinguish maltreating families more than their lack of ties to friends or neighbors, suggesting that their social isolation may be intergenerational rather than interresidential.

Along with extended kin, long-term friendships (which may or may not be neighborhood based) and workplace associates provide relationships that are knit together by common interests and concerns (which may not be true of friendships with neighbors) and have potentially greater stability than community ties. For children—whose primary social networks are, in fact, likely to be neighborhood based because of peer relationships and school-based associations—interventions that foster friendships with individuals outside the local community may provide children with much needed alternative role models and exposure to new perspectives that are valuable for purposes of developmental remediation. Taken together, therefore, the notion of enlisting informal social support networks for preventing child maltreatment is probably a good idea, but limiting this proposal to neighborhood-based social networks may unduly and unnecessarily constrain the range of potential supportive agents in the lives of maltreating parents and offspring.

The provocative research of Garbarino and Polansky has, of course, provided a far richer portrayal of these neighborhoods than previously existed. As noted earlier, however, both research initiatives have been limited by a failure to examine non-neighborhood-based social supports that may provide the families they studied with alternative sources of emotional sustenance, instrumental assistance, and other resources. It would be valuable, therefore, if future researchers would extend these studies to provide a fuller portrayal of the social networks of maltreating families and the potential network resources on which they can rely.

Different maltreatment subpopulations have different social support needs. The importance of distinguishing among different forms of maltreatment (acknowledging considerable overlap among them) is underscored by research on the social isolation of maltreating families. Although strong generalizations are not supportable, it appears that when research attributes social insularity to a parent's deficits in social skills or competence, it typically focuses on populations in which child neglect is preeminent. Furthermore, neglectful parents are more likely to report loneliness or disappointment in close relationships; that is, they lack perceived support. It appears, therefore, that a subset of maltreating families—predominantly but not exclusively neglectful families—experiences limited personal competence in establishing and maintaining successful social relationships outside the family, and with extended kin. Some researchers have suggested, in fact, that the childrearing problems these parents experience are generalizations from their broader difficulties in maintaining coherent and supportive social relationships with others outside the home (Burgess & Youngblade, 1988): These are "neglected" parents who themselves neglect the meaning and value of social ties, including those related to the caretaking needs of offspring.

There is other research evidence, far less substantial, that suggests that another form of social isolation derives instead from anger and conflict between maltreating parents and social network members, especially extended family. In this case, insularity derives from animosity and suspicion, and it seems that this is more likely to be true of physically abusive families than of neglectful ones. It should be emphasized, however, that this is not a well-documented empirical picture. With respect to emotionally maltreating or sexually abusive parents, there is far less research evidence concerning the nature of their social isolation or, indeed, whether they are insulated at all. Daro (1988), in her intensive intervention program, found that all maltreatment subpopulations were comparably characterized by social isolation, but hers is the only study to make this assessment. If this is so, it may nevertheless be true that the origins and characteristics of the social isolation of emotionally or sexually abusive families are somewhat different from the abusive and neglectful subpopulations about which we know somewhat more.

In addition to distinguishing among varieties of maltreatment, it is important to note that the social support needs of maltreating parents are also defined by other problems that may accompany child abuse or neglect. Parents with a substance abuse problem, for example, or with psychological disorders may be socially isolated for other reasons than those related to child maltreatment. Young adolescent parents may also exhibit social insularity that has reasons different from those for other maltreating parents. It is essential, therefore, that the heterogeneity of causes for social isolation is recognized so that diverse intervention strategies will be well-suited to the constellation of needs that these families experience.

Thus, just as the phenomenon of child maltreatment is not unitary, neither is the need for social support. Earlier in this chapter, alternative functions of social support were outlined, including emotional sustenance, counseling and guidance, skills acquisition, access to information, services, and material resources, as well as social control and developmental remediation. When this section is integrated with the preceding sections concerning the varieties of social isolation of maltreating families, it becomes clear that different kinds of social support are needed for different maltreatment subpopulations. Neglectful families may require diverse, multifaceted forms of social support (perhaps in the context of multidimensional support agents) that provide emotional affirmation, skills acquisition, counseling, and access to information and resources (especially in the context of referrals to social service agencies). Abusive families may require social support that provides counseling and advice, especially in the context of modeling and other guided interventions that help to establish and reinforce new patterns of child treatment. Social support *qua* social control is important for all maltreatment subpopulations, especially in the context of tertiary prevention, but perhaps primarily for physically abusive and sexually abusive families in which child maltreatment is often integrated into a broader pattern of family victimization. The kinds of social support that are most valuable for the offspring of maltreating parents are different from those designed for perpetrators and will depend substantively on the age of the child, the kind of maltreatment, and whether the child is at home or in an out-of-home placement.

The needs of different maltreating families vary not only concerning the necessary functions of social support, but also in the best procedures for enlisting this support from network members. The focus of social support efforts for maltreating families has sometimes been to enhance the size of their social networks, even though this may be the least important feature of natural networks from the standpoint of social support. However, the preceding section on the social isolation of maltreating families paints a far more diverse picture of their social network needs and resources. For many maltreating families, some social network members may be supportive while others are not. For some families, network associates are supportive on some issues (e.g., counseling for personal problems) but unhelpful on others (e.g., tangible child care assistance and parenting support). For some parents, strong ties exist to friends but not to extended kin. This suggests that intervention efforts often should be designed to strengthen the target's access to or reliance on perceived supportive individuals who are already network members, or to enhance the supportive activity of particular network associates, rather than merely adding to network size. In other words, working within existing social network resources to strengthen their functioning or the target individual's reliance on them can potentially provide more effective avenues toward increasing social support—and might be accomplished much more easily than striving to increase network size.

Several research studies—unsubstantiated at present—suggest that one secure, supportive social relationship may be all that is necessary to promote adequate functioning in troubled parents. From the perspective of this "sufficiency model," a parent's capacity to rely on at least one supportive network member may make the difference between stress-reactive child abuse and nonabuse in the family history. Although this provocative idea requires further study, it suggests that the goals of social support interventions need not be expansive to accomplish valuable results in the lives of high-risk families, and it further underscores the potential error of focusing on sheer network size as an intervention target.

An additional consideration in social support intervention is that not all cases of maltreatment are equal in severity. Indeed, one of the striking features of this research review on the social isolation of maltreating families is the realization that different researchers often described much different "maltreating families," partly because of differences in the severity, persistence, and frequency of abuse or neglect itself and partly because of differences in their accompanying socioeconomic, ecological, familial, and personal problems. Differences in severity are associated with differences in needs for social network intervention. For some families, economic assistance and referrals to job-training and employment programs are likely to be enough to restore and remedy a temporarily dysfunctional pattern of family interaction. For other families, long-term efforts involving many different kinds of interventions (substance abuse programs, family therapy, and social skills training) may be necessary. In a sense, therefore, the social support needs of different maltreating families are individualized, based not only on the form of abuse but also its severity and the seriousness of the accompanying life circumstances of the family, as well as the network resources on which families can rely. Although all families are likely to benefit from learning about how to access and maintain social support in their neighborhoods, families will vary significantly in the additional needs for which they require assistance.

The challenge, therefore, is to recognize that because social support is multifaceted and the needs of maltreating families are not homogeneous, different kinds of supportive practices should be fostered for different maltreatment subpopulations. Simply trying to add additional network members to the lives of abusive or neglectful families is unlikely to accomplish any serious prevention goals and, indeed, may exacerbate some of the problems of these families. A far more individually tailored array of strategies is essential. Daro's (1988) research provides a preliminary glimpse at how carefully crafted social support interventions might be framed for different maltreatment subpopulations; more research of this kind is necessary to identify the unique needs of different kinds of maltreating families and the kinds of social support that will best benefit them.

Incorporated within this task, however, is the corollary recognition that these families have other needs besides social support, or, conversely, that social support cannot meet all the needs of maltreating families in the context of preventive efforts. This leads, therefore, to another conclusion from this research review.

Social support alone is unlikely to be an effective preventive intervention. If maltreating families are multiproblem families, and if their social isolation derives partly from a variety of associated socioeconomic, ecological, familial, and personal difficulties, social support interventions must be integrated with other services for these families to provide effective preventive assistance. As suggested earlier, social support programs should be integrated with social skills training for some maltreating families or detoxification and substance abuse treatment programs for others. For adolescent parents, social support that integrates resources from their families of origin and, it is hoped, their school settings will be most beneficial. For children who are the victims of maltreatment, it is necessary to integrate social support into their foster care placements and draw on their preexisting support networks among peers and nonfamilial adults as well as within the school system (cf. Lewis & Fraser, 1987).

The operative concept to be underscored is "integrated" (cf. Miller & Whittaker, 1988; Tracy & Whittaker, 1987). Social support interventions that exist at the periphery of other ongoing social services are likely to lose their effectiveness because they are not tied to other resources that are of value to target families—which is, of course, an important feature of natural support from network members. On the other hand, when social support is an intrinsic component of other support services, its impact may be enhanced. One of the reasons, for example, for the success of programs like Homebuilders and Hawaii's perinatal visitation program is that systematic and (in the case of Homebuilders) intense social support is provided to high-risk families in the context of information, material assistance, skills training, access to social services, and other interventions from which parents can benefit. Indeed, social support in these contexts may be one of the most important but least visible (in the eyes of target families) contributors to the benefits they experience from these kinds of programs. Other examples of integrated social support programs include Gaudin's Social Network Intervention Project (which combines strategies to enhance informal network supports for neglectful families with the assistance of regular volunteer aides, the enlistment of neighborhood helpers, and social skills training) (Gaudin et al., 1990–1991), Childhaven's efforts to combine quasi-therapeutic full-time day care services with practical parent education, casework support, parent support, family therapy groups, and social agency referrals (Durkin, 1986; Miller & Whittaker, 1988), and Powell's (1979, 1987, 1988) cooperative child care resource center for high-risk urban families (which combines regular child care with the development of mutual-aid support groups among parents together with community referrals). In each case, the integration of social support with other elements of the program design means that intervention agents at all levels can contribute to the success of the social support component.

More broadly, it is important to recognize that the lack of integration of social support interventions with other services to high-risk families in many circumstances derives from the organization of public welfare systems in this country. In particular, the lack of integration between public welfare and public health programs is sometimes a barrier to coordinated service delivery, despite the fact that many family problems require both kinds of services at the same time. When a single mother with a young infant in stressful life circumstances is at risk for child abuse, for example, she requires not only the efforts of child protection agents but also those in maternal and child health. It is arguable that the effective integration of services for high-risk families will remain wishful thinking until serious efforts to surmount these institutional obstacles in public policy are undertaken.

The integration of social support interventions into preexisting service programs to high-risk families provides useful avenues for effective assistance. As indicated previously, fostering network support alone is unlikely to be an effective preventive intervention unless it is combined with other services that benefit maltreating families. This suggests, however, that grafting efforts to enlist and enhance network support onto preexisting social services might be especially helpful because of how families already recognize the benefits of the accompanying services. Moreover, the stigma that might be attached to carefully targeted social support interventions for maltreating families would be undermined by their integration with social service programs that assist high-risk families under an entitlement model, provide services to broadly defined needy families, or offer universal benefits.

Under recent welfare reforms, for example, the federal government has assumed an expanded role in supporting child care services to welfare recipients and enlisting the states in enhancing and regulating the quality of these services. The Family Support Act of 1988 requires participation in job-training programs for welfare recipients but entitles the parents of young children to child care subsidies associated with their participation in the program as well as for educational and related activities and maintains these subsidies for one year after welfare eligibility has ended. The Act authorizes funds using entitlement-based language to pay for these child care subsidies, which may be used to purchase care from relatives as well as from unrelated caregivers. Moreover, the Act also enlists states more directly in the provision of child care services than has previously been true, recognizing the links between child care quality and children's development (e.g., Phillips, Howes, & Whitebook, 1992).

Given the strong association between socioeconomic distress and child maltreatment, multiple avenues exist for using these provisions to enhance the detection of child maltreatment (through state-regulated training of child care workers in subsidized care settings) as well as for assisting the victims of maltreatment. Special quasi-therapeutic day care services can be created for the offspring of parents who were adjudicated for child abuse or neglect, or for other low-income parents who requested such services with the concurrence of social service agents, to assist high-risk children in the context of programs that seek to support parents and enhance their ties to community agencies. Incentives can be incorporated into the job-training component of the Act to enhance the involvement of welfare recipients with their offspring and to foster their ties to the community, for example, by including them as paid aides in the neighborhood child care settings where their offspring are located, by fostering time-management and other personal skills as well as job-related capabilities, or through more systematic parent-training efforts (such as the Home Instruction Program for Pre-school Youngsters inaugurated by Arkansas Governor Bill Clinton to train welfare mothers to teach their children basic skills). Moreover, the provisions of the Act can be used to place welfare recipients in service jobs within their local communities and, thus, to further integrate them with community agents and resources. Other provisions of the Act can be used to integrate extended kin into a more active supportive role in the lives of maltreating families by enlisting them as child care providers with wage incentives to enhance their training as family support agents.

Other targeted programs may also include social support components that can be enlisted for high-risk families. The WIC (Women, Infants, and Children) program has long been recognized as an important avenue for enhancing the nutritional adequacy of lower-income families, and the benefits it provides are, on the whole, nonstigmatizing to recipients. It is possible that WIC could be used as an avenue for identifying and accessing high-risk families for additional services, such as child care support or informal parent or neighborhood networking. The EPSDT (Early Periodic Screening, Diagnosis, and Treatment) program could be modified to include interventions specifically targeted toward lower-income families that would enhance its role in the early detection of child maltreatment.

Schools are another social institution that can include important social support incentives for maltreating families. As the success of Head Start programs has shown, parent involvement in early childhood education provides overall benefits for parents and offspring alike. Similarly, enfranchising high-risk families into the curricular and extracurricular activities of children at their schools might reduce the social insularity of these families by strengthening their links to community resources and agents. Moreover, their involvement in extracurricular activities (including after-school programs) is one means of keeping low-achieving and needy children tied to the school and, thus, to reliable sources of social support. Schools are, therefore, perhaps one of the most important community-based social institutions to which social support efforts can be linked.

Schools can be helpful in several ways. First, just as the availability of affordable, high-quality (and, on occasion, quasi-therapeutic) child care services can provide support to maltreated children and also assist their parents by reducing child care demands, the availability of after-school programs at schools in high-risk neighborhoods can mutually benefit children and their parents. For parents, reliable after-school care provides relief from stressful child care responsibilities and removes children from the domestic demands and stresses that can contribute to abuse. After-school programs can also provide the kinds of assistance to maltreated and other needy children that may be more difficult to obtain in more structured, curricular contexts. After-school programs can be oriented around the activities and interests that children find attractive and engaging, such as sports, music, hobbies, and social activities (Medrich et al., 1982). Partly because they are local and school based, they do not require parents' active efforts to facilitate children's involvement, at which some parents are more deficient (O'Donnell & Steuve, 1983). Activities can be more easily structured to foster the kinds of social skills and successful peer relations that maltreated children often lack. They can also be designed to enhance self-esteem and perceptions of self-competence through the use of noncompetitive, mastery-oriented programs. Moreover, the adult directors of these activities are more likely to be perceived by children as sources of social support because of their informal, recreational roles. Teachers, by contrast, are not regarded by children as supportive figures, perhaps because of other elements of their role definition (Furman & Buhrmester, 1985, 1992; Reid, Landesman, Treder, & Jaccard, 1989); the same is likely to be true of school counselors and administrators. The peer associations fostered by after-school programs may extend into children's other noncurricular social activities, fostering the development of extended peer support networks for maltreated children that do not depend on parental networks (Hirsch & Dubois, 1989), and this may become especially important in preadolescence when peer networks become more independent of the family system (Berndt, 1989).

Second, schools can be helpful sources of social support for children as forums for peer counseling as well as peer tutoring programs for maltreated children with academic and personal difficulties. There is considerable research evidence that peer tutoring programs not only foster intellectual skills, but are also sources of mutual support that can enhance self-esteem and self-confidence (Asp & Garbarino, 1983). Peer counseling, in turn, is effective for strengthening social support among age-mates. Moreover, the fact that

counselors and tutors themselves reap considerable benefits from peer counseling and peer tutoring programs means that assistance is experienced as
mutual, which can contribute to strengthening supportive peer networks for
targeted children and can help to reduce the social isolation that maltreated
children may experience at school, as well as the stigma that may derive from
receiving assistance from friends.

Third, there are a variety of other means that schools can provide social
support to children with many needs: through special academic/counseling/
parenting programs for teen parents who face the challenge of childrearing
in the context of their own developmental needs; through academic curricula
focused on health, parenting, and self-esteem; through information about
community and recreational agencies that can provide additional sources of
social support; and through opportunities to develop relationships with
nonkin adults who are alternative models of healthy behavioral functioning
(cf. Asp & Garbarino, 1983; Vondra, 1990).

Fourth, schools can be supportive resources for parents also, especially
as parents become enlisted into adult neighborhood networks through their
association with their child's academic and extracurricular activities. Doing
so requires, however, considerable efforts by school personnel to enfranchise
and welcome parents—especially marginal, lower-income parents—into the
academic environment (Cochran & Riley, 1988). This is a difficult task and
cannot be easily accomplished by overworked school personnel.

This portrayal of schools as sources of social support to high-risk families resembles Zigler's (1989) "School of the 21st Century" concept, which
is also intended, in part, to involve schools in neighborhood support networks.
Others have suggested that schools should become locations for neighborhood family resource centers that provide community referrals and networking, sponsor parent education and informal family support groups, coordinate resource sharing (e.g., a toy or book lending library), and sponsor other
activities. Each approach is built on the rather tenuous assumption that
schools have the capacity—as well as being uniquely suited—to assume a
central role in neighborhood-based social support systems. There are good
reasons for questioning this assumption, especially in a contemporary social
context of growing criticism of schools for failing at their basic educational
tasks and a history of efforts to incorporate broadly defined goals into the
mission of local school systems without enhanced funding or other resources.
Certainly it is foolish to expect schools to assume centralized community
support functions without thoughtful consideration of how such school-based
programs should be designed, the personnel to staff them, the implications
of these programs for the school's identity within the community, the consequences of integrating these programs into institutions with an educational
mandate, and the space and other resources necessary for their effective
operation. Moreover, it is wise to organize such programs around—rather
than within—the central academic activities of local schools to avoid con-

flicts with the needs and goals of teachers who must already assume diverse scholastic responsibilities, and that is why this discussion has focused on after-school programs, extracurricular peer counseling and tutoring approaches, and other nonacademic strategies.

However, schools *are* uniquely suited to become central neighborhood resources of social support, especially in distressed neighborhoods where other institutional resources may be deficient; therefore, schools merit thoughtful consideration in the development of a neighborhood-based strategy of social support to maltreating families. Moreover, overburdened school personnel need not assume exclusive, or major, responsibility for the administration of such support services. Increasingly school systems are engaging in partnership models involving outside agencies that, in collaboration with school personnel, design and direct cooperative programs for needy children and their families. School-based programs to enhance social support to high-risk families should use such partnership programs as their model.

The potential for other social institutions as social support resources is mixed for high-risk families. Churches and other religious institutions have social support as a central goal and usually sponsor a variety of services that assist high-risk families (including community food pantries, subsidized counseling services, outreach to local mission projects, clothing and food drives for neighborhood groups, and related activities). Religious institutions may, however, be regarded skeptically by maltreating families (cf. Giovannoni & Billingsley, 1970) whose lack of community involvement is likely to extend to church activities as well. Consequently, church-based social support problems might emphasize outreach to high-risk families in their homes and neighborhoods rather than trying to foster their participation in church-based activities, which is a challenging task. Efforts to enlist community and recreational centers as neighborhood social support resources face similar problems. Because maltreating mothers often do not schedule and encourage their children's involvement in recreational activities and other community events—perhaps as a result of their own lack of planning and participation in community groups—their children are frequently denied access to community activities from which they might benefit. Thus, community and recreational programs must either emphasize local neighborhood activities to which children (and parents) can achieve easy access or supplement their activities with transportation to and from the sites for needy families.

Besides enhancing access to high-risk families, there is another benefit to the efforts of churches, community organizations, and recreational groups to organize outreach activities in the neighborhoods where these families live. Insofar as many people engage in social distancing from high-risk families, the involvement of untroubled, advantaged families in the neighborhoods of high-risk families through church and community organizations helps to diminish their stereotypes about these families, undermine their effortful unfamiliarity with their life circumstances, and, it is hoped, enhance their empathy for their conditions. Consequently, church, community, and recreational groups can assume an important mediational role between needy families and other families in the community that might provide various forms of assistance.

There are many advantages to grafting social support resources onto preexisting social services from which high-risk families already benefit rather than developing network resources de novo. Although integrating social supports in this manner requires thoughtful consideration of how the additional support functions might alter the nature of these service institutions— whether they involve local schools, churches, community, or welfare programs—in most cases social support is a complementary task to those already assumed by these agencies. The more important challenge is designing support programs that exploit the unique roles of these institutions in the communities in which they are embedded, compensate for their potential problems in providing social support (e.g., problems with access and conflicting institutional commitments and goals), and provide the needed resources to make support programs function effectively.

Coordination of social support to children and parents within high-risk families is essential to helping each. Because family life entails overlapping and integrated social connections with the outside world, social support provided to one family member may have complex consequences for the rest of the family. As indicated earlier, support for parents may yield beneficial consequences for offspring but in different circumstances may exacerbate their problems. Assistance to offspring that is intended to help them may do so, but also may provoke negative reactions from other family members. Consequently, the designers of social support interventions for maltreating families must thoughtfully consider how social support has direct and indirect consequences for different family members and, if possible, create interventions that simultaneously benefit multiple family members.

The research on maltreating families indicates, for example, that child care and childrearing demands are among the greatest stresses of family life from which relief is sought among extended kin, neighbors, friends, and other network associates. As a consequence, supportive programs that address child care needs can mutually benefit parents and offspring. The availability of good-quality, quasi-therapeutic day care services for specially targeted high-risk families could provide therapeutic gains for maltreated infants and children and provide them with alternative attachment figures for emotional support (Howes, Rodning, Galluzzo, & Myers, 1988). Such services would also reduce the reliance of lower-income families on informal care from extended kin (which may add stress to relationships with extended family members), neighborhood family day care arrangements (which may be of poor quality), or ad hoc arrangements with live-in companions, friends, or neighbors (of uncertain quality or reliability). Parents would benefit from such arrangements by having a reliable source of affordable, good-quality care available for offspring, and their links to community networks might also be strengthened through their contacts with caregivers and other activities integrated into the child care program (Long, 1983). The same benefits can also be obtained through other kinds of child care supports, such as after-school programs (as discussed above), drop-in and in-home respite care, cooperative neighborhood child care groups (cf. Powell, 1987, 1988), and other resources.

When children are in out-of-home placements, the coordination of the child's social network with those of the foster family as well as the child's family of origin can become especially complicated (Whittaker, 1983). Temporary foster care placements have the goals of providing relief for child victims of maltreatment and simultaneously preserving relationships with the family of origin, and these goals may conflict with each other or with the foster family's own values and interests. Possessiveness and competitiveness between family units and the generation of loyalty conflicts in the child can undermine the child's experience of support in out-of-home placements, even if (and, perhaps, especially when) the foster family is a member of the extended family or neighborhood (Lewis & Fraser, 1987). Moreover, social supports that existed in the family of origin may not be maintained in the foster home, or, conversely, new foster family supportive networks for children may not be continued when the child is returned home. In these cases, the child protection caseworker has a unique responsibility for maintaining supportive network ties for maltreated children across care settings so that the benefits of social support are not lost in multiple transitions, and seeing that supportive assistance from one family network does not create conflict for the child in the alternative family setting. An adult in the child's community may also assume this "brokering" function, especially if the foster home is in the same neighborhood in which the child's family lives.

As these examples suggest, the coordination of supportive interventions to parents and offspring is important to ensuring that the benefits of assistance are shared or, at the least, do not indirectly undermine the needs of other family members. On the other hand, well-integrated supportive services in a neighborhood context have the potential of providing multiple benefits for parents and offspring alike.

Social support is often best achieved by targeting support providers rather than recipients alone. In their insightful analysis of natural helpers, Collins and Pancoast (1976) emphasized the importance of lay support providers in neighborhoods and communities as a supplement to the efforts of formal social service agents. Because of their informal role definitions and their connections to the values and norms of the community, natural helpers can provide multifaceted forms of support that may be more accessible, meaningful and stable than formal assistance agents can provide. Consequently, the value of natural helpers is intrinsic to efforts to develop neighborhood-based social support for maltreating families.

As discussed above, however, the coordination of formal and informal support systems is an important challenge to the development of neighborhood-based resources. Informal helpers may define problems differently from the way professional helpers do, and they may seek different kinds of solutions that are not as oriented toward professional norms and responsibilities (Froland et al., 1981). Defining the nature and limits of their roles vis-à-vis those of professional helpers can sometimes create mutual conflict, and formalization of the roles of "natural helpers" is likely to undermine their efficacy. As a result, it is important that formal support agents respect and support the efforts of natural helpers, not only to maintain their effectiveness as community aides but also because such informal helping networks are one of the defining elements of neighborhood as it is experienced in relational terms (cf. Unger & A. Wandersman, 1985).

In the high-risk neighborhoods in which maltreating families can be found, however, there are additional challenges to the efficacy of natural helpers. First, it may be hard to find central figures with "freedom from drain" (Collins & Pancoast, 1976)—that is, helpers who are not themselves overwhelmed by the stresses of their socioeconomic, ecological, and personal circumstances. Indeed, the identification and enlistment of such individuals to provide social support may impose added demands that helpers will eventually find overwhelming. Insofar as professional helpers seek to coordinate their efforts with and through informal helpers, it may be necessary to "support the supporters" by providing material assistance, emotional sustenance, and other kinds of tangible support to those who are providing assistance to target families. Organizing mutual support groups of natural helpers may also provide a much needed source of social support for those providing social support. Second, because child abuse and neglect elicits such uniform disapproval in our culture, it may also be difficult to find informal helpers who are willing to become supportively involved with parents who maltreat their children (especially when sexual abuse is alleged). This is especially likely if these parents have other undesirable characteristics, such as their suspicion of others, limited social skills, a disinterest in maintaining social relationships with helpers, or a lack of reciprocity in help giving that make them unrewarding targets of help. In these circumstances as well, formal support agents may need to aid informal helpers in providing assistance to families who offer few rewards for doing so, and whose conduct in relation to their offspring evokes strong emotion.

More broadly, it is worth remembering that natural helpers—especially in high-risk, distressed neighborhoods—may not always be the best informal support agents to provide aid to maltreating families. As indicated earlier, the anonymity entailed in many informal social encounters—ranging from casual conversations at a bar to counseling in a crisis line—may permit far more candid disclosure and effective assistance than the kinds of information that can be exchanged with ongoing social network members. Similarly, assistance in the context of self-help groups like Parents Anonymous can be valuable precisely because the individuals with whom one discloses problems and difficulties are similarly afflicted and also because the counseling they provide does not necessarily occur in the context of continuing, everyday social relationships (although, by mutual consent, they may expand beyond the scope of the self-help group). In these circumstances, supporting help providers is a somewhat easier task because natural helpers are not necessarily drawn from the same distressed communities that maltreating families live in and are, thus, not subject to the same stresses and drains on their own socioemotional resources.

Considering the complexity of recipient reactions to aid will enhance the efficacy of social support interventions. Providing assistance—material or social—to needy families can be a perplexing experience when, instead of gratitude, recipients respond with resentment, denigration of the aid, rejection of the benefactor, and/or an unwillingness to receive further assistance. Such reactions often contribute to the "drain" experienced by natural and formal helpers and undermine their motivation to provide future aid. However, an extensive literature on recipient reactions to aid, reviewed earlier in this chapter, indicates that such reactions are not only normative but rational responses to the experience of helplessness, vulnerability, failure, dependency, and/or indebtedness that may derive from receiving assistance from others. Accepting aid often implies personal failure, invokes expectations of reciprocity that may be impossible to fulfill, and evokes fears of exploitation or stigmatization, especially in vulnerable or needy recipients, that accompany the gratitude and relief that are also normative responses to accepting aid. In short, receiving assistance is complex, mingling positive and negative perceptions of the benefactor, the assistance, the recipient, and the circumstances in which help is offered and received.

Social support is distinguished from other kinds of assistance because it is meant to be an ongoing—rather than a one-time—resource to troubled families. These complex recipient reactions to aid suggest that the manner in which social support is provided may be as important as the kind of assistance in predicting their willingness to accept future support. To ensure that troubled families will continue to accept the support offered them, social support interventions should be designed to include several features that will reduce perceptions of stigma, vulnerability, or failure. First, interventions should offer recipients the opportunity to reciprocate the assistance they have received by providing help to others in ways that are consistent with their skills, resources, and motivation. Although some adults may not take the opportunity to do so, such an offer provides a means of restoring equity in the mutual obligations entailed in a help-giving relationship and can also contribute to self-esteem in recipients. Social support programs should identify a range of neighborhood-based projects to which recipient adults can contribute, including home-based assistance to older populations (e.g., Meals on Wheels programs), nonprofessional local housing construction projects (e.g., Habitat for Humanity homes), community-based child care and recreational programs, and related activities. A recipient's participation in programs like these not only satisfies the cultural reciprocity obligations of receiving assistance but also contributes to the positive integration of recipient families into the neighborhood and community and may contribute to altering unfavorable stereotypes of recipients by members of the larger community.

Second, social support should be available to recipient families if they desire it rather than as a requirement for other assistance. Although it seems paradoxical that a social support program might require recipient parents to establish helpful relationships with support agents (as social support cannot easily be coerced), such a requirement would be consistent with the efforts of program planners to better integrate these families into beneficial social networks, especially if doing so was part of a program of social monitoring and control of the parenting practices of high-risk adults. However, as this review has documented, some of the most effective social support interventions occur incognito—that is, as part of activities that have other explicit goals (e.g., perinatal home visitation) or no goals at all (e.g., a casual conversation at a bar or a bus station). The effectiveness of these informal interventions depends partly on the acceptance of assistance as entirely voluntary and self-initiated, which also reduces perceptions of failure, dependency, or indebtedness in a helping relationship. Moreover, allowing the recipient to calibrate the acceptance of social support according to self-perceived need also enhances the probability that support will be meaningfully received because it is desired.

Third, social support should be offered in the context of interventions that are as widely targeted as possible and, conversely, do not distinguish recipients as dysfunctional or needy. One of the more humiliating features of current public welfare policies is the stigmatization of recipient populations by delivery modes and eligibility requirements that denigrate them in public contexts. When benefits are universalized, however, or are available to a wide range of individuals with various needs and backgrounds, accepting social and material support does not necessarily confer undesirable status. One of the attractive features of informal social support networks in neighborhoods and communities is that they are undiscriminating: All individuals enjoy social assistance from others whether or not they are at risk, and, thus, accepting support from neighborhood associates does not designate recipients as different from others. To the extent to which formalized social support interventions can emulate the nonstigmatizing features of these informal support networks, they will contribute to the willingness of needy parents and families to benefit from the services they offer.

Finally, social support should be provided in a context of mutual respect. That is, support should not be accepted as a necessary cost to personal privacy, autonomy, or self-reliance. Insofar as program design is intended to increase the recipient's acceptance of support as an ongoing resource, efforts to pre-serve the recipient's self-esteem by portraying assistance as an entitlement (rather than a bestowal), the benefactor's intentions as partly self-interested (rather than entirely altruistic), and the recipient's needs as extrinsically insti-gated (rather than due to personal inadequacy or failure) will advance this goal. Furthermore, the acceptance of support should not entail greater intru-sions on personal privacy than are necessary to achieve program goals, even if the purpose of social support is to curtail the risk of child maltreatment, because threats to privacy can lead to an unwillingness to receive further aid. In a sense, respect for recipients is a basic corrective to the features of help giving that recipients find denigrating.

Effective social support interventions can involve simple as well as com-plex strategies. This discussion has emphasized the complexities and uncer-tainties in the design of effective social support programs in neighborhoods. Such emphasis is necessary because of a tendency to simplify the nature of "social support" or "natural support networks" and to regard them as a readily available panacea for the complex problem of child maltreatment. The tension throughout this discussion underscores the multidimensional considerations entailed in the use of social support for the prevention of child maltreatment while also identifying helpful avenues for potential intervention.

However, there are also some fairly simple, straightforward interven-tion strategies that can potentially enhance the social supports available to maltreating families. If a high proportion of socioeconomically distressed high-risk families are socially isolated, in part because they have no access to a telephone, subsidizing telephone service may be a straightforward inter-vention with surprising benefits. If anonymous self-disclosure is sometimes a benefit to socially isolated parents or offspring, enhancing access to com-munity telephone support services as well as crisis hot lines may be valuable (cf. Peterson, 1990). If limited access to transportation contributes to im-poverished community associations, incorporating free transportation to and from recreational and parenting activities—or, for that matter, lowering the cost and accessibility of public transportation for economically distressed communities—may be an important key to intervention success. If there is limited popular awareness of the needs of socioeconomically distressed fami-lies or the community resources that exist to address those needs, grocery-bag inserts and milk-carton displays can help to remedy this problem. If child neglect derives in part from the inability of impoverished families to heat their apartments or afford child care while parents work, subsidizing these activities may be an important (and remarkably cost-effective) ingredient of social support.

In the end, of course, for most maltreating families, access to well-paying, affirming employment may be the most valuable social support intervention of all. A job at a reasonable wage reduces poverty, heightens access to social networks that can assume a supportive role in a parent's life, enhances self-esteem, strengthens residential stability and one's integration into a community, and provides material benefits to the family. The availability of jobs at reasonable wages also benefits neighborhoods by curbing the downward spiral of many high-risk communities and strengthening the economic base for community planning. If one singular intervention were to be recommended to curb child maltreatment, adequate employment for needy families would be the answer.

Much more research is needed. This phrase is the default conclusion of most research reviews in the behavioral sciences, but in this case it reflects the enormous gaps in the literatures surveyed. The capacity of the U.S. Advisory Board on Child Abuse and Neglect to design effective neighborhood-based social support systems hinges on the development of essential new knowledge germane to this goal. First, we need to know much more about the characteristics of different maltreatment subpopulations and their social support (and other) needs. Despite the fact that different forms of maltreatment overlap considerably, characterizing the population of maltreating adults and their victims heterogeneously rather than homogeneously in this manner enables us to think of social support as a resource that is carefully tailored to the specific needs of troubled families. Second, we need considerably more information about the nature of the social networks of troubled and untroubled families and how the structural and affiliational features of these networks contribute to perceptions of available social support in potential recipients and enacted support in the experience of high-risk families. This information is critical to understanding the aspects of individual and familial social networks that are the most important targets for social support interventions. Third, we must know much more about the factors affecting the efficacy of potential social support interventions, including the stresses that drain support providers, the overlapping consequences of support provided to different members of the family, and the characteristics of social networks that contribute to their supportive and stressful roles in the lives of individuals and families. Basic theoretical and limited empirical work currently exists concerning these factors in untroubled families, but there remains little understanding of how these predictive factors influence the efficacy of support interventions in high-risk families, which constitutes a pressing research need. Fourth, we desperately need well-evaluated, thoughtfully designed demonstration projects exploring various avenues for providing and heightening natural supports in the lives of high-risk and maltreating families. Even if the Board were to aggressively advance the importance of social support interventions for troubled families for preventing child maltreatment, discouragingly few program models exist to draw on. These four goals are among many that have been identified in this chapter, but they constitute an ambitious research agenda.

More important than all these goals, however, is greater knowledge of the social isolation of maltreating families. I was surprised, in view of the consensus among researchers that abusive and neglectful families are socially isolated, to discover how shallow current information is concerning the nature of their isolation and its consequences. This is particularly striking in light of the rich conceptual portrayal of social networks and social integration that exists in current literatures in family sociology and community psychology, which has been applied only haphazardly to research on the social isolation of maltreating families. Existing studies provide an inconsistent portrayal of maltreating families as differing from others in any aspect of their social networks except their limited embeddedness, which is among the least sensitive indicia of social integration. Findings vary considerably or are lacking altogether about whether high-risk families experience satisfaction with their support agents (and which ones are perceived to be most helpful), whether they report that they actually receive tangible assistance from those on whom they rely in their social networks, and in how they perceive the support resources that may exist within their neighborhoods and larger communities. At the same time, provocative conceptual analyses of social isolation exist from researchers like Garbarino and Polansky that highlight a number of important hypotheses meriting further investigation. Any effort to address the social support needs of maltreating families must rely on detailed information concerning their purported social isolation. At present, that information does not exist.

There is nothing simple about the social circumstances of maltreating families or the enlistment of social support to assist them. Quite clearly, an enduring multistrategy approach is required to address the needs and challenges of these multiproblem families.

ACKNOWLEDGMENTS

I am grateful to the following colleagues for valuable suggestions and ideas during personal meetings, telephone conversations, or an exchange of letters about this chapter: Marcia Allen, Paul Amato, Frank Barry, Urie Bronfenbrenner, Dante Cicchetti, Deborah Daro, Richard Dienstbier, Byron Egeland, Laura Finken, Mary Fran Flood, James Gaudin, Robert Halpern, Scotty Hargrove, Patricia Hashima, Jeffrey Haugaard, Heidi Inderbitzen-Pisaruk, Mary Kenning, Michael Lamb, Susan Limber, Gary Melton, Edward Mulvey, D. Wayne Osgood, Diana Prescott, N. Dickon Reppucci, Michael Rutter, Ira Schwartz, Donald Unger, Michael Wald, James Whittaker, Brian Wilcox, and Diane Willis, as well as the other authors of papers for the U.S. Advisory Board on Child Abuse and Neglect: James Garbarino, Jill Korbin, Paul Lerman, Leroy Pelton, and David Wolfe.

REFERENCES

Aber, J. L., & Cicchetti, D. (1984). The socio-emotional development of maltreated children: An empirical and theoretical analysis. In H. E. Fitzgerald, B. M. Lester,

& M. W. Yogman (Eds.), *Theory and research in behavioral pediatrics* (Vol. 2, pp. 147–205). New York: Plenum Press.

Asp, E., & Garbarino, J. (1983). Social support networks and the schools. In J. Whittaker & J. Garbarino (Eds.), *Social support networks: Informal helping in the human services* (pp. 251–297). New York: Aldine.

Barrera, M. (1986). Distinctions between social support concepts, measures, and models. *American Journal of Community Psychology, 14,* 413–445.

Belle, D. (1982). Social ties and social support. In D. Belle (Ed.), *Lives in stress* (pp. 133–144). Beverly Hills, CA: Sage.

Berndt, T. J. (1989). Obtaining support from friends during childhood and adolescence. In D. Belle (Ed.), *Children's social networks and social supports* (pp. 308–331). New York: Wiley.

Blyth, D. A., Hill, J. P., & Thiel, K. S. (1982). Early adolescents' significant others: Grade and gender differences in perceived relationships with familial and nonfamilial adults and young people. *Journal of Youth and Adolescence, 11,* 425–450.

Blyth, D. A., & Traeger, C. (1988). Adolescent self-esteem and perceived relationships with parents and peers. In S. Salzinger, J. Antrobus, & M. Hammer (Eds.), *Social networks of children, adolescents, and college students* (pp. 171–194). Hillsdale, NJ: Erlbaum.

Brownell, A., & Shumaker, S. A. (1984). Social support: an introduction to a complex phenomenon. *Journal of Social Issues, 40,* 1–9.

Bryant, B. K. (1985). The neighborhood walk: Sources of support in middle childhood. *Monographs of the Society for Research in Child Development, 50* (Serial No. 210).

Bryant, H. D., Billingsley, A., Kerry, G. A., Leefman, W. V., Merrill, E. J., Senecal, G. R., & Walsh, B. A. (1963). Physical abuse of children—An agency study. *Child Welfare, 42,* 125–130.

Burgess, R. L., & Youngblade, L. M. (1988). Social incompetence and the intergenerational transmission of abusive parental practices. In G. T. Hotaling, D. Finkelhor, J. T. Kirkpatrick, & M. A. Straus (Eds.), *Family abuse and its consequences: New directions in family violence research* (pp. 38–60). Newbury Park, CA: Sage.

Cassel, J. (1974a). An epidemiological perspective of psychosocial factors in disease etiology. *American Journal of Public Health, 64,* 1040–1043.

Cassel, J. (1974b). Psychosocial processes and "stress": Theoretical formulations. *International Journal of Health Services, 4,* 471–482.

Cassel, J. (1976). The contribution of the social environment to host resistance. *American Journal of Epidemiology, 102,* 107–123.

Cazenave, N. A., & Straus, M. A. (1979). Race, class, network embeddedness and family violence: A search for potent support systems. *Journal of Comparative Family Studies, 10,* 281–300.

Cicchetti, D. (1990). The organization and coherence of socioemotional, cognitive, and representational development: Illustrations through a developmental psychopathology perspective on Down syndrome and child maltreatment. In R. A. Thompson (Ed.), *Socioemotional development: Nebraska Symposium on Motivation* (Vol. 36, pp. 259–366). Lincoln: University of Nebraska Press.

Cobb, S. (1976). Social support as a moderator of life stress. *Psychosomatic Medicine*, *38*, 300–314.

Cochran, M. M. (1990a). Personal networks in the ecology of human development. In M. Cochran, M. Larner, D. Riley, L. Gunnarsson, & C. R. Henderson (Eds.), *Extending families: The social networks of parents and their children* (pp. 3–32). Cambridge, England: Cambridge University Press.

Cochran, M. M. (1990b). The network as an environment for human development. In M. Cochran, M. Larner, D. Riley, L. Gunnarsson, & C. R. Henderson (Eds.), *Extending families: The social networks of parents and their children* (pp. 265–276). Cambridge, England: Cambridge University Press.

Cochran, M. M. (1990c). Environmental factors constraining network development. In M. Cochran, M. Larner, D. Riley, L. Gunnarsson, & C. R. Henderson (Eds.), *Extending families: The social networks of parents and their children* (pp. 277–296). Cambridge, England: Cambridge University Press.

Cochran, M. M., & Brassard, J. A. (1979). Child development and personal social networks. *Child Development*, *50*, 601–616.

Cochran, M. M., Gunnarsson, L., Grabe, S., & Lewis, J. (1990). The social networks of coupled mothers in four cultures. In M. Cochran, M. Larner, D. Riley, L. Gunnarsson, & C. R. Henderson (Eds.), *Extending families: The social networks of parents and their children* (pp. 86–104). Cambridge, England: Cambridge University Press.

Cochran, M., & Henderson, C. R. (1990). Illustrations. In M. Cochran, M. Larner, D. Riley, L. Gunnarsson, & C. R. Henderson (Eds.), *Extending families: The social networks of parents and their children* (pp. 58–64). Cambridge, England: Cambridge University Press.

Cochran, M., Larner, M., Riley, D., Gunnarsson, L., & Henderson, C. R. (Eds.) (1990). *Extending families: The social networks of parents and their children*. Cambridge, England: Cambridge University Press.

Cochran, M., & Riley, D. (1988). Mother reports of children's personal networks: Antecedents, concomitants, and consequences. In S. Salzinger, J. Antrobus, & M. Hammer (Eds.), *Social networks of children, adolescents, and college students* (pp. 113–147). Hillsdale, NJ: Erlbaum.

Cochran, M., & Riley, D. (1990). The social networks of six-year-olds: Context, content, and consequence. In M. Cochran, M. Larner, D. Riley, L. Gunnarsson, & C. R. Henderson (Eds.), *Extending families: The social networks of parents and their children* (pp. 154–177). Cambridge, England: Cambridge University Press.

Cohen, S., & Wills, T. A. (1985). Stress, social support, and the buffering hypothesis. *Psychological Bulletin*, *98*, 310–357.

Colletta, N. D. (1979). Support systems after divorce: Incidence and impact. *Journal of Marriage and the Family*, *41*, 837–846.

Collins, A. H., & Pancoast, D. L. (1976). *Natural helping networks: A strategy for prevention*. Washington, DC: National Association of Social Workers.

Corse, S. J., Schmid, K., & Trickett, P. K. (1990). Social network characteristics of mothers in abusing and nonabusing families and their relationships to parenting beliefs. *Journal of Community Psychology*, *18*, 44–59.

Cotterell, J. L. (1986). Work and community influences on the quality of childrearing. *Child Development*, *57*, 362–374.

Crittenden, P. M. (1985). Social networks, quality of child rearing, and child development. *Child Development*, 56, 1299–1313.

Crnic, K. A., Greenberg, M. T., Ragozin, A. S., Robinson, N. M., & Basham, R. B. (1983). Effects of stress and social support on mothers and premature and full-term infants. *Child Development*, 54, 209–217.

Crnic, K. A., Greenberg, M. T., Robinson, N. M., & Ragozin, A. S. (1984). Maternal stress and social support: Effects on the mother–infant relationship from birth to 18 months. *American Journal of Orthopsychiatry*, 54, 224–235.

Cross, W. E., (1990). Race and ethnicity: Effects on social networks. In M. Cochran, M. Larner, D. Riley, L. Gunnarsson, & C. R. Henderson (Eds.), *Extending families: The social networks of parents and their children* (pp. 67–85). Cambridge, England: Cambridge University Press.

Cutrona, C. E. (1984). Social support and stress in the transition to parenthood. *Journal of Abnormal Psychology*, 93, 378–390.

Daro, D. (1988). *Confronting child abuse*. New York: Free Press.

Daro, D. (1993). Child maltreatment research: Implications for program design. In D. Cicchetti & S. Toth (Eds.), *Child abuse, child development and social policy* (pp. 331–367). Norwood, NJ: Ablex.

Dornbusch, S. M., Carlsmith, J. M., Bushwall, S. J., Ritter, P. L., Leiderman, H., Hastorf, A. H., & Gross, R. T. (1985). Single parents, extended households, and the control of adolescents. *Child Development*, 56, 326–341.

Durkin, R. (1986). The use of therapeutic day care to resolve the legal dilemma of protecting the rights of both children and parents in equivocal cases of abuse and neglect. *Child Care Quarterly*, 15, 138–140.

Egeland, B., & Sroufe, L. A. (1981). Developmental sequelae of maltreatment in infancy. In R. Rizley & D. Cicchetti (Eds.), *Developmental perspectives on child maltreatment*. San Francisco: Jossey-Bass.

Egeland, B., Sroufe, L. A., & Erickson, M. (1983). The developmental consequence of different patterns of maltreatment. *Child Abuse and Neglect*, 7, 459–469.

Eisenberg, N. (1983). Developmental aspects of recipients' reactions to aid. In J. D. Fisher, A. Nadler, & B. M. DePaulo (Eds.), *New directions in helping: Recipient reactions to aid* (Vol. 1, pp. 189–222). New York: Academic Press.

Elmer, E. (1967). *Children in jeopardy*. Pittsburgh: University of Pittsburgh Press.

Elmer, E. (1977). *Fragile families, troubled children*. Pittsburgh: University of Pittsburgh Press.

Erickson, M. F., Egeland, B., & Pianta, R. (1989). The effects of maltreatment on the development of young children. In D. Cicchetti & V. Carlson (Eds.), *Child maltreatment* (pp. 647–684). Cambridge, England: Cambridge University Press.

Feiring, C., & Lewis, M. (1988). The child's social network from three to six years: The effects of age, sex, and socioeconomic status. In S. Salzinger, J. Antrobus, & M. Hammer (Eds.), *Social networks of children, adolescents, and college students* (pp. 93–112). Hillsdale, NJ: Erlbaum.

Feiring, C., & Lewis, M. (1989). The social networks of girls and boys from early through middle childhood. In D. Belle (Ed.), *Children's social networks and social supports* (pp. 119–150). New York: Wiley.

Ferleger, N., Glenwick, D. S., Gaines, R. R. W., & Green, A. H. (1988). Identifying correlates of reabuse in maltreating families. *Child Abuse and Neglect*, 12, 41–49.

Fischer, C. S. (1982). *To dwell among friends: Personal networks in town and city*. Chicago: University of Chicago Press.

Fisher, J. D., Nadler, A., & Witcher-Alagna, S. (1982). Recipient reactions to aid. *Psychological Bulletin, 91*, 27–54.

Froland, C., Pancoast, D. L., Chapman, N. J., & Kimboko, P. J. (1981). Linking formal and informal support systems. In B. H. Gottlieb (Ed.), *Social networks and social support* (pp. 259–275). Beverly Hills, CA: Sage.

Furman, W., & Buhrmester, D. (1985). Children's perceptions of the personal relationships in their social networks. *Developmental Psychology, 21*, 1016–1024.

Furman, W., & Buhrmester, D. (1992). Age and sex differences in perceptions of networks of personal relationships. *Child Development, 63*, 103–115.

Garbarino, J. (1976). A preliminary study of some ecological correlates of child abuse: The impact of socioeconomic stress on mothers. *Child Development, 47*, 178–185.

Garbarino, J. (1977a). The price of privacy in the social dynamics of child abuse. *Child Welfare, 56*, 565–575.

Garbarino, J. (1977b). The human ecology of child maltreatment: A conceptual model for research. *Journal of Marriage and the Family, 39*, 721–735.

Garbarino, J. (1980). What kind of society permits child abuse? *Infant Mental Health Journal, 1*, 270–280.

Garbarino, J. (1989). Troubled youth, troubled families: The dynamics of adolescent maltreatment. In D. Cicchetti & V. Carlson (Eds.), *Child maltreatment* (pp. 685–706). Cambridge, England: Cambridge University Press.

Garbarino, J., Burston, N., Raber, S., Russell, R., & Crouter, A. C. (1978). The social maps of children approaching adolescence: Studying the ecology of youth development. *Journal of Youth and Adolescence, 7*, 417–428.

Garbarino, J., & Crouter, A. (1978). Defining the community context of parent–child relations: The correlates of child maltreatment. *Child Development, 49*, 604–616.

Garbarino, J., & Gilliam, G. (1980). *Understanding abusive families*. Lexington, MA: Heath.

Garbarino, J., & Kostelny, K. (1991). *Child maltreatment as a community problem*. Unpublished manuscript, Erikson Institute for Advanced Study in Child Development, Chicago, IL.

Garbarino, J., & Sherman, D. (1980a). High-risk neighborhoods and high-risk families: The human ecology of child maltreatment. *Child Development, 51*, 188–198.

Garbarino, J., & Sherman, D. (1980b). Identifying high-risk neighborhoods. In J. Garbarino & S. H. Stocking (Eds.), *Protecting children from abuse and neglect* (pp. 94–108). San Francisco: Jossey-Bass.

Gaudin, J. M., & Polansky, N. A. (1986). Social distancing of the neglectful family: Sex, race, and social class influences. *Child and Youth Services Review, 8*, 1–12.

Gaudin, J. M., & Pollane, L. (1983). Social networks, stress and child abuse. *Child and Youth Services Review, 5*, 91–102.

Gaudin, J. M., Wodarski, J. S., Arkinson, M. K., & Avery, L. S. (1990–1991). Remedying child neglect: Effectiveness of social network interventions. *Journal of Applied Social Sciences, 15*, 97–123.

Gil, D. G. (1970). *Violence against children: Physical child abuse in the United States.* Cambridge, MA: Harvard University Press.

Giovannoni, J. M., & Billingsley, A. (1970). Child neglect among the poor: A study of parental adequacy in families of three ethnic groups. *Child Welfare, 49,* 196–204.

Gelles, R. J., & Cornell, C. P. (1990). *Intimate violence in families* (2nd ed.). Newbury Park, CA: Sage.

Gottlieb, B. H. (1983). *Social support strategies.* Beverly Hills, CA: Sage.

Gottlieb, B. (1985). Theory into practice: Issues that surface in planning interventions which mobilize support. In I. G. Sarason & B. R. Sarason (Eds.), *Social support: Theory, research and applications* (pp. 417–437). The Hague: Martinus Nijhoff.

Granovetter, M. (1973). The strength of weak ties. *American Journal of Sociology, 78,* 1360–1380.

Greenberg, M. S. (1980). A theory of indebtedness. In K. Gergen, M. S. Greenberg, & R. Willis (Eds.), *Social exchange: Advances in theory and research.* New York: Plenum Press.

Greenberg, M. S., & Westcott, D. R. (1983). Indebtedness as a mediator of reactions to aid. In J. D. Fisher, A. Nadler, & B. M. DePaulo (Eds.), *New directions in helping: Recipient reactions to aid* (Vol. 1, pp. 85–112). New York: Academic Press.

Gunnarsson, L., & Cochran, M. (1990). The support networks of single parents: Sweden and the United States. In M. Cochran, M. Larner, D. Riley, L. Gunnarsson, & C. R. Henderson, *Extending families: The social networks of parents and their children* (pp. 105–116). Cambridge, England: Cambridge University Press.

Hartup, W. W. (1983). Peer relations. In P. H. Mussen (Ed.), *Handbook of child psychology: Socialization, personality, and social development* (4th ed., Vol. 4, pp. 103–196). New York: Wiley.

Hatfield, E., & Sprecher, S. (1983). Equity theory and recipient reactions to aid. In J. D. Fisher, A. Nadler, & B. M. DePaulo (Eds.), *New directions in helping: Recipient reactions to aid* (Vol. 1, pp. 113–141). New York: Academic Press.

Helfer, R. E. (1982). A review of the literature on the prevention of child abuse and neglect. *Child Abuse and Neglect, 6,* 251–261.

Heller, K. (1979). The effects of social support: Prevention and treatment implications. In A. P. Goldstein & F. H. Kanfer (Eds.), *Maximizing treatment gains.* New York: Academic Press.

Heller, K., & Swindle, R. W. (1983). Social networks, perceived social support, and coping with stress. In R. D. Felner, L. A. Jason, J. N. Moritsugu, & S. S. Farber (Eds.), *Preventive psychology: Theory, research, and practice* (pp. 87–103). New York: Pergamon Press.

Herrenkohl, R. C., Herrenkohl, E. C., & Egolf, B. P. (1983). Circumstances surrounding the occurrence of child maltreatment. *Journal of Consulting and Clinical Psychology, 51,* 424–431.

Herrenkohl, R. C., Herrenkohl, E. C., Egolf, B., & Seech, M. (1979). The repetition of child abuse: How frequently does it occur? *Child Abuse and Neglect, 3,* 67–72.

Hirsch, B. J., & DuBois, D. L. (1989). The school–nonschool ecology of early adolescent friendships. In D. Belle (Ed.), *Children's social networks and social supports* (pp. 260–274). New York: Wiley.

Homel, R., Burns, A., & Goodnow, J. (1987). Parental social networks and child development. *Journal of Social and Personal Relationships, 4,* 159–177.

House, J. H., Umberson, D., & Landis, K. R. (1988). Structures and processes of social support. In W. R. Scott & J. Blake (Eds.), *Annual Review of Sociology* (Vol. 14, pp. 293–318). Palo Alto, CA: Annual Reviews.

Howes, C., Rodning, C., Galluzzo, D., & Meyers, L. (1988). Attachment and child care: Relationships with mother and caregiver. *Early Childhood Research Quarterly, 3,* 403–416.

Hoyt, D., & Babchuk, N. (1983). Adult kinship networks: The selective formation of intimate ties with kin. *Social Forces, 62,* 84–101.

Hunter, R. S., & Kilstrom, N. (1979). Breaking the cycle in abusive families. *American Journal of Psychiatry, 136,* 1320–1322.

Jensen, D. E., Prandoni, J. R., Hagenau, H. R., Wisdom, P. A., & Riley, E. A. (1977). Child abuse in a court referred, inner city population. *Journal of Clinical Child Psychology, 6,* 59–62.

Kotelchuck, M. (1982). Child abuse and neglect: Prediction and misclassification. In R. H. Starr (Ed.), *Child abuse prediction* (pp. 67–104). Cambridge, MA: Ballinger.

Ladd, G. W., Hart, C. H., Wadsworth, E. M., & Golter, B. S. (1988). Preschoolers' peer networks in nonschool settings: Relationship to family characteristics and school adjustment. In S. Salzinger, J. Antrobus, & M. Hammer (Eds.), *Social networks of children, adolescents, and college students* (pp. 61–92). Hillsdale, NJ: Erlbaum.

Larner, M. (1990a). Changes in network resources and relationships over time. In M. Cochran, M. Larner, D. Riley, L. Gunnarsson, & C. R. Henderson (Eds.), *Extending families: The social networks of parents and their children* (pp. 181–204). Cambridge, England: Cambridge University Press.

Larner, M. (1990b). Local residential mobility and its effects on social networks: A cross-cultural comparison. In M. Cochran, M. Larner, D. Riley, L. Gunnarsson, & C. R. Henderson (Eds.), *Extending families: The social networks of parents and their children* (pp. 205–229). Cambridge, England: Cambridge University Press.

Lazarus, R., & Folkman, S. (1984). *Stress, appraisal and coping.* New York: Springer.

Leslie, L., & Grady, K. (1985). Changes in mothers' social networks and social support following divorce. *Journal of Marriage and the Family, 47,* 663–673.

Lewis, M., Feiring, C., & Kotsonis, M. (1984). The social network of the young child: A developmental perspective. In M. Lewis (Ed.), *Beyond the dyad* (pp. 129–160). New York: Plenum Press.

Lewis, R. E., & Fraser, M. (1987). Blending informal and formal helping networks in foster care. *Child and Youth Services Review, 9,* 153–169.

Litwak, E., & Szelenyi, I. (1969). Primary group structures and their function: Kin, neighborhoods and friends. *American Sociological Review, 34,* 465–481.

Long, F. (1983). Social support networks in day care and early child development. In J. K. Whittaker & J. Garbarino (Eds.), *Social support networks: Informal helping in the human services* (pp. 189–217). New York: Aldine.

Lovell, M. L., & Hawkins, J. D. (1988). An evaluation of a group intervention to increase the personal social networks of abusive mothers. *Children and Youth Services Review, 10,* 175–188.

McAdoo, H. P. (1980). Black mothers and the extended family support network. In L. Rodgers-Rose (Ed.), *The black woman* (pp. 125–144). Beverly Hills, CA: Sage.

Medrich, E. A., Roizen, J. A., Rubin, V., & Buckley, S. (1982). *The serious business of growing up: A study of children's lives outside school.* Berkeley: University of California Press.

Meyer, C. H. (1985). Social supports and social workers: Collaboration or conflict? *Social Work, 30,* 291.

Miller, J. L., & Whittaker, J. K. (1988). Social services and social support: Blended programs for families at risk for child maltreatment. *Child Welfare, 67,* 161–174.

Mitchell, R. E., & Trickett, E. J. (1980). Task force report: Social networks as mediators of social support: An analysis of the effects and determinants of social networks. *Community Mental Health Journal, 16,* 27–44.

Newberger, E. H., Reed, R. B., Daniel, J. H., Hyde, J. N., Jr., & Kotelchuck, M. (1977). Pediatric social illness: Toward an etiologic classification. *Pediatrics, 60,* 178–185.

Nurse, S. M. (1964). Familial patterns of parents who abuse their children. *Smith College Studies in Social Work, 35,* 9–25.

O'Donnell, L., & Steuve, A. (1983). Mothers as social agents: Structuring the community activities of school aged children. In H. Lopata & J. H. Pleck (Eds.), *Research on the interweave of social roles: Jobs and families, families and jobs* (Vol. 3, pp. 113–129). Greenwich, CT: JAI Press.

Ory, M. G., & Earp. J. A. L. (1980). Child maltreatment: An analysis of familial and institutional predictors. *Journal of Family Issues, 1,* 339–356.

Parke, R. D., & Bhavnagri, N. P. (1989). Parents as managers of children's peer relationships. In D. Belle (Ed.), *Children's social networks and social supports* (pp. 241–259). New York: Wiley.

Parke, R. D., & Collmer, C. W. (1975). Child abuse: An interdisciplinary analysis. In E. M. Hetherington (Ed.), *Review of child development research* (Vol. 5, pp. 509–590). Chicago: University of Chicago Press.

Pelton, L. H. (1978). Child abuse and neglect: The myth of classlessness. *American Journal of Orthopsychiatry, 48,* 608–617.

Peterson, L. (1990). PhoneFriend: A developmental description of needs expressed by child callers to a community telephone support system for children. *Journal of Applied Developmental Psychology, 11,* 105–122.

Pettigrew, T. G. (1983). Seeking public assistance: A stigma analysis. In A. Nadler, J. D. Fisher, & B. M. DePaulo (Eds.), *New directions in helping: Applied perspectives on help-seeking and -receiving* (Vol. 3, pp. 273–292). New York: Academic Press.

Phillips, D. A., Howes, C., & Whitebook, M. (1992). The social policy context of child care: Effects on quality. *American Journal of Community Psychology, 20,* 25–51.

Pianta, R., Egeland, B., & Erickson, M. F. (1989). The antecedents of maltreatment: Results of the Mother–Child Interaction Research Project. In D. Cicchetti &

V. Carlson (Eds.), *Child maltreatment* (pp. 203–253). Cambridge, England: Cambridge University Press.

Polansky, N. A., Ammons, P. W., & Gaudin, J. M. (1985). Loneliness and isolation in child neglect. *Social Casework, 66,* 38–47.

Polansky, N. A., Chalmers, M. A., Buttenwieser, E., & Williams, D. P. (1981). *Damaged parents: An anatomy of child neglect.* Chicago: University of Chicago Press.

Polansky, N. A., & Gaudin, J. M. (1983). Social distancing of the neglectful family. *Social Service Review, 57,* 196–208.

Polansky, N. A., Gaudin, J. M., Ammons, P. W., & David, K. B. (1985). The psychological ecology of the neglectful mother. *Child Abuse and Neglect, 9,* 265–275.

Powell, D. R. (1979). Family-environment relations and early childrearing: The role of social networks and neighborhoods. *Journal of Research and Development in Education, 13,* 1–11.

Powell, D. R. (1987). A neighborhood approach to parent support groups. *Journal of Community Psychology, 15,* 51–62.

Powell, D. R. (1988). Client characteristics and the design of community-based intervention programs. In A. R. Pence (Ed.), *Ecological research with children and families: From concepts to methodology* (pp. 122–142). New York: Teachers College Press.

President's Commission on Mental Health. (1978). *Task force report on community support systems.* Washington, DC: U.S. Government Printing Office.

Reid, M., Landesman, S., Treder, R., & Jaccard, J. (1989). "My family and friends": Six- to twelve-year-old children's perceptions of social support. *Child Development, 60,* 896–910.

Robertson, E. B., Elder, G. H., Jr., Skinner, M. L., & Conger, R. D. (1991). The costs and benefits of social support in families. *Journal of Marriage and the Family, 53,* 403–416.

Robertson, J. F. (1975). Interaction in three generation families, parents as mediators: Toward a theoretical perspective. *International Journal of Aging and Human Development, 6,* 103–110.

Rook, K. S., & Dooley, D. (1985). Applying social support research: Theoretical problems and future directions. *Journal of Social Issues, 41,* 5–28.

Salzinger, S., Kaplan, S., & Artemyeff, C. (1983). Mothers' personal social networks and child maltreatment. *Journal of Abnormal Psychology, 92,* 68–76.

Seagull, E. A. W. (1987). Social support and child maltreatment: A review of the evidence. *Child Abuse and Neglect, 11,* 41–52.

Shinn, M., Lehmann, S., & Wong, N. W. (1984). Social interaction and social support. *Journal of Social Issues, 40,* 55–76.

Shumaker, S. A., & Brownell, A. (1984). Toward a theory of social support: Closing conceptual gaps. *Journal of Social Issues, 40,* 11–36.

Smith, S. (1975). *The battered child syndrome.* London: Butterworths.

Smith, S. M., Hanson, R., & Noble, S. (1974). Social aspects of the battered baby syndrome. *British Journal of Psychiatry, 125,* 588–582.

Stack, C. (1974). *All our kin: Strategies for survival in a black community.* New York: Harper & Row.

Starr, R. H. (1982). A research-based approach to the prediction of child abuse. In

R. H. Starr (Ed.), *Child abuse prediction* (pp. 105–134). Cambridge, MA: Ballinger.

Straus, M. A. (1980). Stress and physical abuse. *Child Abuse and Neglect, 4,* 75–88.

Straus, M. A., Gelles, R. J., & Steinmetz, S. (1980). *Behind closed doors: Violence in the American family.* Garden City, NY: Doubleday/Anchor.

Straus, M. A., & Kantor, G. K. (1987). Stress and child abuse. In R. E. Helfer & R. S. Kempe (Eds.), *The battered child* (4th ed., pp. 42–59). Chicago: University of Chicago Press.

Thompson, R. A., Scalora, M. J., Castrianno, L., & Limber, S. P. (1992). Grandparent visitation rights: Emergent psychological and psycholegal issues. In D. Kagehiro & W. Laufer (Eds.), *Handbook of psychology and law* (pp. 292–317). New York: Springer-Verlag.

Tinsley, B. R., & Parke, R. D. (1984). Grandparents as support and socialization agents. In M. Lewis (Ed.), *Beyond the dyad* (pp. 161–194). New York: Plenum Press.

Toro, P. A. (1982). Developmental effects of child abuse: A review. *Child Abuse and Neglect, 6,* 423–431.

Tracy, E. M. (1990). Identifying social support resources of at-risk families. *Social Work, 35,* 252–258.

Tracy, E. M., & Whittaker, J. K. (1987). The evidence base for social support interventions in child and family practice: Emerging issues for research and practice. *Child and Youth Services Review, 9,* 249–270.

Unger, D. G., & Powell, D. R. (1980). Supporting families under stress: The role of social networks. *Family Relations, 29,* 566–574.

Unger, D. G., & Powell, D. R. (1990). Families as nurturing systems: An introduction. In D. G. Unger & D. R. Powell (Eds.), *Families as nurturing systems: Support across the life span* (pp. 1–17). New York: Haworth.

Unger, D. G., & Wandersman, A. (1985). The importance of neighbors: The social, cognitive, and affective components of neighboring. *American Journal of Community Psychology, 13,* 139–169.

Unger, D. G., & Wandersman, L. P. (1985). Social support and adolescent mothers: Action research contributions to theory and application. *Journal of Social Issues, 41,* 29–45.

U.S. Advisory Board on Child Abuse and Neglect. (1990). *Child abuse and neglect: Critical first steps in response to a national emergency* (Stock No. 017-092-00104-5). Washington, DC: U.S. Government Printing Office.

Vaux, A. (1985). Variations in social support associated with gender, ethnicity, and age. *Journal of Social Issues, 41,* 89–110.

Vaux, A. (1988). *Social support: Theory, research, and intervention.* New York: Praeger.

Vondra, J. I. (1990). The community context of child abuse and neglect. In D. G. Unger & M. B. Sussman (Eds.), *Families in community settings: Interdisciplinary perspectives. Marriage and Family Review, 15,* 19–38.

Wahler, R. G. (1980). The insular mother: Her problems in parent–child treatment. *Journal of Applied Behavior Analysis, 13,* 207–219.

Wahler, R. G., & Hann, D. M. (1984). The communication patterns of troubled mothers: In search of a keystone in the generalization of parenting skills. *Education and Treatment of Children, 7,* 335–350.

Weinraub, M., & Wolf, B. M. (1983). Effects of stress and social supports on mother–child interactions in single- and two-parent families. *Child Development*, *54*, 1297–1311.

Whittaker, J. K. (1983). Social support networks in child welfare. In J. Whittaker & J. Garbarino (Eds.), *Social support networks: Informal helping in the human services* (pp. 167–187). New York: Aldine.

Whittaker, J. K., Schinke, S. P., & Gilchrist, L. D. (1986). The ecological paradigm in child, youth, and family services: Implications for policy and practice. *Social Service Review*, *60*, 483–503.

Wolock, I., & Horowitz, B. (1979). Child maltreatment and material deprivation among AFDC-recipient families. *Social Service Review*, *53*, 175–194.

Young, G., & Gately, T. (1988). Neighborhood impoverishment and child maltreatment: An analysis from the ecological perspective. *Journal of Family Issues*, *9*, 240–254.

Young, L. (1964). *Wednesday's children: A study of child neglect and abuse*. New York: McGraw-Hill.

Zigler, E. F. (1989). Addressing the nation's child care crisis: The school of the twenty-first century. *American Journal of Orthopsychiatry*, *59*, 484–491.

Chapter 4

The Role of Material Factors in Child Abuse and Neglect

Leroy H. Pelton

After years of study and research, there is no single fact about child abuse and neglect that has been better documented and established than their strong relationship to poverty and low income. In attempting to understand the possible dynamics of this relationship, one obvious line of reasoning is that child abuse and neglect may be somehow mediated by the material hardships and stresses that poverty and low income cause. If this seems likely, remedies to be considered would include ways to reduce poverty and specific material hardships.

We must keep in mind, however, that poverty refers to level of income and not directly to impact on families and children. Income is a strong but only imperfect indicator of material hardship (Mayer & Jencks, 1989). It is also likely that income is only imperfectly related to stress. Moreover, it is important to note at the outset that only a small proportion of poor people (although large in number) are even alleged to abuse or neglect their children (Pelton, 1981a). The fact of a strong relationship between poverty and child abuse and neglect means that children from impoverished and low-income families are *extremely overrepresented* in the incidence of child abuse and neglect. Thus, reason directs us to contemplate the importance of poverty and low income as a context for child abuse and neglect and to examine the possible mediating physical, social, and personal factors that enhance or reduce the likelihood of child abuse and neglect within that context. All these considerations are explored here, but the emphasis is on the material factors that may contribute to child abuse and neglect or their prevention.

MATERIAL DEFICITS AND CHILD ABUSE AND NEGLECT

Poverty and Low Income

The great majority of families to which child abuse and neglect have been attributed live in poverty or near-poverty circumstances. The finding that poor children are vastly overrepresented among incidents of abuse and neglect has been obtained across a range of methodologies and definitions, forms of abuse and neglect, and levels of severity.

Every national survey of officially reported child abuse and neglect incidents, most of which were conducted by the American Humane Association (AHA) between the years 1975 and 1986, has indicated that the preponderance of the reports involved families from the lowest socioeconomic levels. Data collected by AHA for the year 1976, for example, showed that the median income of families involved in validated reports that year was only $5,051, which was below the 1976 poverty level ($5,815) for a non-farm family of four, compared with a median income of $14,958 for all U.S. families in that year (AHA, 1978; U.S. Bureau of the Census, 1991). About two thirds of the families in validated reports had incomes under $7,000, and only 9% of the families had incomes of $13,000 or more. For reports of neglect only, which were almost twice as numerous as reports of abuse only, the median income was somewhat lower ($4,250) than for abuse only ($6,886).

The AHA data for the year 1977 indicated that 47% of the families involved in substantiated reports had annual incomes of less than $5,000, while only 6% had incomes of at least $16,000, which was the median family income for all U.S. families in 1977 (AHA, 1979a; U.S. Bureau of the Census, 1991). About three quarters of the involved families had incomes under $9,000. Indications that these same trends have continued year after year in a rather stable fashion are reviewed further in the section on public assistance.

It is true, as has often been argued, that poor people are more susceptible to public scrutiny and are thus more likely than others to be *reported* for abuse and neglect. There is also some evidence that, apart from the issue of surveillance, even when incidents are identified, there may be systemic or personal biases (on the part of hospital personnel) leading to lower rates of official reports of those incidents among higher-income than lower-income families, and that race is also a factor (Hampton & Newberger, 1985).

An experimental study employing vignettes found that physicians' recognition and reporting of child abuse were influenced by the socioeconomic status and race of the families involved, although less so the more serious the injury. At a high level of injury, physicians' reporting was not affected by socioeconomic status. Moreover, nurses' recognition and reporting were unaffected by socioeconomic status or race (Nalepka, O'Toole, & Turbett,

1981). In a more recent survey of mandated reporters' responses to vignettes, the socioeconomic status of the involved family was experimentally varied in six vignettes. In three, a statistically significant greater likelihood to recognize the incident as abuse or neglect and to report the case was found when a lower-status family was involved. However, in one of these three vignettes, the likelihood to report was found to be greater for the lower-status perpetrator when the incident was portrayed as less severe in the vignette but greater for the higher-status perpetrator when the incident was portrayed as more severe. In none of another three vignettes in which race was varied was there a statistically significant impact on professionals' recognition of a case as abuse or neglect, or on their intention to report (Zellman, 1992).

Be that as it may, there is substantial evidence that the strong relationship between poverty and child abuse and neglect is not just an anomaly of reporting systems or personal biases (Pelton, 1978). First, while greater public awareness and new reporting laws led to a significant increase in official reporting over the years, the socioeconomic pattern of these reports has not changed appreciably. We might have expected an expanded and more vigilant public watch to produce an increased proportion of reports from above the lower class, but this has not happened.

Second, neither the public scrutiny argument nor personal recognition and reporting biases can explain the evidence that among families living in poverty, child abuse and neglect are related to the extent of material hardships encountered by those families (Giovannoni & Billingsley, 1970; Wolock & Horowitz, 1979). In the Wolock and Horowitz (1979) study, families receiving Aid to Families with Dependent Children (AFDC) who were involved in child abuse and neglect cases were found to be living in more crowded and dilapidated households, to have been more likely to have gone hungry, and, in general, to be existing at a lower material level of living than the other AFDC families studied.

Third, neither the public scrutiny argument nor personal recognition and reporting biases can explain why, among the reported cases, the severest injuries have occurred within the poorest families. In his nationwide survey of child abuse reports made to central registries, Gil (1970) found that injuries were more likely to be fatal or serious among families whose annual income was below $3,500. Thus, poverty is related not only to child abuse, but to the severity of maltreatment. The most severe and least easily hidden maltreatment of children is that which results in death. The public scrutiny argument cannot explain why child homicide studies have consistently indicated that the vast majority of the fatal victims of child abuse and neglect have been from poor families (Weston, 1974; Kaplun & Reich, 1976; Mayor's Task Force, 1983, 1987).

The Westat National Incidence Study was designed to go beyond the officially reported cases of child abuse and neglect known to child protective service agencies (U.S. Department of Health and Human Services

[DHHS], 1981). It did so by also gathering information on abuse and neglect incidents directly from other agencies, such as police and public health departments, and from professionals in hospitals, mental health facilities, other social service agencies, and public schools. The study found that the annual income of the families of 43% of the victims in the year beginning May 1, 1979, and ending April 30, 1980, was under $7,000 (the poverty level for a nonfarm family of four was $7,412 in 1979), compared with an estimated 17% of all American children who lived in a family with an income that low. Fully 82% of the victims were from families with incomes below $15,000, in comparison with 45% of all American children in that year. Only 6% of the victims were from families with incomes of $25,000 or more. The relationship between low income and child maltreatment was less pronounced for abuse than for neglect but still strong. The study concluded that the strong relationship between poverty and child abuse and neglect is not largely explainable in terms of reporting biases because the relationship "is almost as strong for unreported cases as for those which are reported to Child Protective Services" (DHHS, 1981, p. 38). The second National Incidence Study showed that, in the year 1986, the relationship between low income and child abuse and neglect continued to be strong (DHHS, 1988; Sedlak, 1991a). In fact, the incidence rate of child abuse and neglect was more than five times higher among children from families with annual incomes less than $15,000 (the poverty level for a nonfarm family of four was $11,203 in 1986) than from families with incomes of $15,000 or more, and in only 6% of the cases was the family income $30,000 (which was roughly the median income for all U.S. families in that year) or more. (It is important to be clear about the meaning of the term "incidence rate." It refers to the ratio of abused and neglected children in a particular category to all children within that category. Thus, in the foregoing finding, a child in a family whose income was below $15,000 was more than five times more likely to have been abused and/or neglected than a child in a family whose income was $15,000 or more.)

The National Incidence Studies clearly show that strong income-related differences hold for all specific forms of abuse and neglect. For example, in 1986, the incidence rate of physical abuse was three and a half times greater among children from families with annual incomes less than $15,000 than from families with incomes of $15,000 or more, and the incidence rate of emotional abuse was four times greater (Sedlak, 1991a). In fact, family income was the only factor found to be consistently related to risk for all categories of child abuse and neglect (Sedlak, 1991b). In 1979, looked at in a different way, 35% of all children involved in physical abuse incidents were from families with incomes below $7,000, and an additional 44% were from families with incomes between $7,000 and $15,000; the figures for emotional abuse were 31% and 46%, respectively (DHHS, 1981).

In 1986, the incidence rate of physical neglect was nine times greater, and that of emotional neglect almost five times greater, within the lower-income group (less than $15,000) than within the higher-income group ($15,000 or more) (Sedlak, 1991a). In 1979, 57% of all children involved in physical neglect incidents were from families with incomes below $7,000, and an additional 34% were from families with incomes between $7,000 and $15,000; the figures for emotional neglect were 45% and 31%, respectively (DHHS, 1981).

Even sexual abuse is strongly related to poverty and low income. The first National Incidence Study found the relationship between low income and sexual abuse to be just as strong as that between low income and overall child abuse and neglect in that 38% of the families of sexual abuse victims in 1979 had annual incomes under $7,000, and 80% had incomes under $15,000. Only 2% had incomes of $25,000 or more (DHHS, 1981). The second National Incidence Study showed that in 1986, the low-income relationship continued to be strong for sexual abuse. The incidence rate of sexual abuse was six times higher among children from families with incomes less than $15,000 than among those from families with incomes of $15,000 or more (Sedlak, 1991a).

These studies focused on genital contact and included incidents not involving genital contact in their definitions of sexual abuse only when there was evidence that such noncontact experiences might have caused at least some physical or emotional trauma to the child. Other studies, employing broader definitions and a variety of methodologies, have sometimes, but sometimes not, found this low-income relationship to obtain (see Finkelhor, 1984, 1986). Because the preponderance of the incidents counted in the National Incidence Studies did involve genital contact, it is clear that the low-income relationship holds for these more severe forms of sexual abuse. It is likely that the relationship between low income and sexual abuse has been "washed out" in some studies through the inclusion of higher proportions of incidents not involving genital contact and through the inclusion of incidents, such as being exposed to an instance of "flashing," whose labeling as sexual abuse would elicit considerable disagreement and questioning among both experts and laypersons. Any adequate plans to combat sexual abuse will have to take the socioeconomic facts into account.

Severity of the "abusive" *behavior*, often (though not always) corresponding to the severity of the physical or emotional *injury* that might occur, is certainly an important consideration in defining child abuse. Definitions by their nature are arbitrary, and "abuse" can be more narrowly or broadly defined. We can view such definitions as constituting a continuum, and depending on how much we wish to stretch our definitions, we could indeed reach a point at which we could conclude that abuse is rampant throughout society and not class related. For example, if we were to include any instances of physical punishment, such as the occasional spanking of a child, within our definition, we certainly could include larger portions of parents above the low-income classes in our statistics. Most, if not all, parents have behaved hostilely toward their children on occasion, either verbally or physically.

Many people, including myself, would view working to reduce all physical discipline of children in our society and to improve all parenting behavior (for there is always room for improvement) as laudable missions. But the origins of our attention to child abuse are tied to concerns about children who were placed in serious danger of severe harm or who were severely harmed. Although definitions of abuse may vary, the anchor point of our concerns must be the severity of the impact or potential impact on children, in terms of either their harm or their exploitation.

Thus, when we say that abuse is class related, we are really saying that it is the severity of abuse that is class related. This is often clear by definition itself. Both of the National Incidence Studies used definitions of physical and emotional abuse and neglect that only included children believed to have suffered significant physical, mental, or emotional injury or impairment. For example, physical abuse included corporal punishment only if excessive and if it resulted in observable symptoms of bodily injury lasting at least 48 hours. Consistent or extreme inattention to a child's physical or emotional needs was included under neglect, but only if it resulted in serious injury or impairment. Some extreme behaviors, such as abandonment, were assumed to cause serious emotional injury and so were included in the definitions. It is in accordance with this "harm standard" that the findings cited above from these two studies were obtained.

In the second National Incidence Study, however, two sets of findings were produced. Whereas the first was collected in accordance with the harm standard, the second was collected in accordance with an endangerment standard that broadened the criterion of demonstrable significant injury or impairment to endangerment for such harm. Under these revised definitions, still anchored in the concept of harm or potential harm, the relationships between low income and child abuse and neglect did not change very much. The incidence rate of physical abuse became more than four times greater (rather than three and a half times greater) among children from families with incomes less than $15,000 than from families with incomes of $15,000 or more, and the incidence rate of emotional abuse became almost five (rather than four) times greater. The incidence of sexual abuse became five and a half (rather than six) times higher for the low-income group as compared with the higher-income group. The ratio for emotional neglect did not change much either. The largest change pertained to physical neglect: It became 11 (rather than 9) times greater for the low-income group as compared with the higher-income group (Sedlak, 1991a).

Going beyond the definitions to the actual injuries, it was found that the incidence rate of serious injuries was seven times greater for the low-income than the higher-income group, and the incidence rate of moderate injury was five and a half times greater. This finding seems to support the hypothesis of an income-severity relationship. However, the incidence rate of fatalities was only four times greater for the low-income group than for the higher-income group. But this is a puzzling finding. For 1979, the first National Incidence Study found that, using the income cutoff point of $15,000 (which at that time was a little below the median family income level, rather than about half of the median family income level as it was in 1986), the incidence rate of fatalities was 111 times greater for the lower-income group than for the higher-income group. Indeed, 98% of all fatalities occurred in the lower-income group (Sedlak, 1991c).

Another approach to ascertaining the dimensions of child abuse (though not neglect) in the United States has been to survey parents in their homes, eliciting self-reports through use of the Conflict Tactics Scales (CTS). In 1976, a national survey was conducted of couples with a child between 3 and 17 years old. One parent in each of the families was asked whether he or she had directed certain actions, specified by the CTS, toward that child (Gelles, 1978). Of the 1,146 parents who were interviewed, 10% admitted to ever having thrown something at the child, and 5% said they had done so within the past year; 46% admitted to ever having pushed, grabbed, or shoved the child, and 41% indicated that they had done so within the past year; and 71% admitted to ever having slapped or spanked the child, while 58% said that they had done so within the past year. Eight percent of the parents acknowledged ever having kicked, bit, or hit the child with a fist, and 3% confessed to having done so within the past year; 20% admitted to ever having hit the child with something, and 13% to having done so within the past year; and 4% admitted that they had ever "beat up" the child, while 1% confessed to having done so within the past year. Finally, *one* parent (0.1%) confessed to having threatened the child with a knife or gun within the past year and one parent (perhaps the same parent) to having "used" a knife or gun on the child within the past year. Three percent said that they had ever threatened the child with a knife or gun, and the same percentage (perhaps the same parents referring to the same incidents) acknowledged ever having "used" a knife or gun on the child.

When all the aforementioned acts were lumped together into a single index of violence, it was found that the incidence rate of such acts was only 1.12 times higher among families with annual incomes less than $6,000 (which was $500 above the poverty level for a nonfarm family of four in 1975) than among families with incomes of $6,000 or above (Gelles, 1992). (It is not specified in the report whether the index referred to "ever," "within the past year," or a combination of both.) Because having "pushed, grabbed, or shoved" and "slapped or spanked" the child were acts that were reported far more frequently than any of the others, this income relationship obviously pertains largely to these acts. When only the acts of "kicked, bit, or hit with a fist," "beat up," and "threatened with a knife or gun" and "used a knife or gun" were isolated and combined into one index, which the investigators chose to call child abuse (Straus & Gelles, 1986), the incidence rate of such acts was found to be three and a half times higher among the lower-income group than among the higher-income group (Gelles, 1992). Since having "kicked, bit, or hit with a fist" were acts that were reported more frequently than any of the others within the narrower index, this income relationship was strongly influenced by these acts. In a similar survey conducted in 1985, the incidence rate of the acts that were combined into the overall index was scarcely greater among families with annual incomes of $10,000 or less (the poverty level for a nonfarm family of four was $10,989 in 1985) than among families with incomes above $10,000 (Gelles, 1992). However, the incidence rate of the acts combined into the narrower index was twice as great within the lower-income group than within the higher-income group.

In interpreting these findings, especially in relation to the other findings reviewed previously, considerable caution is necessary. "Kicked, bit, or hit with a fist," acts that contributed most heavily to measures acquired from the narrow index the researchers labeled "abuse" (although we do not know which of the three; for example, "kicked" might have been the most prevalent of these acts), would not necessarily meet the harm or endangerment standards of the National Incidence Studies for physical abuse. Nor would they likely constitute reports that would be validated by child protection agencies, or even "screened in" for investigation by such agencies, at least without further information pertaining to the individual acts, the events surrounding them, and their impact or potential impact upon the child. Thus, neither would they have been counted in the AHA surveys. The same can be said about "beat up," which might signify the repeated severe hitting of a child in a manner that leaves injuries; then again, to some parents (who were the interpreters of the meaning of these phrases in the CTS surveys), it might mean spanking the child a few times on the rear (Pelton, 1979). Without additional information, individual acts in this category might not get included in either the National Incidence or AHA studies. We do not even know if the parents who responded affirmatively to having "used a knife or gun" meant that they had once brandished a knife or gun, hit the child on the rear with the butt of an unloaded pistol, rapped the child's knuckles with a butter knife, or in fact shot at or stabbed the child (Pelton, 1979). Indeed, it is enlightening that Gil (1970), in a similar self-report survey of a nationally representative sample conducted a few years earlier, was able to find only 6 of 1,520 respondents, or 0.4%, who acknowledged ever having *injured* a child.

Thus, even with the findings pertaining to the narrower index in the CTS surveys, we are dealing with a less severe level of both acts and potential or real impact on the "abuse" continuum than in the findings related to the National Incidence and AHA surveys. Despite the fact that such acts as "threatened with" or "used a knife or gun" were included in the scales, their relative infrequency of occurrence in the actual data collected pertaining to either the overall or narrower indices means that the overall index is chiefly represented by "slapped or spanked" and "pushed, grabbed, or shoved," and the narrower index by "kicked, bit, or hit with a fist." Thus, in effect, we really have three levels here: the least severe level represented by the overall index in the CTS surveys, the next level by the narrower index in these same surveys (which the CTS investigators chose to call child abuse), and the third, which the term "child abuse" has been more commonly limited to in professional discourse, represented by the incidents included in the National Incidence (by both the harm and endangerment standards) and AHA surveys. Interpreted in this light, and given the frequencies of occurrence of the various action groupings and the income relationships found in the CTS surveys, a most important conclusion that can be drawn from these surveys is that a large proportion of American parents admit to ever having slapped, spanked, pushed, grabbed, or shoved their children, and a substantial minority to ever having hit them with something, and that these forms of physical "discipline" might be rampant throughout our society without regard to class. Moreover, a relatively more severe but far less frequent form of physical "punishment," represented largely by parents admitting to ever having kicked, bit, hit with a fist, or "beat up" their children, is strongly income related. Thus, even within an attenuated continuum that does not include the third level, severity is found to be related to income.

In fact, the small category of families that contains a highly disproportionate number of the families involved in official reports, and the most severe cases of child abuse (and neglect)—the category of families existing at the lowest material levels of living in our society—was evidently excluded from both the 1976 and 1985 CTS surveys. To counter a claim by Stocks (1988) that the two surveys were not comparable because the second was conducted through telephone interviews and, thus, families without telephones, who are likely to be low-income families, were not represented, while the first survey was conducted through in-person house interviews, Gelles, Straus, and Harrop (1988, p. 286) noted that even in-person interviewers are frequently unsuccessful in completing interviews in the same "lower-income and minority households that do not have telephones." Thus, Gelles et al. (1988) argue that the samples were comparable since the "category of households excluded from the second survey were in all likelihood not reached in the first survey either" (p. 286). In fact, while the median income of families involved in official child abuse and neglect reports is far below the median national income, that of the families in the CTS surveys was actually above the median national income in 1975. For black families, the median income of families in the CTS surveys was above the median national income for black families in both 1975 and 1985 (Hampton, Gelles, & Harrop, 1989; U.S. Bureau of the Census, 1990; Pelton, 1991b). Moreover, in a study of families receiving AFDC in northern New Jersey in 1976, Wolock and Horowitz (1979) found that 53% of the AFDC families known to the state child protection agency for child abuse and neglect did not have telephones, and 31% of the other AFDC families did not have telephones. In a study of parents who killed their children in Detroit between 1982 and 1986, Goetting (1988) found that 36% of them did not have telephones, compared to 10% of all Detroit residences without telephones in 1986.

Indeed, by looking at the third level, operationally defining child abuse *and neglect* in terms of the National Incidence Studies and AHA surveys, and focusing on these studies, we see a rough outline of a funneling effect in relation to income. More than 90% of child abuse and neglect incidents at this level occur in the 50% of all families who have incomes below the median income for all U.S. families. In addition, the closer down toward the poverty line a below-median-income family is, the greater the risk its children are at for child abuse and neglect. But further, roughly 40% to 50% of child abuse and neglect incidents occur within the approximately 15% of American families with children who live below the poverty line. This funneling effect is more dramatic when looked at for neglect apart from abuse and neglect. When we use all other studies cited here to further complement this rough outline, we find some reason to believe that the most severe incidents of child abuse and neglect, those that result in fatalities, are even more highly and deeply concentrated within poverty. In addition, going in the other direction of severity, a level of physical "punishment" below that which we are operationally defining here as physical abuse shows a clear funneling effect with income, but one not as strong as for physical abuse as defined here. Finally, an even milder level of "punishment," characterized by slapping, spanking, pushing, grabbing, and shoving children, is quite widespread and shows little if any funneling effect in relation to family income. Thus, overall, the relationship between family income and the *severity* of negative actions (and omissions) toward children, across a wide range of negative actions, is quite clear and dramatic.

This funneling effect is fine-tuned. For example, in 1977, when the poverty level for a family of four was about $6,000, and the median income for all families was $16,000, 28% of the families involved in validated reports of child abuse and neglect had incomes below $3,000; another 19% had incomes between $3,000 and under $5,000; and another 16% had incomes between $5,000 and under $7,000. As we go up the income scale, there is, in fact, a perfect inverse relationship between income bracket and the percentage of validated reports an income bracket accounts for. Another 11% of the families involved in validated reports of child abuse and neglect had incomes between $7,000 and under $9,000, another 8% between $9,000 and under $11,000, another 6% between $11,000 and under $13,000, and another 5% between $13,000 and under $16,000 (the median income), for a total of 94.2% (without rounding) under the median income. An additional 3% had incomes between $16,000 and under $20,000, and another 2% had incomes between $20,000 and under $25,000. Finally, only 1% had incomes between $25,000 and under $40,000, and only 3/10 of 1% had incomes of $40,000 or above (AHA, 1979a). The first National Incidence Study also indicated a perfect inverse relationship between income bracket and the percentage of abused and neglected children accounted for (DHHS, 1981). Such a relationship would be truly difficult to explain in terms of personal biases: It is hard to imagine that prejudices are that fine-tuned.

Given the strong relationship between low income and child abuse and neglect, we should fully expect to find that as poverty rates for children go up, as they have for the past two decades (with some ups and downs along the way), child abuse and neglect rates would also rise. Unfortunately, the available national data do not permit us to test this reasonable hypothesis. Although the AHA surveys of official reports, which were performed annually from 1976 through 1986, show a dramatic and rather steady rise in reporting rates throughout that period, there are many factors that contributed to that rise (AHA, 1988). Indeed, many experts believe that it represents increased detection of child abuse and neglect incidents and not an increase in the incidents themselves. In any event, it is virtually impossible to disentangle the possible role of the poverty factor from other factors that have contributed to the reporting rate increases nationally.

The National Incidence Studies cannot help us much in this regard in that they have been performed at only two points in time—1979 and 1986—and two points cannot establish a trend. However, under the same definitions for both years, a considerably higher child abuse and neglect incidence rate was found for 1986, when the child poverty rate was substantially higher, than for 1979 (Sedlak, 1991a). Yet this increase was largely due to a significant increase in the incidence rate of child abuse and neglect causing moderate injury, rather than to the increase in the incidence of serious injury, which was not statistically significant. This pattern led the investigators to speculate that the overall increase may reflect increased recognition of child abuse and neglect by professionals rather than an increase in the rate of actual incidence (DHHS, 1988; Sedlak, 1991a). On the other hand, the estimated number of fatalities was 10% higher in 1986 than in 1979, although this difference was not statistically significant.

The CTS surveys have also been performed only twice. A statistically significant decline was found in the incidence rate of the narrower index, from 1975 as compared with 1985 (Straus & Gelles, 1986). This apparent decline might be due to a possible noncomparability of samples alluded to before in that the second survey used telephone interviews, an approach that might have reached fewer families existing at the lowest material levels of living within poverty than did the in-person interviews of the first survey. More likely, however, *both* surveys excluded or undersampled families at this lowest economic rung within the poverty range, and the findings, which were due largely to a statistically significant decline in the incidence rate of the "kicked, bit, or hit with a fist" action grouping, may reflect a true decrease within the larger society. Such progress might have been brought about by increased public awareness, attributable to public and private efforts surrounding child abuse, which has led to greater sensitivity and self-reflection among many parents in regard to the disciplining of their children. At the same time, however, we must remember that in regard to more severe forms of child maltreatment, the evidence indicates no decline: The National Incidence Studies show no decline in the incidence rates of serious injuries and fatalities due to child abuse and neglect (Sedlak, 1991a).

To confirm the hypothesis that increments in child poverty rates over time correspond to increments in child abuse and neglect rates, we need to perform studies that examine data considerably below the national scope, preferably on the neighborhood level. From one point of view, such studies are not really necessary, given the overwhelming evidence of the relationship between poverty and child abuse and neglect. Such studies, however, may uncover additional intricacies of this relationship. For example, we may find that increases in poverty rates are more disastrous in terms of child abuse and neglect in neighborhoods that are already largely poor.

A study on the county level does provide some evidence, reported in the next section, that increases in poverty, when indicated by increases in the rates of food stamp recipients, are associated with increases in child abuse and neglect reports (McNicoll, 1989).

Public Assistance and Food Stamps

AFDC payments, together with other government aids that AFDC recipients are eligible to receive, such as food stamps and Medicaid, provide income and other material supports. Thus, we might expect their receipt to be associated with reduced incidence of child abuse and neglect, and, indeed, we might speculate that the incidence of abuse and neglect in the United States would be much higher than it is if these programs were nonexistent. At the same time, however, the fact is that AFDC allowances to families are universally below the poverty level and so maintain eligible families within poverty. For this reason, AFDC status is used by researchers merely as an indicator of poverty.

In his nationwide survey of child abuse reports made to central registries, Gil (1970) found that nearly 60% of the involved families (he studied abuse only) received some form of public assistance during or prior to the study year of 1967, and 34% of the involved families were receiving AFDC (and an additional 3% were receiving other forms of public assistance) at the time of the incident. The AHA data for 1976, based on approximately 18,000 validated reports of child abuse and neglect, indicated that 42% of the families were receiving public assistance, mostly AFDC (AHA, 1978). In 1977, based on more than 32,000 validated reports, 44% of the families were found to be receiving AFDC or other forms of public assistance (AHA, 1979a). In 1979, the proportion was 48% (AHA, 1981a); in 1980, 44% (AHA, 1981b). In 1981, based on about 117,000 reports (before substantiation), the proportion was 43% (AHA, 1983). The proportion was 43% in 1982 and 48% in 1984 (AHA, 1988). Finally, in 1986, the proportion of all reported families (before substantiation) that were receiving public assistance was 49%, which was about four times the proportion of all U.S. families receiving such assistance (AHA, 1988).

Note that these percentages have remained remarkably stable over time, and that the percentages of families who had *ever* received public assistance, rather than of those that were receiving it at the time of the incident, would no doubt be substantially higher. A study of abused and neglected children on the case load of the state child protection agency in Mercer County, New Jersey, found that the families of at least 81% of these children had received public welfare benefits at some time (Pelton, 1981a). Overall, these facts merely reinforce the findings on the relationship between poverty/low income and child abuse and neglect reviewed earlier.

A study of county rates (or more precisely, rates at 27 offices corresponding to the 39 counties of Washington State) of child abuse and neglect reports in the state of Washington from 1983 through 1986 found that, across counties, they were significantly and positively correlated with the rates of food stamp recipients per county (McNicoll, 1989). Moreover, month-by-month analyses over time indicated that increases in the rates of food stamp recipients were associated with increases in the rates of child abuse and neglect, at least for two of the five individual counties for which separate analyses were reported.

Housing

The AHA data for 1976 indicate that, based on child protection workers' judgments, inadequate housing was a factor present for families involved in 26% of substantiated neglect-only reports and 9% of abuse-only reports (AHA, 1978). For 1977, the proportions were 23% and 8%, for neglect-only and abuse-only substantiated reports, respectively (AHA, 1979a). For 1978, the proportions were 28% and 10%, respectively (AHA, 1979b). The relationship between inadequate housing and child abuse and neglect is not surprising given the prevalence of poverty among abusing and neglecting families, although one might have expected a greater proportion of abuse cases to be associated with inadequate housing.

In a study involving hundreds of families in northern New Jersey, comparing AFDC recipient families known to the state child protection agency and identified as having abused and/or neglected their children with AFDC families not known to that agency, the maltreating families were found to be living in more crowded and dilapidated households than were the other AFDC families (Wolock & Horowitz, 1977, 1979). The maltreating families had significantly more individuals per room, with their children more likely to share a bed, than did other AFDC families. Interviewers were more likely to describe the state of repair of the maltreating families' rooms as poor or very poor (28% vs. 18% for the other AFDC families). The maltreating families were less likely to have a shower, air conditioner, or telephone in their homes. In fact, as indicated previously, only 47% had telephones (the study was performed in 1976–1977), compared to 69% of other AFDC families. The maltreating families were more likely to report ever having been evicted than were other AFDC families. A third of all of the families said that they had seen rats in their home, and 14% said that they had been without heat for most of the winter, but these factors did not distinguish maltreating families from the other AFDC families.

In a further analysis of a random subset of families drawn from the sample of maltreating AFDC families only, Horowitz and Wolock (1981) found that families living in the *most* deprived material circumstances, a measure of which in good part referred to housing conditions, tended to contain the most *severe* maltreatment.

In the Wolock and Horowitz (1979) study, a large majority of the maltreating families showed evidence of neglect only, and a considerable proportion involved both neglect and abuse. Few cases in the sample involved abuse only. Zuravin's (1985) review of the research literature led her to conclude that there is little evidence that housing inadequacies are related to abuse when socioeconomic status is controlled for. However, in a later study Zuravin (1986) found that household overcrowding, as measured by the percentage of housing units in Baltimore census tracts containing more than 1.5 persons per room, was associated with reporting rate differentials for abuse as well as neglect among those tracts after controlling for race and class. This measure of overcrowding was, though, more strongly associated with neglect than with abuse.

Finally, Zuravin and Taylor (1989) found that child abuse and neglect reporting rates were no higher in urban neighborhoods in Baltimore in which the predominant proportion of households with children are in public housing projects than in comparably poor neighborhoods in which few households with children are located in public housing projects. Assuming greater social stress in public housing projects, the authors expected to find higher reporting rates in public housing project neighborhoods. To explain the finding of no difference, they suggest that because public housing families pay low rents, they may be better off financially, although poor, than their nonpublic housing counterparts, and their better financial situations may offset the impact of whatever greater social stresses (such as crime) might exist in the public housing project environment.

Thus, we can conclude from the research literature that within the context of poverty, material hardships indicated by inadequate housing are independently related to abuse and neglect, although more strongly to neglect than to abuse. Moreover, housing environment arrangements may not be as important as those housing factors that contribute to measures of material level of living.

Food

In the Wolock and Horowitz (1977, 1979) study, respondents from the maltreating AFDC families were significantly more likely than those from the other AFDC families to report that they or someone else in the family had gone hungry for a day or more during the past month because there was not enough food in the house (14% vs. 7%).

Health

The AHA data for 1986 indicate that, based on child protection workers' judgments, health problems (including alcohol/drug dependency, medical and physical disabilities of the caretaker or child, and mental retardation or mental health problems of the caretaker or child) were factors present for families involved in 43% of child abuse and neglect reports (both substantiated and not) (AHA, 1988). The percentage was about the same for physical abuse as for physical neglect.

Elmer (1981) found a high frequency of chronic illness among three groups of lower-class children—abused, accidentally traumatized, and nontraumatized children—with little difference between the groups.

Wolock and Horowitz (1977, 1979) found that the respondents in the maltreating AFDC families reported approximately the same types and number of parental physical illnesses as the other AFDC families, and their children had similar rates of illness and developmental disabilities. However, in their further analysis (including case record reviews) of a subset of the maltreating AFDC families, Horowitz and Wolock (1981) found that in 53% of the families, the main caretaker had a severe physical illness or condition, and 33% of the main caretakers had a severe mental or emotional problem, most frequently severe depression. Moreover, 60% of the families included an adult member who used alcohol excessively, and 20% contained a member who was a heroin user. In addition, 76% of the families had at least one child with serious health problems, and 24% of the families had at least one child who is mentally retarded.

In this further analysis, Horowitz and Wolock (1981) found the extent of material deprivation to be related to the severity of maltreatment. They also found that families living in the poorest material conditions were more likely to have a retarded child than were the other maltreating AFDC families and to have a child with a severe physical illness. The parents in these families were more likely to have physical health problems, although parents living in the *less* deprived material condition were more likely to have emotional problems. Material level of living was not related to alcohol abuse.

Race/Ethnicity

It has been difficult to discern the relationship between race/ethnicity and child abuse and neglect. The AHA data for 1977 indicated that 17% of the alleged perpetrators were black (not including Hispanic blacks), as compared with 11% of the general population who were black (including Hispanic blacks), and 9% were Hispanic, compared with 5% of the general population (AHA, 1979a). The AHA data for 1986 indicated that 21% of the alleged child victims were black (not including Hispanic blacks), as compared with about 15% of the entire child population (including Hispanic blacks), and 11% were Hispanic (AHA, 1988).

In the first National Incidence Study, it was found that the incidence rate of child abuse and neglect was essentially the same for black and white children (DHHS, 1981). When income level was taken into account, the incidence rate was found to be similar for white and nonwhite children for families with annual incomes of $15,000 or more, whereas the incidence rate for white children was higher than for nonwhite children in families with lower incomes. In the second National Incidence Study, no statistically significant relationships were found between the incidence of child abuse and neglect and children's race/ethnicity (Sedlak, 1991a). Yet, three marginal findings indicated that nonwhite children may be at higher risk than white children for fatalities, physical abuse, and physical neglect. However, when income is controlled for, most racial differences disappear, leaving only older black and Hispanic children at greater risk of physical abuse than older white children (Sedlak, 1991b). No racial differences remain for physical neglect.

Thus, most racial differences that have been found from time to time (such as the moderate overrepresentation of blacks in the AHA data) are very likely a function of income rather than of race per se. For example, in the Wolock and Horowitz (1979) study, although the proportion of maltreating AFDC families that were black was found to be high (60%), it was no higher than the proportion of nonmaltreating AFDC families who were black (63%). Because disproportionately greater percentages of black than white families are submerged in poverty, and because the relationship between family income and child abuse and neglect is so strong, we would actually expect the incidence rate of child abuse and neglect to be greater among black families, based on income alone. Beyond income measures, and within poverty, Horowitz and Wolock (1981) found that the *level* of material deprivation, which was related to severity of maltreatment, was also strongly related to race. This finding is consistent with the overrepresentation of black children among child abuse and neglect fatalities (Goetting, 1988). However, in his secondary analysis of the data from the first National Incidence Study, Hampton (1987a) found the proportion of abuse and neglect incidents that resulted in "serious" injury to be about the same among black families as among white families, even though three quarters of the black families as opposed to half the white families had annual incomes of less than $7,000. This leaves open the question whether something about being black does or does not buffer the relationship between severity of maltreatment and material level of living established in this chapter.

In regard to the "kicking, biting, or hitting with a fist" and "beating up" of the CTS surveys (this time with "hitting or trying to hit with something" added), the incidence rates of such actions toward children in 1975 were found to be about the same among black families as among white families (Straus, Gelles, & Steinmetz, 1980). For the year 1985, however, the CTS survey indicated that the incidence rate was twice as great in black families as in white families (Hampton et al., 1989). This difference might be attributable to a decline in such acts among white families only, possibly indicating a greater impact of public awareness campaigns on the self-consciousness of white parents. Such campaigns might "speak to" them more than to black parents, but yet do not effect more severe levels of child abuse and neglect examined in other studies.

The point of this discussion for the purposes of this chapter is that the strong relationship between poverty/low income and child abuse and neglect is certainly not an artifact of the relationship between race/ethnicity and child abuse and neglect. Findings in regard to the latter are often an artifact of the former, even though differences in ethnic patterns in regard to child abuse and neglect may indeed exist (Hampton, 1987a, 1987b; Garbarino & Ebata, 1987).

Unemployment

There is substantial evidence that unemployment is strongly related to child abuse and neglect. In his nationwide survey of child abuse reports made to central registries in 1967, Gil (1970) found that only 53% of the fathers of the involved children had been employed throughout the year. The AHA data for the year 1981 indicated that no caretaker was currently employed in 40% of the families officially reported for child abuse and neglect (based on 26,730 substantiated and unsubstantiated reports combined, that is, on reports before substantiation), as compared with a national unemployment rate of 13% at that time for families with children under 18 years of age (AHA, 1983). Data collected by AHA for the year 1986 showed that no caretaker was currently employed in 35% of the families reported for child abuse and neglect (based on reports before substantiation) (AHA, 1988). This proportion varied somewhat for specific forms of abuse and neglect, from 26% for sexual abuse to 42% for neglect involving "deprivation of necessities."

In a study of the relationship between unemployment and child abuse and neglect reporting based on data from nine states comprising 599 counties, it was found that county unemployment rates were significantly correlated with reporting rates based on the AHA annual reporting data (Bycer, Breed, Fluke, & Costello, 1983). That is, counties that had the highest unemployment rates also had the highest reporting rates for each of the three years (1979, 1980, and 1981) studied.

The foregoing findings are not surprising in light of the facts that low income levels are strongly associated with child abuse and neglect, because we would expect poverty to be related to high unemployment rates. To learn more about the possible effects of unemployment, we can examine the relationship between *change* in unemployment and *change* in child abuse and neglect rates. The findings cited thus far do not address this issue.

The relationship between economic change, as indexed by unemployment rates, and a variety of behavioral and health consequences, has been rather extensively studied for some time now. Rises in unemployment rates have been linked to subsequent increases in rates of suicide, mental hospital admissions, alcohol abuse, cirrhosis mortality, homicide, deaths resulting from motor vehicle accidents, incidence of and mortality from heart disease, infant mortality, prison admissions, and delinquency (Brenner, 1984). However, very few studies have examined the possible link between economic change and child abuse and neglect. All are based on official reports of child abuse and neglect.

The one relevant finding from the Bycer et al. (1983) study cited above was a slight positive correlation of .089 between a change in county unemployment rates between the years 1979 and 1981 and a change in county child abuse and neglect reporting rates over the same 2-year period. This correlation was statistically significantly different from zero at only the 10% level of confidence. (Bycer et al. found a stronger positive correlation between county unemployment rates for 1979 and county reporting rates for the following year, but this finding does not address *change*. It merely means that counties with high unemployment rates continue to have high reporting rates and this, in turn, might reflect the possibility that the highest unemployment rates are occurring in the poorest counties.)

In another study, the relationship between job loss and child abuse and neglect reports was examined for Los Angeles and Orange counties in California over a 30-month period between 1975 and 1977 (Steinberg, Catalano, & Dooley, 1981). No significant relationship was found between increases in the monthly unemployment rate and concurrent or subsequent increases in child abuse or child neglect reports in either county. However, using a different measure of job loss, the authors found declines in size of the work force to be significantly related to increases in child abuse reports 2 months later in both counties. The authors note that size of the work force might be a more sensitive measure of job loss than unemployment rates because the latter do not include people who have stopped looking for work. Curiously, however, the same relationship was not found with child neglect reports in either county. Rather, declines in the size of the work force were discovered to be significantly related to *concurrent* increases in child neglect reports in Los Angeles County only.

Judging from these two studies, we would have to conclude thus far that the relationship between increases in job loss levels and increase in child abuse and neglect reports is fragile indeed. Despite the use of massive databases, one study indicates a weak and questionable correlation with unemployment rates. The other study finds no relationship with unemployment rates but, in resorting to what is presumed to be a more sensitive measure of job loss, reveals mixed and somewhat confusing results. Yet another study has even found some evidence of a puzzling inverse relationship between changes in month-by-month county unemployment rates and child abuse and neglect report rates (McNicoll, 1989).

However, the findings of one report, stemming from a rather simple statistical analysis of changes in county unemployment rates during 1981 (taking the rates in January 1982 as compared with those in January 1981) and in annual child abuse and neglect reporting figures during that same year (comparing the total figures for the year of 1981 with those of 1980) in the state of Wisconsin, are quite impressive (Mills, 1982). Of the 10 counties in the state that had the greatest unemployment rate increases, 9 had concurrent rises in child abuse and neglect reporting; of the 10 counties with the greatest decreases in unemployment rate, 8 had declines in child abuse and neglect reporting. Furthermore, of the 51 counties in the state that showed increased unemployment rates, 35, or 68.6%, had increases in child abuse and neglect reporting, whereas only 4, or 19%, of the 21 counties with unemployment rate decreases had increases in child abuse and neglect reporting.

The report's identification of the 10 counties with the highest unemployment rate increases permitted me to do a further simple analysis utilizing the unemployment and child abuse and neglect change rates provided in the report (Pelton, 1984). Based on census statistics for the year 1979 (U.S. Bureau of the Census, 1983), I found that the average percentagewise increase in child abuse and neglect reporting was almost 13 times greater for the six counties that had at least 8.5% of its families with incomes below the poverty level than for the four remaining counties, which had 5.9% or less of its families with incomes below the poverty level. (The statewide family poverty rate for Wisconsin in 1979 was 6.3%.) This was true despite the fact that the two subsets of six and four counties had a similar average increase in unemployment rate (up an additional 4.75% and 4.35%, respectively).

This additional finding permits the tentative conclusion that unemployment increases in the poorest communities are likely to beget greater increases in child abuse and neglect reporting than are unemployment increases, even of similar magnitude, in other communities. Thus, considering the two previous studies, we can conclude that the relationship of *magnitudes* of unemployment rate change and child abuse and neglect reporting change is weak only when the original economic status of the community is not taken into account. A county with a high increase in unemployment can have either a high or a relatively low increase in child abuse and neglect reporting, depending, in part, on how poor that community is.

A likely key mediating factor in this relationship is material hardship. In their surveys of Chicago families to investigate the relationship between income and material hardship (the latter measured by respondents' answers to questions pertaining to their ability to afford food, adequate housing, and medical care), Mayer and Jencks (1989) found that "families whose incomes dropped in 1984 did not experience as much hardship as families with the same 1984 income whose 1983 income had also been low" (p. 111). They speculate that families with relatively high incomes in the previous year "had accumulated either savings or informal credit with others, against which they drew when the need arose" (pp. 110–111). Indeed, when the authors asked respondents in their survey if they could borrow $500 when they needed it, only 34% of those with incomes below the poverty level said that they could, whereas 79% of those with incomes two to three times the poverty level, and 96% of those with incomes more than three times the poverty level, said that they could. As Mayer and Jencks (1989) suggest, "past affluence provides some cushion against the effects of current poverty" (p. 111).

Job loss can have direct material effects on an entire household. Indeed, many reports of child neglect actually involve a "deprivation of necessities" (AHA, 1983, p. 7). However, a family's existing economic resources can negate the material impact of job loss. The direct material effects of job loss are dependent on the extent of savings (or ability to borrow) that a family has to cushion the loss of job income. Since middle- and upper-class families are more likely to have a cushion of savings (or ability to borrow) than are the poor, the material impact of job loss will be most immediate and severe for families who are already poor. In the long run, of course, rising and enduring unemployment would impoverish more and more families. Thus, based on the few studies currently available, it is suggested that the relationship between increases in unemployment and increases in child abuse and neglect is mediated by material hardship and is dependent on the economic status of the community. (It is noteworthy that in the above survey, low-income families who said that they could borrow usually said that they would do so from a relative or a friend.) That is, unemployment increases in the poorest communities are likely to beget the greatest increases in child abuse and neglect reports. The effects of unemployment rate increases on children are greatest among the poor.

MEDIATING FACTORS BETWEEN POVERTY/LOW INCOME
AND CHILD ABUSE AND NEGLECT

The strong relationship between poverty and the incidence and severity of child abuse and neglect is a fact but not an explanation. Although the conclusion that problems of poverty might be partial determinants of child abuse and neglect is compelling, we need to understand the dynamics of the relationship. We need to examine the mediating factors that lead to individual variation, especially since we know that although as much as 5% of poor children are considered to be abused or neglected within a given year, most poor people do not abuse or neglect their children.

The first step is to recognize that while most studies have examined the relationship between poverty, rather than material hardship, and child abuse and neglect, poverty is defined in terms of income rather than impact and is only a rough indicant of the extent of material hardship. Yet, poverty has its impact on families through the imposition of material hardships or, in other words, through the conditions that poverty gives rise to; thus, material hardships are themselves important mediating factors.

As is argued later, there is a *direct* way in which the material conditions of living in poverty can give rise to what we call child abuse and neglect, as well as to the severity of harm done. However, the relationship between material hardships and child abuse and neglect, although probably even stronger than the poverty relationship, is far from perfect. Thus, the search for explanation and mediating factors has led theorists to consider the individual experiences and qualities of people, which, being more variable, may help to explain, for example, why individuals living at the same material level may differ in regard to abusive and neglectful behavior.

A major concept has been the experience of stress. As Gil (1970) has pointed out, the living conditions of poverty generate stressful experiences that may become precipitating factors in child abuse, and the poor have little means by which to escape from such stress. According to Gil (1970), environmental stress factors "may weaken a person's psychological mechanisms of self-control" and may contribute to "the uninhibited discharge of aggressive and destructive impulses" (p. 136) toward children. Under these circumstances, even minor misbehaviors of and annoyances by powerless children may trigger abuse. Such poverty-related factors as unemployment; dilapidated and overcrowded housing; and insufficient money, food, recreation, or hope can provide the stressful context for neglect as well as abuse (Pelton, 1978). Such potentially stressful conditions and events can provoke the anger that may lead to abuse as well as the despair that may lead to neglect when, for example, parents attempt to raise a large family in cramped and unsafe living quarters with no help and little money. This discussion is consistent with the conceptualization of psychological stress by Cohen and Wills (1985), which posits that "stress arises when one appraises a situation as threatening or otherwise demanding and does not have an appropriate coping response" (p. 312), that a characteristic effect of stress appraisal is negative affect, and that appraised stress may give rise to feelings of helplessness and possible loss of self-esteem.

In fact, both income and social class have been found to be inversely correlated with psychological distress (Bradburn, 1969; Dohrenwend & Dohrenwend, 1969; Srole, Langner, Michael, Opler, & Rennie, 1962; Kleiner & Parker, 1970). Unemployment has been found to be related to increased anxiety, depression, and hostility (Liem & Liem, 1988). In this study, financial strain (as measured by the amount of unpaid bills) was discovered to be correlated with the initial impact of unemployment on depressive mood. Increased somatic complaints, hostility, depression, and anxiety were also found among the wives of the men who had experienced job loss.

There is evidence suggesting that household overcrowding is experienced by individuals in terms of excessive demands and lack of privacy and is reacted to by physical and psychological withdrawal, inability to plan, ineffective thinking and action, and feelings of emotional drain (Gove, Hughes, & Galle, 1979). Moreover, crowding and its experience are related to psychological distress, hostility and physical violence within the home, feelings of being annoyed or harassed by one's children, and not getting along with the children (Gove et al., 1979).

Some evidence suggests that stressful events in the lives of low-income mothers, aside from low socioeconomic status itself, are indeed associated with child abuse and neglect (e.g., Gaines, Sandgrund, Green, & Power, 1978; Egeland, Breitenbucher, & Rosenberg, 1980).

Early clinical studies identified a variety of personality factors that were thought to distinguish abusing and neglecting parents from other parents. In a review of these studies, Gelles (1973) found that abusing parents were said to have personality deficits ranging from pervasive anger, poor emotional control, and immaturity to sadomasochism, narcissism, and "transference psychosis." He identified several problems regarding the validity of these trait attributions. There was little agreement among the studies in regard to the traits identified; most of the discussions were inconsistent and contradictory as to the nature and presence of various personality deficits. Most studies did not test the assumptions they made: Attributions were made simply on the basis of the abusing behavior and were then offered as explanations. Finally, inadequate sampling procedures were used, and these were coupled with the absence of comparable control groups of nonabusers. Thus, we would have no way of knowing whether the proposed attributions could be generalized to all abusers or whether they differentiate abusers from nonabusers.

In a review of more recent and better controlled research, Wolfe (1985) concluded that "studies using measures of underlying personality attributes or traits have been unable to detect any patterns associated with child abuse beyond general descriptions of displeasure in the parenting role and stress-related complaints" (p. 465). Evidence from other studies allowed him to conclude that abusive parents "display stress-related symptoms such as depression and health problems that likely impair their parental competence" (p. 471).

Recent studies have found that maltreating AFDC mothers are more likely to suffer from depression than are nonmaltreating AFDC mothers, and that depression is even more strongly related to neglect than to abuse (Zuravin, 1988; Zuravin & Greif, 1989). Moreover, the maltreating AFDC mothers were found to have a lower level of self-esteem and were less likely to feel in control of their lives (Zuravin & Greif, 1989).

Such depression may be due to differential stressful events or material hardships among maltreating and nonmaltreating low-income families or differential stress appraisal, which may, in turn, as Cohen and Wills (1985) suggest, give rise to feelings of helplessness and low self-esteem. Lack of social support may adversely affect the appraisal of stress or the stress reaction. It is still possible, however, that the depression reported in the studies is more a personality characteristic than a situational reaction to stressful events and conditions. Such a characteristic, in turn, can arise from a low level of inner resources for the purpose of making appropriate coping responses to life situations. It has been shown that high levels of inner resources of self-esteem and mastery may help reduce the depressing effects of economic strain (Kessler & Essex, 1982). On the other hand, neglecting mothers describe their neighborhoods as less friendly and helpful than their neighbors do (Polansky, Gaudin, Ammons, & Davis, 1985). It is possible that their own personal inadequacies reduce their access to available support.

Thus, we may conclude that no matter what their sources, the only personal differences that have been found (depression, self-esteem, a sense of mastery) are those directly relevant to one's ability or inability to cope with poverty and its stressors, which include its material hardships. Even if we were to entertain the possibility that for some individuals these personal factors did not arise from the stressors of poverty but contributed to their falling into poverty in the first place, and contribute to preventing them from rising out of poverty, my basic conclusion would not change. For people living in poverty, the probability of child abuse and neglect is largely dependent on the extent of one's ability to cope with poverty and its stressors.

Other factors frequently associated with child abuse and neglect include health problems, social isolation, family discord, family size, and alcohol and drug dependence (AHA, 1978, 1981b, 1988; Pelton, 1981b; Sedlak, 1991a). These factors, too, whether or not arising from poverty and its stressors, affect one's ability to cope with poverty and its stressors. The stressors of poverty can engender individual modes of dysfunctional "coping," such as alcohol and drug abuse, that can destroy parental competence.

Lack of knowledge of parenting skills is relevant to relatively few cases of child abuse and neglect (Pelton, 1981a; Wolock & Horowitz, 1977, 1979) and is not the issue here. I speak of the ability to cope with *poverty*, and this cognitive coping ability may or may not involve specific knowledge of particular cognitive coping skills. It may well be akin to a personal cognitive style. We do not understand it too well because research has focused on the consequences of the negative end of the continuum of such ability, such as child abuse and neglect, or on families in which the ability is nearly absent, rather than on the positive end. Thus, for example, we do not understand what inner resources allow some mothers—living on welfare with many children, in crowded and dilapidated housing in dangerous neighborhoods with high crime rates and schools with inadequate resources—to raise their children in a manner (far from abusing or neglecting them) that protects the children from the hazards within and outside the home, provides excellent care and nurturance, gets the children educated, and allows these mothers to see their children go on to college and rise out of poverty. This is the other end of the continuum, involving as it does heroic rather than deficient parenting, but the point is that I am talking about a continuum. For the purposes of this chapter, however, I am concerned only with the lower end of the continuum, insofar as low levels of ability to cope with poverty may be a factor involved in many child abuse and neglect cases.

This discussion then, which began with the *indirect* way in which poverty may lead to child abuse and neglect, through the stresses that poverty may produce, has returned us to a consideration of the *direct* way, only briefly mentioned at the outset, in which the material conditions of living in poverty can give rise to what we call child abuse and neglect, as well as to the severity of the harm done.

The most frequent form of child abuse and neglect is neglect, and most incidents of neglect involve "deprivation of necessities" and/or "inadequate supervision" (AHA, 1978, 1981b, 1988; Pelton, 1981a; Sedlak, 1991a). In fact, the majority of incidents involve neglect (Sedlak, 1991a). In 1986, more than half of all reports indicated deprivation of necessities, a category including inadequate supervision and neglecting to provide nourishment, shelter, clothing, and health care (AHA, 1988). Leaving a child alone or unattended for excessive periods of time may be the most prevalent form of child neglect (Pelton, 1981a).

Thus, most neglect is defined or characterized in terms of availability of physical necessities to the child, if the parents had some control over such availability, and the adequacy of supervision in protecting the child from potential harm. Both concepts make direct reference to material conditions but implicate the responsibility of parents as well. The incident need only have been avoidable on the part of the caretakers or permitted by them (Sedlak, 1991a, 1991c).

The term "neglect" is applied to incidents in an all-or-none fashion. It is employed as a dichotomous concept; neglect is present or it is not, meaning that the caretakers are responsible for the incident or they are not. The concept forces us to view responsibility in an all-or-none manner when, in fact, responsibility is a matter of degree in most neglect incidents. In most incidents, both the caretakers and material conditions contribute to the incident. We need only determine that the parents did make some contribution to call it neglect. The proportion of responsibility borne by the caretakers need not be taken into account—some is equivalent to all. Yet responsibility is not all-or-none, and material conditions play a major role, as can be easily shown. Likewise, it can be shown that although "inadequate supervision" is a concept employed in an absolute manner in regard to neglect incidents, the adequacy of supervision is relative to the material conditions of the environment. Although these comments may seem to be excessively philosophical, they are directly relevant to the ultimate practical question concerning the extent to which material supports can contribute to the prevention of harm and potential harm to children that we currently view as due to child neglect.

There is little doubt that poverty is associated with dangerous conditions in and around the home. The physical home and neighborhood environments of children from low-income families are far more dangerous than others. For example, studies have confirmed that the rate of residential fires as well as the fatality rate from such fires is far greater in low-income areas than it is in middle-class neighborhoods (Gunther, 1981; Mierley & Baker, 1983). One study found that children from impoverished families were five times more likely to die from fire than were children from other families (Nersesian, Petit, Shaper, Lemieux, & Naor, 1985). In New York City, cases of childhood lead poisoning have been concentrated in the poorest neighborhoods; children's falls from windows have been concentrated among AFDC families (Pelton, 1989; Spiegel & Lindaman, 1977). Children are more likely to be hit by motor vehicles in low-income areas (Rivara & Barber, 1985).

Impoverished families tend to live, though not by choice, in neighborhoods with the highest crime rates, in apartments that are not secure, and in homes made dangerous by lack of heating, poor wiring, and exposed lead paint, to name only a few of the health and safety hazards associated with poverty. These conditions, the same ones that may cause indirect danger to children by generating stressful experiences for the parents, cause direct danger as well, for which it becomes possible to implicate the parents for not preventing. Moreover, in the presence of these conditions, impoverished parents have little leeway for lapses in responsibility, whereas in middle-class families, there is some leeway for irresponsibility, a luxury that poverty does not afford.

Poverty is dangerous to children, and, in fact, to counter this endangerment, impoverished parents need to be *more* diligent than middle-class parents are in the supervision of their children. Because the adequacy of supervision cannot be judged without reference to the dangerousness of the environment in which the child is supervised, identical behavior may be judged neglectful or nonneglectful, depending on the context in which it occurs. In fact, this is what happens in practice. Whereas occasional lapses in responsibility are normal for most parents (as there are few perfect parents), these lapses are more dangerous when committed by impoverished parents and are more amenable to being construed as neglect.

Definitions of neglect, in effect, by their very nature and in their inability to address adequate supervision as a concept that is interactional with the environment—that is, relative to or dependent on the adequacy of the environment—are more likely to attribute neglect to the behavior of impoverished parents than to the same behavior on the part of middle-class parents, since in the former case the behavior can cause serious endangerment, while in the latter the home and neighborhood are not as drastically beset with the health and safety hazards that would make that behavior dangerous. Because the behavior need only *contribute* to the endangerment, no matter to what degree, any lapse of responsibility or less than optimal behavior in a dangerous environment can be deemed neglectful.

Moreover, middle-class parents can be careless with their money and squander some of it but still have enough so that their children will not be deprived of basic necessities. Because their children are not deprived, there is no way that the parents' behavior can be called neglectful. Yet, an identical degree of squandering of money on the part of impoverished parents may cause their children to go hungry during the last few days of the month. This same behavior can now be called, and often has been called, neglect. The less money one has, the better manager of money one has to be in order to avoid depriving children of necessities. Thus, poor people have very little margin for mismanagement of either time or money.

Indeed, no squandering or mismanagement need even be involved. Many families that receive AFDC run out of money before the end of the month (Wolock & Horowitz, 1977, 1979), simply due to the insufficiency of AFDC grants, and are thus exposed to the potential of being called neglectful.

In some cases a mother does not have much choice but to provide her children with inadequate supervision or to deprive them of necessities. A low-income mother with many children cannot easily obtain or pay for a babysitter every time she wants or needs to leave the house. If she leaves her children alone, she is gambling with their safety; if she stays with them, she may be unable to do her shopping in order to provide food and other necessities. Thus, she may be caught up in a difficult situation that has less to do with her adequacy and responsibility as a parent than with the hard circumstances of her life. It is not uncommon for such a mother to leave younger children in the temporary care of a 12- or 13-year-old sibling and to be charged with neglect for it. Because of the hazards of her home environment, her children may indeed be in greater danger than those left in the care of a 12- or 13-year-old babysitter by a middle-class mother.

Financial hardship, physical and emotional problems of children and parents, large families, health and safety hazards associated with deteriorated housing and neighborhoods, family tensions, and social isolation all are factors that may increase the likelihood of inadequate supervision. That is, these factors either decrease the capability of parents to maintain proper supervision or heighten the diligence or closeness of the supervision necessary to maintain the children's safety. Financial hardship makes it difficult not to play a role in depriving one's children of necessities.

Yet, as concluded earlier, people vary in their ability to cope with poverty and its stressors. Some poor people do exceptionally well given their circumstances, and this is reflected in the care of their children. For people living in poverty, adequacy of child care is dependent on one's ability to cope with poverty. Most poor people are not accused of abuse or neglect, but some are. The ability to cope with poverty is not an all-or-none matter. It constitutes a continuum and allows some people to give more adequate care to their children than others. Given the dangerousness of the poverty environment, no amount of care and supervision is entirely adequate, and adequacy of care itself constitutes a continuum, not the on-or-off switch that the concept of neglect would have us conceptualize it as. Those few poor people who fall at the lower end of the first continuum tend to fall at the lower end of the second, and through their inability to cope with poverty, they are likely to be involved in incidents we call neglect. Therefore, it is not surprising that in one study, for example, children hospitalized for lead poisoning were found to have caretakers who provide more inadequate child care than do caretakers of children who did not have lead poisoning (Hunt, Hepner, & Seaton, 1982).

At a material level of living at which daily life is a struggle, some will win out over that struggle, many will barely and minimally survive, and others will be defeated. It would not be surprising to learn that individual differences in coping capacities (i.e., personal differences) are a factor involved in distinguishing those who win from those who survive and those who are defeated.

It should be noted that much sexual abuse involves inadequate supervision in a dangerous neighborhood environment, in that the alleged perpetrator is someone other than a parent or stepparent in 58% of sexual abuse reports and the child is entirely unrelated to the alleged perpetrator in 35% of such reports (AHA, 1988). It is probable that because of the recent intense public and professional focus on sexual abuse, many of the incidents now called sexual abuse used to be called neglect.

Moreover, as Tertinger, Greene, and Lutzker (1984) suggest, even physical abuse may be directly related to material deficits in the environment in that parents may resort to physical abuse in their anxious attempts to keep children away from safety hazards. Indeed, dangerous neighborhoods and living environments may elicit extreme anxiety and fear for the well-being of their children on the part of parents, who may, ironically, be driven by intense concern for their children's safety to physically or emotionally abuse them in attempts to control their children's behavior.

I argue here that a combination of poverty-related conditions and less than optimal behavior on the part of the parents is responsible for the incidents that we call neglect and, to some extent, abuse. The concepts and definitions of both abuse and neglect focus our attention on the contribution of the parents to their children's endangerment, however large or small the role of the parents' responsibility may be. Yet, in most cases, there is multiple causation of the risk of harm to children and multiple sources of responsibility. Thus, the risk of harm is amenable to preventive efforts aimed at one or several elements of the configuration of multiple causation. Even just one factor, if addressed, can defuse a dangerous situation, and the most effective way to defuse dangerous situations may be to address the environmental factors involved.

Implied here, especially in neglect cases, is the parents' lack of ability to cope with poverty and its stressors without outside supports. A key deficiency is lack of resources.

Studies at the neighborhood level of analysis have clearly shown that although children are at greater risk of child abuse and neglect in poorer than in wealthier neighborhoods, their risk in low-income neighborhoods is related to the level of environmental supports existing in those neighborhoods (Garbarino & Crouter, 1978; Garbarino & Sherman, 1980; Garbarino, 1981). They are at greater risk in neighborhoods that have high concentrations of economically impoverished families and low levels of environmental supports than they are in neighborhoods containing high concentrations of economically impoverished families but higher levels of environmental supports. Many of the supportive resources found to be related are social in nature, but many also have a material aspect, such as the availability of child care, as well as of family members, neighbors, and professionals to provide help (presumably material help as well as social support). A recent study indicates that of two economically impoverished Chicago communities having similar child abuse and neglect rates in 1980, the one whose maltreatment rate had soared to twice that of the other by 1986 also had considerably fewer human service agencies available to it at that time (Garbarino & Kostelny, 1992). It is conceivable that the agency resources available to the first community may have *declined* during that period, and that its poverty rate might have increased relative to the other community, with its increased maltreatment rate being due to a combination of increasing poverty and reduced agency supports. Other studies have indicated that the withdrawal of supportive services (in the form of fire-fighting resources) from an impoverished community can precipitate the further decline and destruction of that community and the growth of homelessness (Wallace, 1989).

As Garbarino (1981) suggests, a dearth of personal resources, which include personal characteristics that make for competence as well as personal financial resources, increases the importance of social resources for adequate child care. "Personally impoverished families clustered in socially impoverished places" produce neighborhoods and situations in which "the conditions of life conspire to compound rather than counteract the deficiencies and vulnerabilities of parents" (Garbarino, 1981, pp. 234, 237). Without denying the significance of the social aspects of social supports, the question can be raised as to the importance of the material supports that may be embedded within social supports in achieving reduced risk of child maltreatment. For the purposes of this chapter, I focus on material supports only.

MATERIAL SUPPORTS AS PREVENTIVE FACTORS IN CHILD ABUSE AND NEGLECT

When we take into account the overwhelming evidence of a strong relationship between poverty (and its material hardships) and child abuse and neglect, together with the evidence that poverty and its material hardships are associated with stress and that stress is associated with child abuse and neglect, and add the logic of the analysis of the *direct* way that the material hardships of poverty can give rise to what we call child neglect, the conclusion that, at the very least, is highly suggestible is that the most effective way to reduce child abuse and neglect in the United States may be to reduce poverty and its attendant material hardships. In fact, in terms of general impact on the overall reduction of the incidence of child abuse and neglect, there is no single hypothesis that is better supported by the available evidence, research, and logical analysis than this one.

Yet all the research evidence reviewed here has been of a correlational nature, not permitting conclusive establishment of a cause–effect relationship. Moreover, most of the evidence pertains to covariation of factors, such as income and child abuse and neglect, at a single point in time. That is, the evidence comes from cross-sectional studies. Only in regard to unemployment (and number of food stamp recipients) and child abuse and neglect do we have evidence of a change relationship, with increases in abuse and neglect rates corresponding to or following upon increases in unemployment rates (especially in communities with relatively high poverty rates). Such a temporal correlation more convincingly suggests that the relationship may be causal but is no substitute for experimental evidence. For obvious ethical reasons, it is not possible to perform controlled experiments in which the independent variable would be one or another form of material deprivation to be imposed on the experimental group and not on the control group.

We must look further, then, to the evidence for the relationship between material *supports* and child abuse and neglect. Even here, however, we have no experimental evidence. That is, no research has been performed in which material supports of one form or another were provided to an experimental group to observe the effects on child abuse and neglect in comparison with a control group to which the material supports were not provided—at least not as a separate independent variable. Given the promise of the hypothesis suggested by the overwhelming correlational evidence pertaining to the relationship between material deprivation and child abuse and neglect, the absence of experiments employing material supports as the independent variables represents a disappointing and glaring gap in past and present research and research strategies concerning child abuse and neglect and their prevention. However, even positive evidence of a correlational nature concerning material provision would bolster the convincingness of our prevention hypothesis over and above its convincingness based on correlational evidence involving material deprivation alone. Some fragmentary evidence does exist, which will be discussed shortly.

The New Jersey Income Maintenance Experiment, involving 1,350 families and lasting several years, does provide some experimental evidence of the social psychological effects of income provision, although child abuse and neglect were not studied. Increased income provided through the experiment was not found to have significant impact (relative to the controls) on the responses of male heads of families to questions and scales pertaining to general happiness; psychosomatic and nervous symptoms; self-esteem; boredom; anomy; quality of life; and worry about money, own health, bringing up children, or losing a job (Middleton & Allen, 1977). Even when data were analyzed separately for the families receiving the most generous plan, amounting to about $45 per week and constituting about 40% of weekly family earnings, no effect on psychological well-being was found. This plan, however, guaranteed income at only 125% of the poverty level, and it is possible that greater increases might have had an effect. Using a different measure of psychological distress, a study of the adult heads of households participating in the Seattle and Denver Income Maintenance Experiments found that increased income provided through the experiments did not reduce psychological distress relative to controls (Thoits & Hannan, 1979). The income increases examined were as moderate as in the previous study. In the rural North Carolina–Iowa Income Maintenance Experiment, a statistically significant, though mild, positive effect on psychological well-being was found for two of the three more generous, although moderate, guaranteed income plans (Hannan, 1978). Yet these findings, at the very least, should promote caution in our acceptance of the stress hypothesis in our attempts to explain the relationship between poverty and child abuse and neglect. Although the stress hypothesis has been quite popular in the child abuse and neglect literature, perhaps it has been overemphasized. It is time to generate new hypotheses and to examine other routes and intervening variables that might link poverty to child abuse and neglect in a causative manner, as I have attempted in this chapter.

However, the New Jersey Income Maintenance Experiment did show that increased income induced experimental families to improve their housing by moving to higher-cost accommodations (Wooldridge, 1977). If we assume that the housing they moved to provided safer environments than their previous housing, we would expect a reduction in child neglect based on our analysis of how inadequate environments impact on the adequacy of supervision and, hence, neglect. Again, however, it should be emphasized that the experiment did not include any measures of child abuse and neglect (nor did any of the other income-maintenance experiments conducted in various parts of the country during the 1970s).

In a correlational study of Texas counties, Spearly and Lauderdale (1983) found that after controlling for the socioeconomic status of the counties, those counties providing higher average monthly AFDC expenditures per child had lower child abuse reporting rates, although the relationship was not found for child neglect. Spearly and Lauderdale suggest that future studies should examine the relationship between other types of family support programs, such as day care and child nutrition programs, and child maltreatment rates. Unfortunately, few such studies exist. However, Kotch and Thomas (1986) did find that among families reported for child abuse and neglect, the use of child care on a regular basis was related to a considerably lower substantiation rate of such reports. McNicoll (1989) found that higher proportions of single-parent AFDC families who received child care income deductions corresponded to lower child neglect reporting rates, across counties. One study indicated that neglecting mothers reported less material supports available to them through informal networks than did nonneglecting mothers of comparably low socioeconomic status (Polansky et al., 1985).

Other studies evaluated mixed interventions (that combine material support, social support, and rehabilitation efforts) in a manner such that the independent effects of each component could not be determined. For example, one experimental study showed that unmarried teenage mothers of low socioeconomic status who were provided with a nurse home visitor for the first 2 years of the child's life were less likely to be involved in substantiated reports of child abuse and neglect during that time than were comparable mothers who were not provided with this service (Olds, Henderson, Chamberlin, & Tatelbaum, 1986). They were also observed in their homes to punish and restrict their children less frequently than were the comparable mothers in the control condition. Their babies were also seen less frequently in the emergency room during the 1st year of life. During the 2nd year, the larger group of nurse-visited mothers, which included others in addition to the poor unmarried teenagers, differed from comparison mothers in that their babies were seen in the emergency room less frequently and were seen by physicians less frequently for accidents and poisonings. The nurse visitors who accomplished these successes engaged in three major activities. They provided parents with education regarding infant development. They also encouraged the women's close friends and relatives to help with household responsibilities and to aid in child care. In addition, the home visitors linked families with community health and human service agencies and referred parents to such services as vocational training programs, legal aid, and the nutritional supplementation program for women, infants, and children (WIC). Although it is not known which activity—education, encouragement of informal support, and linkage with formal support—was most crucial to success, it is clear that the second and third activities involved the encouragement and procurement of considerable material aid.

In a study of the Homebuilders program, which is largely therapeutically oriented and whose emphasis has been on changing the parents in some way (Pelton, 1992), a significantly higher proportion of mothers whose children remained in the home after intervention, as opposed to those whose children did not, reported the provision of concrete services by therapists (Fraser & Haapala, 1987–1988). The families were referred to Homebuilders to prevent the need for placement, for which the children were at risk due to child abuse and neglect or some other form of family disturbance.

An evaluative study of intensive family preservation services programs based on the Homebuilders model at six sites in the states of Utah and Washington showed that the provision of and help in procuring concrete services was associated with a considerable reduction in the risk of placement (Fraser, Pecora, & Haapala, 1991). Only about half the cases in this study were referred from Child Protective Services, and the rest were juvenile justice or status offense cases usually involving family conflict with adolescents. The study provided some indication that concrete services were more relevant to the child protection cases, especially neglect, and so separate analyses for child protection and juvenile justice cases could be expected to provide even stronger support for the relation between concrete services and reduced risk of placement. The study also showed that the use of concrete services was correlated with the achievement of the treatment goals of establishing trust and functional working relationships with clients, increasing their parenting and anger management/conflict resolution skills, increasing their self-esteem, reducing their depression, and improving the school performance and self-esteem of the children. Thus, the findings suggest that in addition to contributing to the prevention of the need for placement by directly improving the families' situations and environments, concrete services may also have the indirect effect of contributing to positive changes in the parents themselves.

Caution is still necessary in coming to definitive conclusions. Preliminary findings from an experimental evaluation of the Family First time-limited and home-based services placement prevention programs in Illinois indicate that although substantially higher percentages of families in the programs than in the control group received concrete services, the Family First programs did not reduce the incidence of placement or of child abuse and neglect (Staff, 1991). However, analyses performed thus far have not evaluated families who received substantial quantities of concrete services (the median number of services received by families in the programs was four, and although the majority of these families received, for example, financial assistance, we are not told how much) separately from those who did not.

One of the most successful intensive family preservation programs to date in terms of preventing placement (as assessed by experimental evaluation), the New York State Preventive Services Project, provided a high frequency of concrete services across the cases it served, such as financial assistance in 78% of the cases and help with housing in 45% of the cases (Jones, Neuman, & Shyne, 1976). In contrast, a recent study of a Homebuilders program in the Bronx in which few concrete services were provided to families showed no effect of the program on placement prevention (Mitchell, Tovar, & Knitzer, 1989).

The Comprehensive Emergency Services model implemented in Nashville included emergency caregiver and emergency homemaker services and an around-the-clock emergency intake that enabled swift delivery of such services to families in crisis situations. An approximately 50% reduction was reported in the number of children who entered foster care in Nashville during the 1st year of the program as compared with the year preceding the inception of the program (Burt & Balyeat, 1977). However, unlike the evaluation of the New York State Preventive Services Project, no control group was employed; thus, a conclusive verdict on its effectiveness is not possible.

As stated previously, there is a direct way in which the material conditions of living in poverty can give rise to what we call child abuse and neglect as well as to the severity of the harm done. "Adequacy" of supervision is relative to the material conditions of the environment. As Tertinger et al. (1984) suggest, the poor and unsafe conditions of the home are often the basis for referring clients to child protection agencies. Most injuries that occur to children in child protection cases are accidental; that is, they are unintentional. There is much evidence that heightened risk of severe accidental injury to children is strongly related to low socioeconomic status (Gunther, 1981; Mierley & Baker, 1983; Nersesian et al., 1985; Rivara & Barber, 1985; Spiegel & Lindaman, 1977; Pelton, 1989). Such risk is due, in part, to health and safety hazards associated with deteriorated housing and neighborhoods. Such factors increase the diligence of supervision necessary to maintain children's safety. When injury occurs and less than optimal supervision is found to be present, the probability increases that the injury will be attributed to neglect rather than to accident or nonintentional injury. In most cases called neglect, there is multiple causation of the risk of harm to children, yet the focus for blame is the parents themselves. This inordinate emphasis on parental responsibility in child protection laws, policy, and practice has contributed to excessive placement of children in foster care and too little emphasis on remedying dangerous conditions of poverty that contribute to nonintentional injuries and severe harm to children.

Indeed, it is recognized by those who study nonintentional injuries that the most effective way to reduce injuries is not through attempts to change individual behavior but through environmental changes and passive measures (e.g., Dershewitz & Williamson, 1977; Pless & Arsenault, 1987; Wilson & Baker, 1987). In New York City, for example, where about half of all children's falls from windows occurred among families receiving public assistance, a program that included the provision of free window guards to families with preschool children living in tenements in high-risk areas apparently resulted in a sharp decline in falls and in fatalities due to such falls (Spiegel & Lindaman, 1977).

Provisions of material supports, by contributing to reduction of dangers of nonintentional injuries and prevention of harm due to such dangers, can thereby reduce the number of situations that give rise to attributions of "neglect." Nonintentional injuries are multiply caused, but the removal of even one causal element can prevent or reduce the risk of injury. Leaving a child alone in a room cannot result in a window fall if window guardrails have been installed. The degree of supervision that is adequate in a safe environment is not adequate in a dangerous environment, and the dangerous environment provides greater opportunity for detecting "neglect." But it also provides opportunity for implementing preventive modifications of the environment for child protection.

Based on an emergency fund for child protection developed in Union County, New Jersey (Horowitz & Wintermute, 1978), I was instrumental in the establishment of a simple and inexpensive *statewide* emergency cash fund within New Jersey's state child welfare agency. The purpose of the fund was to address concrete needs in child protection cases in order to prevent the need for placement. When looked at on a case-by-case basis, the use of this statewide fund had readily apparent links to the immediate prevention of harm to children, as well as to the immediate prevention of the need for foster care placement (Pelton & Fuccello, 1978). An examination of a random sample of 100 instances of the use of the fund indicated that cash grants to families were used by caseworkers mainly for the emergency purchase of food, the payment of rent, rental security deposits on new apartments (usually after eviction from the old), rent arrears (in order to prevent eviction), the payment of utility bills that were in arrears, the payment of charges involved in turning on utilities, and the purchase of furniture such as cribs and beds (Pelton & Fuccello, 1978). In fact, 79% of all grants, accounting for 92% of all expenditures, were used for the aforementioned needs. The remaining instances included the purchase of a stove, a refrigerator, new door locks, smoke detectors, medical bandages, and disposable diapers. When the circumstances of the cases in which grants were given were examined, the role of the grants in the immediate prevention of danger and placement was often obvious. Crisis situations included lack of money for food, fire hazards created by candles and lanterns used as substitutes for utilities that were turned off, lack of heat during winter, the prospect of eviction leading to homelessness, children not attending school due to lack of warm clothing, the need for new locks to keep an abusive alcoholic father out of the house, and a need for smoke detectors in a home in which one child had been setting fires and, according to the caseworker, would have had to be removed from the home if safety devices were not installed. Most such circumstances could easily have been characterized as "deprivation of necessities" or "inadequate supervision," and thus neglect, if material supports had not been provided. In at least a third of the instances in which grant requests were approved, the caseworkers believed that placement would have been the only alternative.

A follow-up evaluation study of the statewide fund examined the same 100 cases in the Pelton and Fuccello (1978) study in which grants were approved. The follow-up study found that more than 1 year after the grants were given, 60% of the caseworkers believed that the grants had produced long-lasting effects on the families involved (Fuccello & Lowe, 1980). Eighty percent of the caseworkers said that the specific problem that the grant was designed to address had not recurred. Judging from caseworker responses, positive long-term outcomes, including a general improvement in the case situation and/or achievement or maintenance of family integrity, occurred in 69% of the cases. In 39% of the cases, the caseworkers believed that the grant had enabled the family to stay together. According to caseworker responses, the grants were also found to improve worker–client relationships.

Moreover, examination of agency records indicated that 43% of the original sample of 100 cases were terminated within 12 months of receiving the grant, and only 10 children from the 100 families had been placed (Fuccello & Lowe, 1980). Seven of these children were not placed until at least 6 months after the grant. Although one of the guidelines for use of the fund was that the children must be in imminent danger of placement, the findings on placement are merely suggestive because no control group was employed.

Finally, when district office supervisors were interviewed in this follow-up study, their response was overwhelmingly positive. "Supervisors found the fund useful, easy to administer and control, and popular among their caseworkers as a means of gaining trust and confidence with the client family while providing concrete, tangible assistance in times of great need" (Fuccello & Lowe, 1980, p. 11). Most district office supervisors believed that the fund was effective in reducing the rates of placement within their particular counties, although these were opinions not based on hard evidence.

My own further analysis indicated that the start of a decline in the number of children entering foster care in New Jersey coincided with the initiation of the fund in the beginning of 1978, and an acceleration of the decline during 1980 and 1981 in the number of children *in* foster care coincided with the increased availability and use of money in the fund (Pelton, 1982a). The most crucial data concern the number of children *entering* foster care. The fund began operation in early 1978, and approximately 800 families received grants from the fund during that year. Roughly the same number of grants were made during 1979, and thereafter a greater annual amount of money was placed into the fund. The number of children entering foster care in 1977 was almost identical to the number in 1976. During 1978, however, 600 fewer children entered care than in 1977, and this reduction was maintained during 1979 (when the number of children entering care was only 26 above the number entering care in 1978). Again, however, such data are merely suggestive.

Finally, despite the fact that the majority of caseworkers believed that positive long-term outcomes were achieved by grants from the fund, we could expect that an emergency grant would have only temporarily and minimally interrupted the flow of hardships and even stresses of poverty, and that additional grants or other services at later irregular intervals would have been needed to continue to stave off harm and placement. Any permanent solution to the kinds of crises that the emergency fund attempts to address would require a major reassessment of public welfare policies and welfare reform.

Although the provision of material supports is sometimes looked upon as a means of establishing a trusting relationship with the client, for the purpose of "rehabilitating" the client or changing the client in some way, it should be clear from the analyses developed in this chapter that such change might not be necessary for the reduction of child abuse and neglect. The foremost influence of the provision of material supports on the prevention of child abuse and neglect may well be through its direct impact on the environment and conditions in which the family is residing. It has been argued that by changing the *situation*, material supports can reduce the incidence of child abuse and neglect even without any change in the parents themselves ever occurring. The adequacy of parents' supervision of their children is directly dependent on the adequacy of their environments. By improving the environment, the same parenting behaviors, without change, have a reduced probability of being characterized as abusive and neglectful. Put another way, to reduce the health and safety hazards of the environment is to automatically reduce the probability of attributions of abuse and neglect. Moreover, such measures surely reduce the severity of harm that may be due to child maltreatment by reducing the health and safety hazards in the environment that make child neglect so dangerous.

CONCLUSIONS

There is overwhelming and remarkably consistent evidence—across a variety of definitions and methodologies and from studies performed at different times—that poverty and low income are strongly related to child abuse and neglect and to the severity of child maltreatment. Children from impoverished and low-income families are vastly overrepresented in the incidence of child abuse and neglect. The strong relationship between poverty and low income and child abuse and neglect holds not only for child abuse and neglect in general but for every identified form of child abuse and neglect, including emotional abuse, emotional neglect, and sexual abuse.

In fact, there is a strong funneling effect in regard to child abuse and neglect and their severity, with the poorest children in our society being at greatest risk (having the highest incidence rates) and the wealthier children being at least risk (having the lowest incidence rates). Approximately 40–50% of all child abuse and neglect incidents occur within the less than 15% of all U.S. families with children who live below the poverty level. More than 90% of all incidents occur in families below the median income, meaning that another 40–50% of all incidents occur within the roughly 35% of families with incomes above the poverty level but below the median income. Thus, the incidence rate is less than half for children in such families than it is for children living in families below the poverty level. Finally, less than 10% of all incidents occur within families with incomes above the median. Thus, children in families with incomes above the poverty level but below the median income are at 5 to 7 times greater risk than children in families with incomes above the median, and children in families below the poverty level are at 13 to 17 times greater risk.

Not surprisingly, since AFDC status is merely an indicator of poverty, 40–50% of all child abuse and neglect incidents occur within families receiving AFDC at the time of the incident, and the great majority of families involved in such incidents have been on AFDC at some time. For similar reasons, counties with the highest rates of food stamp recipients are also the counties with the highest incidence rates of child abuse and neglect.

Yet, poverty is merely a measure of income, and a rough one at that. Moreover, income is merely a rough indicant of material hardship, but it is through the material hardship that poverty causes that poverty is likely to have an impact on children and families. In fact, evidence has related material hardship directly to child abuse and neglect. AFDC families involved in child abuse and neglect incidents have been found to be existing at lower material levels of living than are other AFDC families. Their comparatively greater material hardships include more overcrowded and dilapidated housing, not enough beds for their children, less likelihood of having basic amenities such as air conditioners and telephones, and greater likelihood of at least occasional hunger. There is an astoundingly high prevalence of a wide range of serious health problems among both parents and children in AFDC families involved in child abuse and neglect, but there is no evidence yet that this prevalence is higher than among other AFDC families.

Unemployment is strongly related to child abuse and neglect but not independently of the extent of the material hardship it might cause. That is, job loss is more strongly related to child abuse and neglect among families who are already poor and do not have the financial resources to cushion the additional blow of job loss (and therefore loss of income) to their material circumstances.

The relationship between poverty and its resultant material hardship, on the one hand, and child abuse and neglect on the other, is a fact but not an explanation. Attempts to explain the connection take us into the realm of theory. The concept of stress, viewed as a mediating factor, was previously regarded as a major key to a reasonable explanation. In fact, some evidence suggests that such stressful events and conditions as unemployment, financial strain, and overcrowded housing can lead to increased anxiety, depression, hostility, and aggressiveness.

Bolstering the stress hypothesis, few personal differences have been found to distinguish abusing and neglecting parents from other parents other than depression, low self-esteem, and feelings of helplessness. On the other hand, although we know that stress can give rise to and exacerbate such differences, we do not know whether or not they more predominantly represent pervasive and enduring personality characteristics. No matter what their genesis, these personal differences—depression, self-esteem, and a sense of mastery—affect future stress appraisal and reaction to stress and are directly related to one's ability or inability to cope with poverty and material hardship. It was concluded that for people living in poverty, the probability of child abuse and neglect largely depends on the extent of one's ability to cope with poverty, its material hardships, and its stressors.

Acknowledgment that such differences in cognitive coping abilities exist led to an examination of the *direct* way in which material hardship and its attendant environmental deficits, quite apart from the stresses such hardship may generate, contribute to child abuse and neglect. Adequacy of child care was suggested to be relative to and interactional with the adequacy of the environment and one's material circumstances. What is adequate child care in one environment may be inadequate in another. In most instances of child abuse and neglect, there is multiple causation of the risk of harm to the child, and any harm is nonintentional. Yet, the concepts of child abuse and neglect do not take into account the role of the environment, attributing responsibility to parents in an all-or-none fashion. An incident need only have been judged "avoidable" by the parents to implicate the parents. But the diligence of care necessary to protect a child in a dangerous environment is greater than in a safer environment. It is not possible to judge adequacy of care apart from the environment in which the care is needed. Thus, poor parents are more susceptible to a judgment of neglect. Yet people vary in their ability to cope with poverty, and those people with the least ability are most likely to be charged with abuse and neglect. However, to the extent that their environments and living conditions are made less dangerous—through the provision of material supports—the quality of care that they are capable of giving, although the same as before, will now be less inadequate. Studies do indeed indicate that comparably impoverished neighborhoods contain more or less child abuse and neglect depending on the level of supportive resources that are available in those neighborhoods. Although a variety of types of supports may be needed, this chapter has focused on the material aspects of deprivations and supports.

It was concluded that the most effective way to reduce child abuse and neglect in the United States may be to reduce poverty and its attendant material hardships. Whereas abundant evidence of the relationship between child abuse and neglect and material deprivation points to this conclusion, the additional need for *experimental* research investigating the role of material *supports* in reducing child abuse and neglect was emphasized.

Some experimental evidence, for example, does not support the hypothesis that moderate income increases beget reduced stress appraisal. These findings should at least promote caution in our acceptance of the stress hypothesis in explaining the relationship between poverty and child abuse and neglect. It was suggested that we more seriously examine other ways in which poverty might cause child abuse and neglect, as I did in this chapter. Experimental evidence does show that increased income induces families to move to higher-cost, presumably safer, housing. According to the analysis provided in this chapter, we would expect such housing moves to reduce child abuse and neglect.

Correlational evidence pertaining to the role of material supports does exist, indicating that higher AFDC payments per child are related to lower child abuse reporting rates, that provision of day care is related to lower substantiation rates of child abuse and neglect reports, and that material supports in general are related to lack of neglect.

One experimental study did show that a nurse home-visitor program, which included a considerable emphasis on material aid, did in fact reduce the risk of child abuse and neglect. Correlational evidence pertaining to the Homebuilders program indicates that the receipt of concrete services within that program distinguishes families in which child placement was successfully prevented from those families in which placement was not prevented. An evaluative study of intensive family preservation services programs based on the Homebuilders model provided correlational evidence of a similar nature. Studies of family preservation programs that provided high levels of concrete services show some success in the prevention of placement.

The interaction among adequacy of supervision, unsafe environments, accidents or nonintentional injuries, and attributions of child neglect was noted, as was the evidence of a relationship between severe accidental injury and low socioeconomic status. It was also noted that the most effective way to reduce nonintentional injuries, which include injuries attributable to neglect, is thought to be through environmental changes and passive measures. Evidence indicates that the provision of passive restraints, such as window guardrails, is effective in reducing nonintentional injuries to children. Evaluations of a statewide emergency fund for child protection cases in New Jersey indicated that the fund was used for the provision of a variety of vital concrete supports, and that it prevented imminent danger of nonintentional injury to children in such cases. In the judgment of caseworkers, use of the fund prevented placement in many cases, led to nonrecurrence of the specific condition addressed, contributed to improvement in the care situation and maintenance of the family unit, and improved worker–client relationships. Moreover, very few children were found to have actually been placed within 1 year after a grant from the fund. Further analysis indicated that the beginning of a decline in the number of children entering foster care in New Jersey coincided with the initiation of the fund.

Such measures, however, can only be expected to temporarily, intermittently, and minimally interrupt the flow of material hardships that result from poverty. Such measures are made necessary only to the extent that national social welfare policies deal inadequately with poverty and its resultant environmental deficits. Social services must include many concrete services if our child welfare agencies are to be responsive to the inadequacies of national social welfare policies.

Child abuse and neglect, as we have seen, are strongly associated with poverty. In general, there are three broad ways in which a society can deal with poverty and its effects in a positive manner. First, it can directly address poverty itself, by reducing or eliminating it. Second, it can directly address specific environmental deficits and material hardships that arise from poverty. Third, it can help people to deal with the stresses that arise from poverty and its resultant deficits. Broad social welfare policy measures, such as a guaranteed minimum annual income above the poverty level, can affect the first plane, and broad social welfare policy measures such as universal national health care and day care can affect the second plane. Social services, however, have the potential to address the second and third planes only, and operate within the ongoing context of poverty.

To the extent that our society's national social welfare policy measures are and remain inadequate to deal with poverty and its resultant material deficits, it is left to social services to deal with those deficits. Current social services, however, are more frequently aimed at the third than the second plane. That is, most social services are aimed at rehabilitation—trying to change people rather than their situations—or attempt to provide emotional and social supports aimed either at changing the client's perceptions of stressful circumstances or reducing the stress reaction. Although all these measures are relevant in light of my overall analysis of the dynamics of child abuse and neglect discussed in an earlier section of this chapter, few social services address the second plane by providing concrete supports that have the potential to directly alleviate the circumstances themselves that might be not only causing stress but contributing directly to the danger of harm to children.

Perhaps an "empowered" and superiorly competent person can ward off poverty, its deficits, and/or the stresses that can arise therefrom. But the environment is real, not just a matter of perception, and can overwhelm people. To put it bluntly, few social services within our child welfare system have been aimed at the conditions that generate the stressful circumstances and the dangers of harm, and thus our child welfare system has not been responsive to the inadequacies of national social welfare policies. Because of this, and because of a similar lack of focus on concrete services on the part of researchers, few studies exist evaluating the effects of material supports as preventive factors in child abuse and neglect.

It is recommended that future research be designed to examine further the relationship between changes in child poverty rates and changes in child abuse and neglect incidence rates over time, at both the county and neighborhood levels. Future research should also examine the interactive effects of unemployment rate increases and poverty on the incidence of child abuse and neglect. The stress hypothesis as it specifically relates to child abuse and neglect requires further examination in research, and it is recommended that the direct ways in which material deficits give rise to child abuse and neglect, as outlined here, be targeted as an area of greater research concern and activity. Further, and most important, experimentally controlled studies should be developed to evaluate the role of a variety of material supports in the prevention of child abuse and neglect. Experiments should be designed to assess the separate effects of different material supports independently of other types of services. Finally, more efforts should be made to study impoverished parents who provide excellent care and nurturance to their children despite the context of an adverse environment in order to discover the specific strengths that enable them to do so.

The conclusion I have drawn is that the relationship between poverty and child abuse and neglect is more likely to be mediated directly by the inadequacies of the environment and living conditions that poverty causes, in interaction with individual variation in cognitive abilities to cope with poverty, its material hardships, and its stresses, than to be mediated indirectly by the impact of the stresses of poverty on parents. If this is so, child abuse and neglect, and especially neglect, can be viewed as a subset of nonintentional injuries, or accidents, which are also related to poverty. Any measures that would reduce material hardships, by reducing the dangerous aspects of environments and living conditions, would reduce harm to children, whether such harm is attributed to child abuse and neglect or to nonintentional injury. Yet, even an emphasis on the stress hypothesis would lead to the same recommendations: To reduce the stress that may lead to child abuse and neglect, we must reduce poverty and its resultant material hardships and dangers.

Of course, in the long term, we must increase the individual competencies and inner resources of all who are deficient, but this is less likely to be achieved through therapy, parenting skills classes, self-help groups, and the like, than through opening up opportunities for decent education, jobs, and careers, and through ensuring the health and safety of children to allow them to take advantage of such opportunities as they grow up. In short, we must address the poverty conditions that leave children abused, neglected, or otherwise harmed in the short run if we are to increase individual competencies and inner resources in the long run.

The unavoidable conclusion is that the most effective way to reduce child abuse and neglect is to reduce poverty and its material hardships by increasing the incomes of families at least to above the poverty level. Various proposals have been set forth for reducing child poverty. They include setting AFDC benefits nationally at or above the poverty level and indexing them to cost-of-living increases; providing a guaranteed minimum annual income, at the poverty level or up to half the national median income; assuring a full-employment economy through the creation, if need be, of government jobs programs; establishing an unconditional right to employment at wages compatible with an adequate level of living; increasing mandated minimum wages; creating a universal children's allowance in the form of a direct cash payment or a refundable tax credit, as is done in all western European countries; promoting full utilization of the Earned Income Tax Credit; and creating a national child support enforcement program coupled with a government-insured minimum benefits plan to address instances in which absent parents do not meet their child support obligations (e.g., Horowitz & Wolock, 1981; Gil, 1981; Garfinkel & McLanahan, 1986; National Commission on Children, 1991). This chapter is not the place to debate the relative merits and drawbacks of one or another of these proposals or combinations thereof, or to recommend one or another means for reducing child poverty by increasing income. The concern of this chapter is simply that there is a direct and intimate relationship between magnitude of family income and incidence rate of child abuse and neglect, and that the most effective way to reduce child abuse and neglect would be to increase family income, especially at the lowest regions of the income scale. It is most important to reduce poverty by increasing income, no matter what means are employed to increase income levels.

When families are wealthy, they need no material supports, or, more precisely, they can purchase the supports they need to address the material conditions and circumstances of their lives. They can buy safe living environments, adequate health care, and day care. Child abuse and neglect are directly and intimately related to material hardship. Deficient material conditions and circumstances form the context in which child abuse and neglect occur, and in the absence of which child abuse and neglect are less likely to occur and less likely to result in severe harm to children. If child abuse and neglect are to be reduced, material supports must be provided to impoverished and low-income families. Some of these supports can best be provided through national policies. Thus, I contend here, recommendations for a national universal health care system, a universal day care system, and renewed federal efforts to provide public housing are directly relevant to a national strategy to reduce child abuse and neglect.

Recommendations for full funding of the WIC program, which currently serves less than 60% of the eligible population, are also consistent with such a strategy (National Commission on Children, 1991). Expansion of Head Start, which currently serves less than 20% of income-eligible 3- to 4-year-old children, or public prekindergarten programs, and the development of parental-leave policies will promote quality of care for children at the same time that the programs enable parents to increase their incomes by holding full-time jobs (Hayes, Palmer, & Zaslow, 1990; McKey et al., 1985).

To the extent that current national social welfare policies deal inadequately with poverty and its resultant material deficits, and to the extent that it is unlikely that such policies will be improved or reformed sufficiently within the near future to adequately deal with poverty, we need social service programs that address the gaps left.

Current public child welfare agencies, whose missions are to protect children and to preserve families, are not adequately equipped to deliver concrete services and programs to address the material hardships of impoverished and low-income families and are not designed to do so. Large portions of the budgets of these agencies are devoted to foster care and the investigation of child abuse and neglect complaints, and few social services are provided in child protection cases. Moreover, because of the prospect of being stigmatized as abusers or neglecters, and the possibility of having one's children taken away, and perhaps because of the unlikelihood of receiving needed concrete services, few parents involve themselves with the agencies voluntarily or through self-referral. The "eligibility requirement" for receiving what few, often inappropriate, services are available is to be involved in substantiated abuse or neglect.

Therefore, it is recommended that in every state, a state child welfare agency be established whose sole function would be to provide social services and programs to all families who want and need such services and cannot afford to purchase them on their own (Pelton, 1989, 1990, 1991a, 1992). Such an agency would not be involved in any way in foster care placement and investigative functions. Based on the analysis of child abuse and neglect developed in this chapter, indicating that most incidents fall within the category of nonintentional injuries and that most parents involved in such incidents do not deliberately endanger their children and would want to protect them if they could, all services and programs would be offered on a voluntary acceptance basis only. Parents would no longer fear coming to such an agency for help.

Studies have shown that the types of services that child welfare clients are most interested in receiving are those of a concrete and materially supportive nature, directed at altering the clients' situations in some way, such as housing assistance, day care, and financial assistance (see Sudia, 1981; Pelton, 1982b, for reviews of this research). Not coincidentally, this chapter demonstrates that these are the same types of services most needed by these clients for the purpose of protecting their children's welfare. If such services are made available, without threat of accusation or child removal, they will come. Our current child abuse and neglect prevention strategies have helped to create the erroneous impression that many impoverished parents (those accused of child abuse and neglect) do not care much about their children's welfare. This false assumption, in turn, has reinforced the coercive approach to child protection that guides our current child welfare system.

The new state child welfare agency recommended here would develop and offer a wide and attractive array of services wanted and needed by families experiencing child welfare difficulties. The agency would not limit itself to concrete services but would offer a broad spectrum of services from concrete services to family counseling. However, the mix or balance of services would be appropriately weighted toward material supports. The new agency would become the focal point for the coordination and provision of such concrete services as emergency caretakers and homemakers, housing assistance (including gaining needed structural repairs for the family's current housing and eliminating certain health and safety hazards, as well as helping the client to locate new housing), emergency cash assistance, installation of window guardrails and smoke detectors, rodent control, lead-based paint removal, day care and night care, in-home babysitter services, provision of cribs and playpens, parent aides, visiting nurses, and transportation. In addition, other services, such as instruction in home safety, money management, and parenting skills; facilitation of self-help support groups; assistance in gaining access to substance abuse treatment, health care, welfare benefits, food stamps, WIC and Head Start programs; crisis intervention counseling; and other forms of counseling, would also be provided.

The new agency would devote its entire budget to services, programs, and advocacy for families and would engage in outreach to families who might need such services. Not all programs would deliver services on a case-by-case basis. Some programs, such as educational campaigns or the development of day care centers, would not. Some programs may target the entire state and others, whether on a casework basis or through some other intervention level, would focus on geographical areas with high concentrations of impoverished and low-income families. Some programs, such as youth recreation programs, would be designed to reduce the dangerousness of high-risk neighborhoods, and thus the agency would reach beyond the scope of household environments to address street and neighborhood environments, all of which can cause danger of child abuse and neglect. Although the agency might operate out of central, regional, and district offices across the state, it would establish neighborhood centers for its operations in areas with high concentrations of impoverished and low-income families.

The foregoing proposals are intimately consistent with the weight of the evidence. The presence of material hardship is so pervasive in child abuse and neglect cases that it is clear that any strategy aimed at significantly reducing the incidence of child abuse and neglect must centrally address this bedrock context in which harm to children thrives. Without a key focus on material hardship, other additionally desirable approaches will not succeed in significantly reducing the incidence and severity of child abuse and neglect within our nation.

REFERENCES

American Humane Association. (1978). *National analysis of official child neglect and abuse reporting*. Denver, CO: Author.

American Humane Association. (1979a). *National analysis of official child abuse and neglect reporting: 1977* (issued by the National Center on Child Abuse and Neglect, U.S. Department of Health, Education, and Welfare). Washington, DC: U.S. Government Printing Office.

American Humane Association. (1979b). *National analysis of official child neglect and abuse reporting: Annual report, 1978*. Denver, CO: Author.

American Humane Association. (1981a). *The national study on child neglect and abuse reporting* [Summary]. Denver, CO: Author.

American Humane Association. (1981b). *National analysis of official child neglect and abuse reporting: Annual report, 1980*. Denver, CO: Author.

American Humane Association. (1983). *Highlights of official child neglect and abuse reporting: Annual report, 1981*. Denver, CO: Author.

American Humane Association. (1987). *Highlights of official child neglect and abuse reporting: 1985*. Denver, CO: Author.

American Humane Association. (1988). *Highlights of official child neglect and abuse reporting: 1986*. Denver, CO: Author.

Bradburn, N. M. (1969). *The structure of psychological well-being*. Chicago: Aldine.

Brenner, M. H. (1984). *Estimating the effects of economic change on national health and social well-being*. Washington, DC: U.S. Government Printing Office.

Burt, M. R., & Balyeat, R. R. (1977). *A Comprehensive Emergency Services system for neglected and abused children*. New York: Vantage Press.

Bycer, A. M., Breed, L. D., Fluke, J. D., & Costello, T. (1983, August). *Unemployment and child abuse and neglect reporting* [Draft report]. Denver, CO: American Humane Association.

Cohen, S., & Wills, T. A. (1985). Stress, social support, and the buffering hypothesis. *Psychological Bulletin, 98*, 310–357.

Dershewitz, R. A., & Williamson, J. W. (1977). Prevention of childhood household injuries: A controlled clinical trial. *American Journal of Public Health, 67*, 1148–1153.

Dohrenwend, B. P., & Dohrenwend, B. S. (1969). *Social status and psychological disorder*. New York: Wiley.

Egeland, B., Breitenbucher, M., & Rosenberg, D. (1980). Prospective study of life stress in the etiology of child abuse. *Journal of Consulting and Clinical Psychology, 48*(2), 195–205.

Elmer, E. (1981). Traumatized children, chronic illness, and poverty. In L. H. Pelton (Ed.), *The social context of child abuse and neglect* (pp. 185–227). New York: Human Sciences Press.

Finkelhor, D. (1984). *Child sexual abuse: New theory and research.* New York: Free Press.

Finkelhor, D. (1986). *A sourcebook on child sexual abuse.* Beverly Hills, CA: Sage.

Fraser, M., & Haapala, D. (1987–1988). Home-based family treatment: A quantitative-qualitative assessment. *Journal of Applied Social Sciences, 12*(1), 1–23.

Fraser, M. W., Pecora, P. J., & Haapala, D. A. (1991). *Families in crisis: The impact of intensive family preservation services.* New York: Aldine de Gruyter.

Fuccello, E., & Lowe, F. (1980, October). *A follow-up evaluation of an emergency cash fund in child protective services.* Trenton, NJ: Bureau of Research, New Jersey Division of Youth and Family Services.

Gaines, R., Sandgrund, A., Green, A. H., & Power, E. (1978). Etiological factors in child maltreatment: A multivariate study of abusing, neglecting, and normal mothers. *Journal of Abnormal Psychology, 87*(5), 531–540.

Garbarino, J. (1981). An ecological approach to child maltreatment. In L. H. Pelton (Ed.), *The social context of child abuse and neglect* (pp. 228–267). New York: Human Sciences Press.

Garbarino, J., & Crouter, A. (1978). Defining the community context of parent–child relations: The correlates of child maltreatment. *Child Development, 49,* 604–616.

Garbarino, J., & Ebata, A. (1987). The significance of ethnic and cultural differences in child maltreatment. In R. L. Hampton (Ed.), *Violence in the black family: Correlates and consequences* (pp. 21–38). Lexington, MA: Lexington Books.

Garbarino, J., & Kostelny, K. (1992). Child maltreatment as a community problem. *Child Abuse and Neglect, 16,* 455–464.

Garbarino, J., & Sherman, D. (1980). High-risk neighborhoods and high-risk families: The human ecology of child maltreatment. *Child Development, 51,* 188–198.

Garfinkel, I., & McLanahan, S. S. (1986). *Single mothers and their children: A new American dilemma.* Washington, DC: Urban Institute Press.

Gelles, R. J. (1973). Child abuse as psychopathology: A sociological critique and reformulation. *American Journal of Orthopsychiatry, 43,* 611–621.

Gelles, R. J. (1978). Violence toward children in the United States. *American Journal of Orthopsychiatry, 48,* 580–592.

Gelles, R. J. (1992). Poverty and violence toward children. *American Behavioral Scientist, 35*(3), 258–274.

Gelles, R. J., Straus, M. A., & Harrop, J. W. (1988). Has family violence decreased? A response to J. Timothy Stocks. *Journal of Marriage and the Family, 50,* 286–291.

Gil, D. G. (1970). *Violence against children.* Cambridge, MA: Harvard University Press.

Gil, D. G. (1981). The United States versus child abuse. In L. H. Pelton (Ed.), *The social context of child abuse and neglect* (pp. 291–324). New York: Human Sciences Press.

Giovannoni, J., & Billingsley, A. (1970). Child neglect among the poor: A study of parental inadequacy in families of three ethnic groups. *Child Welfare, 49,* 196–204.

Goetting, A. (1988). When parents kill their young children: Detroit 1982–1986. *Journal of Family Violence, 3*(4), 339–346.

Gove, W. R., Hughes, M., & Galle, O. R. (1979). Overcrowding in the home: An empirical investigation of its possible pathological consequences. *American Sociological Review, 44,* 59–80.

Gunther, P. (1981, May). Fire-cause patterns for different socioeconomic neighborhoods in Toledo, Ohio. *Fire Journal, 75,* 3–8.

Hampton, R. L. (1987a). Violence against black children: Current knowledge and future research needs. In R. L. Hampton (Ed.), *Violence in the black family: Correlates and consequences* (pp. 3–20). Lexington, MA: Lexington Books.

Hampton, R. L. (1987b). Family violence and homicide in the black community: Are they linked? In R. L. Hampton (Ed.), *Violence in the black family: Correlates and consequences* (pp. 135–156). Lexington, MA: Lexington Books.

Hampton, R. L., Gelles, R. J., & Harrop, J. W. (1989). Is violence in black families increasing? A comparison of 1975 and 1985 national survey rates. *Journal of Marriage and the Family, 51,* 969–980.

Hampton, R. L., & Newberger, E. H. (1985). Child abuse incidence and reporting by hospitals: Significance of severity, class, and race. *American Journal of Public Health, 75*(1), 56–60.

Hannan, M. T. (1978). Noneconomic outcomes. In J. L. Palmer & J. A. Pechman (Eds.), *Welfare in rural areas: The North Carolina–Iowa Income Maintenance Experiment* (pp. 183–210). Washington, DC: The Brookings Institution.

Hayes, C. D., Palmer, J. L., & Zaslow, M. J. (1990). *Who cares for America's children? Child care policy for the 1990s.* Washington, DC: National Academy Press.

Horowitz, B., & Wintermute, W. (1978). Use of an emergency fund in protective services casework. *Child Welfare, 57*(7), 432–437.

Horowitz, B., & Wolock, I. (1981). Material deprivation, child maltreatment, and agency interventions among poor families. In L. H. Pelton (Ed.), *The social context of child abuse and neglect* (pp. 137–184). New York: Human Sciences Press.

Hunt, T. J., Hepner, R., & Seaton, K. W. (1982). Childhood lead poisoning and inadequate child care. *American Journal of Diseases of Children, 136,* 538–542.

Jones, M. A., Neuman, R., & Shyne, A. W. (1976). *A second chance for families: Evaluation of a program to reduce foster care.* New York: Child Welfare League of America.

Kaplun, D., & Reich, R. (1976). The murdered child and his killers. *American Journal of Psychiatry, 133,* 809–813.

Kessler, R. C., & Essex, M. (1982). Marital status and depression: The importance of coping resources. *Social Forces, 61*(2), 484–507.

Kleiner, R. J., & Parker, S. (1970). Social structure and psychological factors in mental disorder: A research review. In H. Wechsler, L. Solomon, & B. M. Kramer (Eds.), *Social psychology and mental health* (pp. 203–218). New York: Holt, Rinehart, & Winston.

Kotch, J. B., & Thomas, L. P. (1986). Family and social factors associated with substantiation of child abuse and neglect reports. *Journal of Family Violence, 1*(2), 167–179.

Liem, R., & Liem, J. H. (1988). Psychological effects of unemployment on workers and their families. *Journal of Social Issues, 44*(4), 87–105.

Mayer, S. E., & Jencks, C. (1989). Poverty and the distribution of material hardship. *Journal of Human Resources, 24*(1), 88–113.

Mayor's Task Force on Child Abuse and Neglect. (1983, November). *Report on the preliminary study of child fatalities in New York City.* New York: Author.

Mayor's Task Force on Child Abuse and Neglect. (1987, January). *High risk factors associated with child maltreatment fatalities.* New York: Author.

McKey, R. H., Condelli, L., Ganson, H., Barrett, B. J., McConkey, C., & Plantz, M. C. (1985, June). *The impact of Head Start on children, families and communities: Final report of the Head Start Evaluation, Synthesis and Utilization Project* (DHHS Publication No. OHDS 85-31193). Washington, DC: U.S. Government Printing Office.

McNicoll, P. (1989). *The social and economic precursors of child maltreatment: A study of the exosystem.* Unpublished doctoral dissertation, University of Washington, Seattle.

Middleton, R., & Allen, V. L. (1977). Social psychological effects. In H. W. Watts & A. Rees (Eds.), *The New Jersey Income Maintenance Experiment: Vol. III. Expenditures, health, and social behavior; and the quality of the evidence* (pp. 151–194). New York: Academic Press.

Mierley, M. C., & Baker, S. P. (1983). Fatal house fires in an urban population. *Journal of the American Medical Association, 249,* 1466–1468.

Mills, D. (1982, July 16). *Child abuse reports in counties of high unemployment* [Memorandum]. Madison, Wisconsin: Wisconsin Department of Health and Social Services, Bureau for Children, Youth and Families.

Mitchell, C., Tovar, P., & Knitzer, J. (1989, December). *The Bronx Homebuilders Program: An evaluation of the first 45 families.* New York: Bank Street College of Education.

Nalepka, C., O'Toole, R., & Turbett, J. P. (1981). Nurses' and physicians' recognition and reporting of child abuse. *Issues in Comprehensive Pediatric Nursing, 5,* 33–44.

National Commission on Children. (1991). *Beyond rhetoric: A new American agenda for children and families.* Washington, DC: U.S. Government Printing Office.

Nersesian, W. S., Petit, M. R., Shaper, R., Lemieux, D., & Naor, E. (1985). Childhood death and poverty: A study of all childhood deaths in Maine, 1976 to 1980. *Pediatrics, 75,* 41–50.

Olds, D. L., Henderson, C. R., Jr., Chamberlin, R., & Tatelbaum, R. (1986). Preventing child abuse and neglect: A randomized trial of nurse home visitation. *Pediatrics, 78*(1), 65–78.

Pelton, L. H. (1978). Child abuse and neglect: The myth of classlessness. *American Journal of Orthopsychiatry, 48,* 608–617.

Pelton, L. H. (1979). Interpreting family violence data [Letter]. *American Journal of Orthopsychiatry, 49,* 194, 372.

Pelton, L. H. (1981a). Child abuse and neglect and protective intervention in Mercer County, New Jersey. In L. H. Pelton (Ed.), *The social context of child abuse and neglect* (pp. 90–136). New York: Human Sciences Press.

Pelton, L. H. (Ed.). (1981b). *The social context of child abuse and neglect.* New York: Human Sciences Press.

Pelton, L. H. (1982a). *Displaced children: Has review made a difference in New Jersey?* [Draft]. Newark, NJ: Association for Children of New Jersey.

Pelton, L. H. (1982b). Personalistic attributions and client perspectives in child welfare cases: Implications for service delivery. In T. A. Wills (Ed.), *Basic processes in helping relationships* (pp. 81–101). New York: Academic Press.

Pelton, L. H. (1984). *Unemployment, poverty, and child abuse and neglect.* Unpublished manuscript.

Pelton, L. H. (1989). *For reasons of poverty: A critical analysis of the public child welfare system in the United States.* New York: Praeger.

Pelton, L. H. (1990). Resolving the crisis in child welfare: Simply expanding the present system is not enough. *Public Welfare, 48*(4), 19–25, 45.

Pelton, L. H. (1991a). Beyond permanency planning: Restructuring the public child welfare system. *Social Work, 36*(4), 337–343.

Pelton, L. H. (1991b). Ideology, terminology, and the politics of family violence. *Readings: A Journal of Reviews and Commentary in Mental Health, 6*(3), 12–17.

Pelton, L. H. (1992). A functional approach to reorganizing family and child welfare interventions. *Children and Youth Services Review, 14,* 289–303.

Pelton, L. H., & Fuccello, E. (1978, December). *An evaluation of the use of an emergency cash fund in child protective services.* Trenton, NJ: Bureau of Research, New Jersey Division of Youth and Family Services.

Pless, I. B., & Arsenault, L. (1987). The role of health education in the prevention of injuries to children. *Journal of Social Issues, 43*(2), 87–103.

Polansky, N. A., Gaudin, J. M., Jr., Ammons, P. W., & Davis, K. B. (1985). The psychological ecology of the neglectful mother. *Child Abuse and Neglect, 9,* 265–275.

Rivara, F. P., & Barber, M. (1985). Demographic analysis of childhood pedestrian injuries. *Pediatrics, 76,* 375–381.

Sedlak, A. J. (1991a). *National incidence and prevalence of child abuse and neglect: 1988. Revised report.* Rockville, MD: Westat.

Sedlak, A. J. (1991b, February 20–21). *National prevalence of child abuse and neglect.* Paper prepared for the Conference on Child Welfare Reform Experiments, American Enterprise Institute, Washington, DC.

Sedlak, A. J. (1991c). *Study of national incidence and prevalence of child abuse and neglect: Final report—Appendices (Revised).* Rockville, MD: Westat.

Spearly, J. L., & Lauderdale, M. (1983). Community characteristics and ethnicity in the prediction of child maltreatment rates. *Child Abuse and Neglect, 7,* 91–105.

Spiegel, C. N., & Lindaman, F. C. (1977). Children can't fly: A program to prevent childhood morbidity and mortality from window falls. *American Journal of Public Health, 67,* 1143–1147.

Srole, L., Langner, T. S., Michael, S. T., Opler, M. K., & Rennie, T. A. C. (1962). *Mental health in the metropolis: The midtown Manhattan study.* New York: McGraw-Hill.

Staff. (1991, June). *Evaluation of the Illinois Family First placement prevention programs: Progress report.* Chicago: Chapin Hall Center for Children, University of Chicago.

Steinberg, L. D., Catalano, R., & Dooley, D. (1981). Economic antecedents of child abuse and neglect. *Child Development, 52,* 975–985.

Stocks, J. T. (1988). Has family violence decreased? A reassessment of the Straus and Gelles data. *Journal of Marriage and the Family, 50,* 281–285.

Straus, M. A., & Gelles, R. J. (1986). Societal change and change in family violence from 1975 to 1985 as revealed by two national surveys. *Journal of Marriage and the Family, 48,* 465–479.

Straus, M. A., Gelles, R. J., & Steinmetz, S. K. (1980). *Behind closed doors.* Garden City, NY: Anchor Press/Doubleday.

Sudia, C. E. (1981). What services do abusive and neglecting families need? In L. H. Pelton (Ed.), *The social context of child abuse and neglect* (pp. 268–290). New York: Human Sciences Press.

Tertinger, D. A., Greene, B. F., & Lutzker, J. R. (1984). Home safety: Development and validation of one component of an ecobehavioral treatment program for abused and neglected children. *Journal of Applied Behavior Analysis, 17,* 159–174.

Thoits, P., & Hannan, M. (1979). Income and psychological distress: The impact of an income-maintenance experiment. *Journal of Health and Social Behavior, 20,* 120–138.

U.S. Bureau of the Census. (1983). *1980 census of population* (General social and economic characteristics; Tables 72, 181). Washington, DC: U.S. Government Printing Office.

U.S. Bureau of the Census. (1990). *Statistical abstract of the United States, 1990* (110th ed., Table No. 727). Washington, DC: U.S. Government Printing Office.

U.S. Bureau of the Census. (1991). *Statistical abstract of the United States: 1991* (111th ed.; Tables 730, 745). Washington, DC: Author.

U.S. Department of Health and Human Services. (1981). *National study of the incidence and severity of child abuse and neglect.* (DHHS Publication No. OHDS 81-30325). Washington, DC: Author.

U.S. Department of Health and Human Services. (1988). *Study of national incidence and prevalence of child abuse and neglect.* Washington, DC: Author.

Wallace, R. (1989). "Homelessness," contagious destruction of housing, and municipal service cuts in New York City: 1. Demographics of a housing deficit. *Environment and Planning A, 21,* 1585–1603.

Weston, J. (1974). The pathology of child abuse. In R. Helfer & C. H. Kempe (Eds.), *The battered child* (2nd ed.). Chicago: University of Chicago Press.

Wilson, M., & Baker, S. (1987). Structural approach to injury control. *Journal of Social Issues, 43*(2), 73–86.

Wolfe, D. A. (1985). Child-abusive parents: An empirical review and analysis. *Psychological Bulletin, 97,* 462–482.

Wolock, I., & Horowitz, B. (1977). *Factors related to levels of child care among families receiving public assistance in New Jersey* (Final report, Vol. 1. Grant No. 90-C-418). Washington, DC: National Center on Child Abuse and Neglect.

Wolock, I., & Horowitz, B. (1979). Child maltreatment and material deprivation among AFDC recipient families. *Social Service Review, 53,* 175–194.

Wooldridge, J. (1977). Housing consumption. In H. W. Watts & A. Rees (Eds.), *The New Jersey income maintenance experiment: Vol. III. Expenditures, health, and social behavior; and the quality of the evidence* (pp. 45–71). New York: Academic Press.

Zellman, G. L. (1992). The impact of case characteristics on child abuse reporting decisions. *Child Abuse and Neglect, 16,* 57–74.

Zuravin, S. J. (1985, November–December). Housing and child maltreatment: Is there a connection? *Children Today,* pp. 8–13.

Zuravin, S. J. (1986). Residential density and urban child maltreatment: An aggregate analysis. *Journal of Family Violence, 1*(4), 307–322.

Zuravin, S. J. (1988). Child abuse, child neglect, and maternal depression: Is there a connection? In National Center on Child Abuse and Neglect (Eds.), *Research symposium on child neglect.* Washington, DC: Clearinghouse on Child Abuse and Neglect Information.

Zuravin, S. J., & Grief, G. L. (1989). Normative and child-maltreating AFDC mothers. *Social Casework: The Journal of Contemporary Social Work, 70*(2), 76–84.

Zuravin, S. J., & Taylor, B. S. (1989). *The connection between urban child maltreatment and the public housing project environment: An exploratory ecological study.* Unpublished manuscript, University of Maryland School of Social Work and Community Planning, Baltimore.

Chapter 5

Sociocultural Factors in Child Maltreatment

Jill E. Korbin

The purpose of this chapter is to assess the importance of sociocultural factors in the development of a successful neighborhood-based child protection strategy (see, e.g., U.S. Advisory Board on Child Abuse and Neglect, 1990). The dual challenge of incorporating culture into child protection is (1) to accommodate cultural diversity while (2) assuring equitable standards of care and protection for all children.

Many unresolved issues remain in elucidating the relationship between culture and child maltreatment. The relationship between ethnically diverse populations in a multicultural society and child protection systems is one that is politically charged and can best be dealt with in context, at a neighborhood level.

SOCIOCULTURAL FACTORS AFFECTING THE DEFINITION OF CHILD ABUSE AND NEGLECT

Incorporating culturally informed definitions of child abuse and neglect into a neighborhood-based strategy has implications for the identification of cases of child maltreatment. The goal of a neighborhood-based strategy should be for congruence on definitions to provide a basis for differentiating what is cultural and what is maltreatment (or the components of each) such that prevention, identification, and intervention can be accomplished on a consensual rather than an adversarial basis.

Culture and child maltreatment are both problematic to define. They are political as well as social and scientific terms that have historical variability. The difficulty in defining these terms is compounded by the reality that they are heterogeneous and not unitary phenomena.

Literature on Cultural Definitions of Child Maltreatment

The literature on culturally informed definitions of child maltreatment has involved three broad approaches. First, theoretical constructions have been offered, based on the cross-cultural literature (Finkelhor & Korbin, 1988; Korbin 1981, 1987a). Second, descriptions of specific cultural/ethnic groups have sought to identify the diversity of conceptions of abuse (e.g., Gray & Cosgrove, 1985). Third, vignette studies (Giovannoni & Becerra, 1979; Hong & Hong, 1991) have sought to study systematically cultural (and professional) diversity and congruence on parameters for the perceived seriousness of abusive incidents.

Each of these three approaches has its strengths and weaknesses. In the first two literatures, definitions are often anecdotal or based on small and nonrepresentative samples. Theoretical models for definitions have been suggested but have not been subjected to empirical verification. Nevertheless, these first two approaches indicate the importance of considering cultural meanings and definitions in child maltreatment. The third approach, vignette studies, is methodologically rigorous, but does not necessarily reflect actual behavior (Garbarino & Ebata, 1983). Vignette studies, however, have suggested cultural differences in childrearing beliefs and values that may impact definitions of child maltreatment (e.g., Hong & Hong, 1991). Vignette studies have also countered the misconception, based on the disproportionate representation of people of color in child abuse reports, that people of color judge child abuse incidents as less serious than do middle-class European Americans.

Definitions: Child Maltreatment

Definitional ambiguity is a major impediment to multicultural work in child maltreatment. Imprecision and variability in definitions have hampered research and precluded valid and reliable comparisons. Although this issue has received considerable attention in the literature, solutions remain to be found (Aber & Zigler, 1981; Besharov, 1981; Gelles, 1982; Giovannoni & Becerra, 1979; Rizley & Cicchetti, 1981). Definitional problems are exacerbated in cross-cultural and multiethnic comparisons. Two definitional problems, the homogeneity with which the term "child abuse and neglect" is employed and the lack of precise operational criteria, have important implications for cross-cultural research. The dynamics involved in various forms of maltreatment do not justify the homogeneous use of the term (Besharov, 1981; Giovannoni & Becerra, 1979; Jason, Williams, Burton, & Rochat, 1982; Polansky, Chalmers, Buttenwieser, & Williams, 1981; Rizley & Cicchetti, 1981).

The label "battered child syndrome" was intentionally chosen to grasp public, professional, and legislative attention. It referred to a "clinical condition in young children who have received serious physical abuse" (Kempe,

Silverman, Droegmueller, & Silver, 1962, p. 105). In 25 years, definitions of child abuse and neglect have expanded to encompass political realities and needs (e.g., Baby Doe regulations) as well as expanded understanding of the problem (e.g., Munchausen's syndrome by proxy and psychological maltreatment). The definition of maltreatment has expanded to include a range of caretaker behaviors and child outcomes as exemplified by the definition employed by the national incidence study:

> A child maltreatment situation is one where, through purposive acts or marked inattention to the child's basic needs, behavior of a parent/substitute or other adult caretaker caused foreseeable and avoidable injury or impairment to a child or materially contributed to unreasonable prolongation or worsening of an existing injury or impairment. (National Center on Child Abuse and Neglect [NCCAN], 1981, p. 4)

In a sense, then, "child abuse and neglect" has come to be used in the singular, encompassing anything deemed "bad" for children for which parents or caretakers can be deemed accountable. This lack of clear definitions that can be operationalized in research and service has been a serious problem. Further, and of critical importance to a neighborhood-based strategy, conceptions of "badness" and "goodness" are culturally bound. There is not a universal ideal parenting strategy, but rather parenting must be viewed within the social and historical context in which it is embedded (e.g., Eisenberg, 1981; Korbin, 1981, 1987a; Sternberg & Lamb, 1991).

Definitions of child abuse and neglect in the United States have been based on identifiable harm to a child that can be attributed to caretaker commission or omission. Neither parental action nor physical injury is adequate in itself as a critical defining element of child maltreatment across cultures. Determinations of maltreatment depend on the interaction of consequences to a child and caretaker action or inaction. This is a complex issue because the same parental behavior may have different meanings and interpretations in different cultural contexts. For example, Gray and Cosgrove (1985) reported that Mexican American clinicians felt that the practice of calling children by names reflecting their physical attributes, for example, *gordito* (fatty), might be interpreted by outsiders to their culture as demeaning or verbally abusive rather than as a sign of affection. Similarly, child outcomes may have different meanings. It does not make sense to equate bruises inflicted on a child by angry parents in the United States with a child who is bruised in the process of the Vietnamese curing practice of "coin rubbing" (Yeatman, Shaw, Barlow, & Bartlett, 1976).

Definitions of child abuse have many gray areas, both within and between cultures, that rely on careful consideration of sociocultural context before being identified as abuse or neglect. A working definition of child maltreatment as "the portion of harm to children that results from human action that is proscribed, proximate, and preventable" (Finkelhor & Korbin, 1988, p. 4) fills two criteria for culturally informed definitions. It distinguishes child abuse from other circumstances that have detrimental consequences for children, and it is flexible enough to encompass a range of cultural contexts.

Efforts must be made to operationalize and cross-culturally validate definitions of caretaker behaviors that result in sufficient actual or potential harm to children to fall within the parameters of child maltreatment. Research should move toward uses of terms more amenable to operationalization that can be employed more validly and reliably across cultural boundaries. Definitions must include a consideration of the type of maltreatment (physical, emotional, sexual) and not simply include all harms to children as homogeneous under the label "child abuse and neglect."

Further, if the goal in definition is to aid in the identification of cases, literature indicates that there is a wide range of diversity and bias in reporting, as discussed in the section on culture/ethnicity. Indeed, two social workers in the same agency may disagree on whether or not a case should be reported as child abuse. These individual differences in the conceptualization of child maltreatment obviously complicate the task of translating definitions across cultural contexts.

Definitions: Culture/Ethnicity

The importance of definitions of culture and ethnicity for a successful neighborhood-based strategy are (1) how people living in a neighborhood identify their own cultural membership or affiliation and that of their neighbors and (2) how people living in a neighborhood are identified by those providing services (both preventive and remedial).

Hundreds of definitions have been offered for the concept of culture. A useful and flexible definition is that culture is the acquired and shared knowledge that individuals use to order their lives and interact with one another. This definition is particularly suited to a neighborhood-based strategy in which diverse individuals must come together for a child protection effort.

Ethnicity as a concept has generally been used to refer to groups living within multicultural societies. Harwood (1981) distinguished between "behavioral" (shared lifestyle, values, beliefs and behaviors) and "ideological" (a more political identification with the group by virtue of common descent) ethnicity. Similarly, Sue (1988) distinguished "ethnic membership" (national or geographic descent) from cultural membership (current identification and commonalities with group in question).

Cultures and ethnic groups are not homogeneous and there is substantial diversity within any group.[1] Culture and ethnicity are too often defined on the basis of large groupings of people based on skin color or geographical area from which descent can be traced. Broad racial identifications (e.g., African American, Asian American, Native American, and European descent) may be useful for some purposes, but they are not capable of accurately identifying the cultural composition of a neighborhood. There are multiple types of Hispanics/Latinos (e.g., Cubans, Puerto Ricans, Mexicans, Mexican Americans, and Guatemalans), blacks (e.g., African Americans, Haitians, and West Indians), Asians (e.g., Chinese, Japanese, Koreans, Thai, Cambodians, and Indians), Pacific Island peoples (e.g., Hawaiians, Samoans, Tahitians, and Maoris), Native Americans (e.g., Navaho and Sioux), and European Americans (e.g., Italians, Germans, and British). Each of these subgroups has been addressed as having a unique culture and therapeutic needs (McGoldrick, Pearce, & Giordano, 1982). Further, there is vast diversity within any one cultural group along the lines of generation, acculturation, education, income, gender, and so on. For example, Mendoza (1984) found that Hispanics or Chicanos could not be identified as a homogeneous group but, instead, were found at varying points along an "acculturation" continuum.

Culture/ethnicity and neighborhoods may or may not overlap. Neighborhoods may be made up of single or multiple ethnic groups that may or may not be amenable to working together. Even within ethnic groups there may be important distinctions (e.g., rival gangs), that preclude successful intervention on the basis of ethnicity alone. There may be important divisions within any ethnic group in a neighborhood. For example, middle-class immigrant generation Chinese who own businesses in any of our cities' Chinatowns may differ markedly from the more recent immigrants from China whose adolescents are forming gangs. Self-identification of ethnicity, therefore, will have to be an important component of a neighborhood-based strategy.

Culturally Competent or Culturally Informed Definitions of Child Maltreatment

Culturally competent definitions of child maltreatment must avoid extreme ethnocentrism or extreme relativism. A general lack of training and knowledge about cultural diversity has hampered child protection efforts and promoted tendencies toward the extremes of both ethnocentrism and relativism.

Ethnocentrism is the belief that one's own cultural beliefs and practices are the superior (and sometimes only) approach. Relativism is the belief that every culture must be viewed in its own right as equal to all others. An exclusive reliance on either position precludes culturally competent judgments in child protection, and both are antithetical to a child-centered, neighborhood-based approach. Instead, what must be achieved is a moderate and context-sensitive position between these two extremes.

An extreme position on ethnocentrism disregards cultural differences and imposes a single standard for child care practices. This is potentially harmful to children in the denigration of their cultural background. It is also potentially harmful to child protection efforts in that one strategy (that of the dominant culture) will be used for all neighborhoods, regardless of their cultural composition. On the other hand, an extreme position on relativism suspends all standards and potentially compromises the well-being of categories of children whose parents have cultural or religious beliefs that are at odds with their well-being.

An extreme position on ethocentrism runs the risk of false positives, or misidentification of cultural practices as child maltreatment. A well-documented example of such a practice is *cao gao*, or coin rubbing, among Southeast Asians. The practice, in which metal coins are pressed forcefully on the child's body, leaving a symmetrical pattern of bruises, is believed to cure illness. Such bruises are indeed nonaccidentally inflicted and may be extensive (sometimes beyond what will result in a report for physical abuse as a result of being hit with a belt). Nonetheless, this is recognized as a cultural practice with good intentions and is generally not reported as a case of child abuse.

On the other hand, an extreme relativist position runs the risk of false negatives, or missed cases. Because a behavior can be grounded in a cultural heritage does not necessarily mean that it is "good" for children (or as good as children from other cultural groups receive). "Just because we have been blind to 'culture' we must not now be blinded by it" (Tharp, 1991, p. 809). Taking the same example, an extreme position on relativism would say that parents who rely solely on coin rubbing or other medical practices, and who, therefore, do not bring their children in for biomedical care, are only following their cultural dictates. Such families usually come to the attention of child protection agencies only if the child becomes seriously ill or permanently disabled, or dies. (Consequences to the parents generally ensue only if it can be demonstrated that the parents had knowledge of alternative strategies, such as Western biomedical care, but refused or did not seek it.) While respecting cultural differences, this position would facilitate a different standard of care (with risk of harm) for some children and not others. The American Academy of Pediatrics (1988) has recommended that religious exemptions that preclude medical treatment for children be prohibited. Several states have adopted this recommendation (Morris, 1979; Singelenberg, 1990). However, in considering this example, it is important to contemplate the position of middle-class white U.S. parents traveling in Southeast Asia with a toddler who becomes ill far away from the U.S. embassy. What would be their reaction to being told that antibiotics were against the law and that instead their child would be treated with coin rubbing? What if they were told that, if they did not comply, their child could be removed from their care? Medical practices and beliefs around the world are based on empirical knowledge grounded in experience of past illness episodes. Because most illnesses resolve on their own, intervention of any kind is likely to "work." In our own society, when the first course of antibiotic therapy does not resolve an ear infection, we do not abandon antibiotics but assume that perhaps a second dose or another antibiotic would resolve the problem. Other medical traditions have similar beliefs, grounded in their empirical evidence.

Potential for Cultural Conflict in Defining Child Maltreatment

Cultural conflict in defining child maltreatment generally arises as a result of disagreement concerning cultural differences in child care. The greater the divergence in child care practices and beliefs, the greater the potential for cultural conflict in definitions of maltreatment (see Figure 5.1).

In reality, practices that can be identified as cultural, such as coin rubbing, are generally not reported as cases of child maltreatment. Such cases become identified as maltreatment when the child suffers an identifiable consequence, such as impairment or death from lack of Western biomedical care. Further, disciplinary techniques, such as excessively long time-outs or spankings, are not usually identified as child maltreatment, again, unless harm can be identified.

Culturally Informed Definitions

How, then, do we begin to define maltreatment in a culturally informed way? Three levels have been suggested for culturally informed definitions of child maltreatment: (1) cultural practices that are viewed as abusive or neglectful

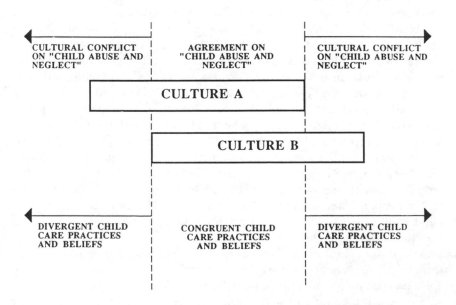

FIGURE 5.1. Cultural conflict in defining child abuse and neglect.

by other cultures, but not by the culture in question; (2) idiosyncratic departure from one's cultural continuum of acceptable behavior; and (3) societally
induced harm to children beyond the control of individual parents and caretakers (Korbin, 1981, 1987a). Definitional ambiguity and confusion in the
cross-cultural literature have arisen from not differentiating these three levels.

Cultural Differences

At the first level, legitimate cultural differences in child care practices must
be respected. Cultural patterns of child care persist through the force of custom and because parents believe that adherence to the dictates of their cultural tradition will enhance their children's, and their own, well-being. The
cultural context of a behavior must be viewed holistically. No single element
of a cultural pattern can be removed from its context and judged in isolation
from other integrated aspects of that culture. The changing nature of childrearing advice in European American societies stands as a caution against
too facile determinations of what is good and bad for children. "Best" child
care advice has varied from one generation to the next as to, for example,
breast versus bottle feeding, scheduled versus demand feeding, and how
quickly to attend to a crying infant. Insider (emic) and outsider (etic) perspectives on what constitutes child maltreatment may vary (Gray & Cosgrove, 1985; Green, 1978, 1982; Korbin, 1977, 1987a).

With respect to cultural diversity in child care practices, a neighborhood-
based child protection effort should follow the model in education and employ a difference rather than a deficiency model. A model emphasizing cultural and ethnic difference has been successfully employed in studies of
education rather than assuming a cultural deficiency in groups of children
who were not succeeding in school (e.g., Gallimore, Boggs, & Jordan, 1974).

Examples of cultural practices may be helpful at this point. Divergent
medical practices may be a source of cultural conflict in identifying child
maltreatment (e.g., Feldman, 1984; Sandler & Haynes, 1978; Trotter,
Ackerman, Rodman, Mattinez, & Sorvillo, 1983; Yeatman et al., 1976). The
example of Vietnamese coin rubbing above must be included here. Another
example concerns infants with colic in the United States. The symptoms of
colic would arouse suspicion of bad child care practices or inflicted trauma
among Hawaiian–Polynesian Americans. Hawaiian–Polynesian Americans
would attribute symptoms of fussiness, indigestion, general discomfort, and
inconsolable crying to jiggling of infants, which causes a condition known
as *opu huli* (turned or twisted stomach). *Opu huli* is diagnosed by seeing
which leg a child pulls up when lying down flat. It can be treated by someone familiar with therapeutic massage. If child maltreatment is to be defined
as an identifiable consequence to a child resulting from parental action (or
inaction), jiggling a child and causing *opu huli* would certainly qualify among
Hawaiian–Polynesian Americans—thereby putting all mainlanders with

colicky infants under suspicion of abuse rather than making them objects of sympathy.

These examples are intended to point out the complexity of the situation. Is the child who experiences coin rubbing accorded a different standard of protection because we respect his parents' rights to practice their own culture? Is the mainland child with *opu huli* accorded a different standard of care than Hawaiian–Polynesian American children would receive if Hawaiian–Polynesian American adults ran child protective services?

At this first level of cultural differences, definitions of child maltreatment have a substantial component of relativity. Cultural practices must be understood within their context. Explanation and understanding, however, do not preclude trying to ensure equitable standards of protection and reduction of suffering for children. It is important at this point to establish that there are different kinds of cultural differences.

First, cultural practices must be viewed in the context of change. What is well suited to one situation may not be suited to another. Ritchie and Ritchie (1981), for example, wrote about the practice of sibling caretaking among Polynesian Maoris in New Zealand. Sibling caretaking involves one child (perhaps 8 to 10 years old through the teenage years) taking care of an infant or toddler. In the indigenous setting, this pattern is highly valued by both children and adults (Gallimore et al., 1974; Korbin, 1978) and is adaptive to a Polynesian socialization pattern. In changing circumstances, however, with a move to urban settings, this practice is misunderstood and indeed becomes dangerous to children who are living in more hazardous circumstances, separated from a larger supportive network.

As a second example, Japanese parents who commit suicide are expected to take their children with them rather than leaving them to face the world alone (Wagatsuma, 1981). Indeed, parents who commit suicide without killing their children are far more likely to be condemned than are those who commit a joint homicide/suicide (Wagatsuma, 1981). In contrast, in the United States, we stoutly condemn parents who kill their children in the context of their own suicides. Is this simply an example of cultural trivia? What happens as Japanese families come to the United States?

In a well-publicized case in California, a Japanese woman accompanied her husband who came to the United States to work. She was so humiliated by his blatant infidelity that she felt she had no option but to kill herself and thus maintain some level of honor. She walked into the Pacific Ocean carrying an infant and holding her other two young children with each hand. Swept away by the waves, she survived, but her children perished. An important component of her defense strategy at trial was that she behaved in a culturally consistent way, which mitigated the consequences she faced. She did not intend to survive her children but to do the best for them by taking them with her. Her misery that she survived but her children did not was immeasurable.

Again, understanding the culturally based rationale for a behavior does not necessarily diminish the consequences to the children. Still, it is not Japanese culture that is at fault or deficient. Clearly, all Japanese individuals who experience shame do not kill themselves and do not kill their children. Is it the marginalized or troubled individuals who are most vulnerable to the extremes of their culture's repertoire of responses and behaviors? The argument is not intended to excuse or justify homicide accompanied by parental suicide. Rather, it is designed to put the issue of defining child maltreatment into context. Wagatsuma's (1981) research indicates that Japanese individuals would be equally disapproving of an American woman living in their midst who became despondent and committed suicide, leaving her children behind with only a note.

Child protection efforts also must acknowledge that some cultural practices may cause injury or be harmful to children. These practices may not be inflicted with malintent but may cause harm nevertheless. Even if not reportable or strictly defined as child maltreatment, intervention can occur.

In the Southwest, for example, lead poisoning in young children was linked to indigenous medications, *azarcon* and *greta*, used to cure *empacho*. *Empacho* is an illness defined by Hispanics as a bolus in the stomach that must be purged. Trotter and his colleagues (1983) found that these indigenous medications were almost pure lead. Educational and community awareness efforts were successful in diminishing the harmful form of these substances, and thus the incidence of lead poisoning, while not minimizing the cultural importance or reality of treating *empacho*.

Finally, in child protection work, a cultural practice must be differentiated as to whether it is a primary or a secondary presenting problem. A legitimate case of child maltreatment may be confused by the entry of cultural information if that information is secondary to the actual abuse. For example, an 8-year-old girl was sexually abused by her father. Her mother reported the abuse as soon as the girl disclosed it to her. The girl's responsibilities for her 2-year-old brother were interpreted as evidence of role reversal, which has been linked in the literature with child abuse and neglect. The treatment plan involved protecting the girl from further sexual assault and relieving her of her babysitting burden to free her to enjoy her childhood. The girl listened to the treatment plan dispassionately until she was told that she would no longer be caring for her younger brother on a daily basis. At this point, she collapsed into sobs. The primary diagnosis of sexual assault was buttressed by the information on her child care responsibilities. However, this secondary issue was culture bound in that the family was Hispanic and sibling caretaking was highly valued. Consistent with sibling caretaking practice cross-culturally, all the girl's peers had younger child charges and they all played together after school in multiage play groups with adults nearby for assistance should a problem arise. Sibling caretaking can be enhancing of self-esteem in children whose cultures value the behavior (Korbin,

1978). This child, then, would have been excluded from a culturally appropriate and valued behavior.

Idiosyncratic Violation of Cultural Norms

At the second level, intracultural diversity, or idiosyncratic departure from cultural standards, is an important domain within which to identify culturally informed definitions of child maltreatment. All cultures contain individuals who deviate from their cultural standards and norms (Edgerton, 1976, 1985), including those concerning parenting and child care. This is found in cultures that are generally indulgent of children as well as in cultures that tend toward harsher treatment of children (Korbin, 1977). The continuum of acceptable and unacceptable behavior within any culture must be understood. This is the level at which cultural practices can best be differentiated from maltreatment.

At the idiosyncratic level of definition and identification, the concept of culture can be misused and the claim of cultural differences can mask true cases of maltreatment. Misuse of culture can take two basic forms.

The first type of misuse is to use culture as an excuse or justification. Similar to abusive parents relying on their own childrearing experiences as justification for their own behavior, so too can parents rely on culture as a justification. In its most blatant form, parents or other perpetrators may simply misrepresent their own culture, whether consciously or unconsciously. For example, among the Navajo, once a girl undergoes a puberty ceremony, she is eligible for marriage. This cultural practice persists but has been used by some perpetrating men to justify the rape of teenage girls who have undergone this ceremony but who are not, in reality, considered ready for marriage (Hauswald, 1987).

Similarly, it has been reported that the Laotian Hmong practice of bride capture has been transformed by some into a justification for the kidnapping and rape of a desired but unwilling bride. Traditionally, the young Hmong groom kidnapped the bride over her culturally required protests. In the traditional context, these culturally prescribed complimentary behaviors were well understood by all participants. The wider network legitimized the union with the exchange of resources, signifying marriage. In the United States, however, this marriage custom has been misused and misrepresented with young girls being kidnapped and raped when they and their families do not consent to marriage ("Asian Tradition," 1988). Cross-culturally, many groups practice bride capture as a legitimate form of marriage. We do not know how often in the indigenous situation the practice is misused and/or misrepresented.

The second type of misuse of the concept of culture is to extend cultural boundaries from the legitimate to the unacceptable. For example, some cultures practice, encourage, and value the fondling and praising of very young children's genitals (Korbin, 1990a; Olson, 1981). This is done either to soothe and quiet infants and young children or to praise their incipient fertility. The behavior is not carried out in secret, is not considered sexually gratifying to the adults involved, and is not regarded as rule breaking or deviant. When one family from a culture with this practice migrated to the United States, the family came to the attention of child protective services. The mother, who was accused of fondling her son, was adamant that this was acceptable in her culture and that she was being persecuted for her cultural heritage. Her husband, a soldier, agreed that this behavior was widely and openly practiced in his wife's home setting and that nobody there seemed to regard it as problematic. However, the son was far beyond his toddler years and was the one who lodged the complaint. Thus, a legitimate cultural practice was extended beyond its acceptable bounds, making it deviant. Child protective services then could address the issue of an inappropriate expression of an appropriate cultural practice rather than condemn the culture.

Difficulties in differentiating cultural differences in childrearing practices from child maltreatment can be resolved at the neighborhood level with input from neighborhood residents and consultants. This differentiation has been hampered in current child protection work largely because child protection workers are usually restricted in their community contacts to problematic individuals and families rather than to the continuum of acceptable and unacceptable behaviors.

Leaving children alone and unattended is a frequent cause of child maltreatment reports among the Navajo (Hauswald, 1987). This practice is justified by the parents who engage in this behavior in terms of traditional Navajo childrearing patterns of sibling caretaking and the high level of responsibility entrusted to children. However, the results of interviews with Navajo mothers ($n = 30$) indicated that none of these mothers thought that young children should be left alone for extended periods with siblings less than 13 years of age. These mothers disapproved of leaving children alone overnight without adult supervision. Still, neglect cases in the community involved children as young as 5 years of age being left for long periods with younger siblings (Hauswald, 1987). This practice, then, is not a cultural pattern but a departure from cultural norms and values exacerbated by problems of poverty and alcoholism on the reservation. As noted earlier, only an in-depth knowledge of the relevant culture allows such an identification.

A cultural practice cannot simply be equated with maltreatment or risk of maltreatment. Providers tend not to see the times that children are cared for by a legitimate sibling caretaker with no increased risk of harm to either child. Indeed, sibling caretaking may be a positive experience for caretakee and caretaker alike. Sibling caretaking, however, needs to be understood as it was meant to be practiced, not in altered circumstances that may make it more dangerous for children.

Similarly, providers tend not to see the times that an object is picked up as a threat of punishment, or the times that children are hit but not harmed. Instead, the cases in which children are left with buckle marks, bruises, welts, and other injuries are more commonly seen by child protection workers. Cultural acceptance of physical discipline cannot necessarily be equated with abuse. The complex relationship between "proper" childrearing practices and the larger cultural context is illustrated in the words of an urban U.S. black woman concerned with the rise in juvenile delinquency:

> Children is not like they was. You never had no juvenile, nothin' like that. . . . And there's a law you can't whup your children, and if you can't whup your children, you look for all this to happen. Everybody should know how to whup 'em without beatin' 'em and bruisin' 'em up. (Snow, 1977, p. 104)

To gain neighborhood support of diverse ethnic and cultural groups for the prevention and treatment of child maltreatment, it is more fruitful to capitalize on the standard in virtually all cultures that children should not be harmed, rather than denigrating deep-seated and long-standing cultural practices that have not been conclusively demonstrated to be harmful across cultural contexts.

Societal Abuse

Societal abuse and neglect of children is the level of deprivation, poverty, discrimination, and danger that societies are willing to tolerate for their children (e.g., poverty, homelessness, institutional abuse, and incidence of firearms deaths). The threshold of tolerance for these conditions varies across societies. These conditions, which affect children and adults alike, are difficult to define as abuse and neglect for which caretakers can be held accountable. Societal and idiosyncratic abuse and neglect may overlap in terms of which children are vulnerable to societal exploitation or deprivation.

Vignette Studies

Systematic efforts to study definitions of child maltreatment have taken the form of vignette studies designed to tap the perceived seriousness of situations that could be defined as maltreatment (Giovannoni & Becerra, 1979; Hong & Hong, 1991). Giovannoni and Becerra (1979) pointed out that ethnically diverse populations judge maltreatment vignettes more seriously than do middle-class whites, who are the model for child protective services. Hong and Hong (1991) found that Chinese judgments of seriousness were influenced by a high value on filial piety that increased tolerance for physical discipline by parents to achieve desired ends. Vignette studies, however, are limited in the conclusions that can be drawn from them (Garbarino & Ebata, 1983). Vignettes do not necessarily evoke or reflect real-world responses that would be involved in a neighborhood-based system.

Definitional congruence is the first step in a culturally informed and culturally competent child protection system. However, definitions of child maltreatment and identification of specific cases of maltreatment may not overlap because of distrust of the child protection system. Long (1986) reported that a community of Native Americans agreed in a case of child maltreatment that the behavior was wrong. Nevertheless, the family who reported the maltreatment was severely criticized for reporting to the white-dominated child protection agency.

SOCIOCULTURAL FACTORS AFFECTING THE RATE OF CHILD MALTREATMENT

There is little empirical basis, at present, to indicate that any cultural, ethnic, or racial group in the United States has greater rates of child maltreatment than any other. Nevertheless, this issue is the topic of much speculation and has obvious implications for service delivery. This section first considers the literature examining rates of reported child maltreatment in diverse cultural/ethnic groups. Results of studies are often contradictory. The discussion then turns to factors in the sociocultural milieu that may promote or impede the occurrence of child maltreatment.

Studies that compare the incidence or prevalence of child maltreatment by race, culture, or ethnicity have been limited in their conclusions for a number of reasons.

First, studies too often rely on broad racial categorizations as the operationalization of culture. Intracultural variation, a promising area of inquiry, has been virtually unexplored. The heterogeneity of broad classifications (e.g., African American, European American, Asian American, Hispanic/Latino, and Native American) was discussed in the preceding section.

Second, the definitional basis for the databases employed are flawed. The definitions of child abuse and neglect are imprecise, precluding valid and reliable comparison across studies. A wide range of maltreatment types, which frequently overlap, must be included in attempts to assess incidence and prevalence rates. Problems in the definition of child abuse and neglect were also discussed in the preceding section.

Third, sampling problems limit the conclusions that can be drawn. Some research employs clinical samples, some official reports to child protection agencies, and some self-reports of violent behaviors. Clinical samples are not necessarily representative, official reporting is subject to biases, and self-reports of behavior are not equivalent to abusive situations.

Fourth, bias in reporting cannot be dismissed. The debate then continues as to whether child abuse and neglect reports represent a detection phenomenon or true incidence.

Fifth, studies rarely consider socioeconomic status or social class. It has been virtually impossible to disaggregate the effects of culture and socioeconomic status.

Finally, with rare exception, studies do not link the cultural practice that is thought to lead to higher incidence or prevalence with child maltreatment rates in a systematic way. This has led to speculation, in the absence of empirical justification, about which cultures are more or less prone to abusive and neglectful behaviors than others. Better research is badly needed on the relationship between childrearing beliefs and practices and abusive behavior.

Incidence and prevalence rates based on official reports usually combine physical abuse, sexual abuse, and neglect. Sexual abuse incidence and prevalence rates are discussed separately.

Physical Abuse and Neglect

Neither of the two national incidence studies (1981, 1988) has found a significant relationship between race, culture, or ethnicity and the incidence, type, or severity of child maltreatment. Both studies classified children as black, white, or other. As discussed in the first section of this chapter, these classifications have little meaning in terms of understanding cultural differences.

Jason, Amereuh, Marks, and Tyler (1982), using data from the Georgia Department of Protective Services, found that blacks were disproportionately reported for child abuse. They did not find reporting bias to be responsible for this finding. Horowitz and Wolock (1981) found that while blacks were overrepresented in the abuse and neglect reports, their distribution was equal to their representation among families receiving Aid to Families with Dependent Children. Garbarino and Ebata (1983) argue that it is under conditions of socioeconomic deprivation and stress that cultural differences are most important. Giovannoni and Billingsley (1970) found that it is the poorest of the poor who neglect across ethnic groups.

Lauderdale, Valiunas, and Anderson (1980) found a racial/ethnic bias in rates of abuse reports in Texas among Anglos, Mexican Americans, and blacks. This research found an overrepresentation for blacks, with whites having the lowest rates. In addition, looking for within-group differences in terms of types of abuse, Anglos had the highest rate of abuse relative to other types of maltreatment, and blacks and Mexican Americans had higher proportions of neglect. Lauderdale et al. (1980) speculated as to the cultural reasons for these differences based on the literature on socialization and personality patterns.

Of more interest than the between-ethnic group comparisons, Lauderdale et al. (1980) found a significant rural–urban difference within ethnic groups. Blacks living in rural areas had the lowest rates of abuse, even though blacks had the highest rates of abuse of all ethnic groups when urban–rural residence was not included in the analysis. Rates for Mexican Americans also were lower than Anglo rates when residence type was included in the analysis. There are, however, multiple possible explanations for and implications of these findings. The most obvious is to look for strengths of rural black communities that diminish as protective factors for child maltreatment with increasing urbanization. One cannot, however, dismiss the possibility of bias in the reports.

Light (1973), more than 20 years ago, reanalyzed Gil's (1970) data, comparing incidence rates for blacks and whites in four northern and four southern states. In the northern states, whites accounted for 27.3% of child abuse and neglect cases, whereas in the southern states, whites accounted for 72.9% of the cases. This discrepancy was not attributable to the proportions of blacks and whites in the population. Rather, at the time the data were gathered, in 1967, services and facilities for black children in the South were extremely scarce. Child abuse and neglect in the black population tended to be handled informally, within kin and community networks, and without recourse to public agencies. In the North, however, most reports comprised poor, ethnically diverse families who utilized public welfare services. What at first examination could have been a difference tied to residence turned out also to be related to service availability.

Wolock (1982) more recently examined judgments about the severity of abuse and neglect situations. She utilized a vignette instrument and found workers to be influenced by the overall severity of cases coming to their agencies. That is, workers in socioeconomically disadvantaged areas with more severe abuse and neglect case loads tended to judge the vignettes less seriously. In contrast, workers in socioeconomically advantaged areas had a lower threshold in judging the severity of abuse vignettes. This has important implications for a neighborhood-based child protection system. Not only are child abuse and neglect cases influenced by reporting bias based on the identity of reporter or the ethnicity of the alleged perpetrator, but they are also influenced by neighborhood and community socioeconomic factors and the severity of an agency's case load.

Wolock (1982) also noted the implications for differential service delivery if the same incident is treated differently in a socioeconomically advantaged neighborhood than it is in a disadvantaged neighborhood. If families are reported for less severe cases in socioeconomically advantaged areas, they may receive more extensive intervention than does a similar family from a disadvantaged neighborhood. The families in the socioeconomically advantaged area, then, may appear more amenable to intervention.

Newberger, Reed, Daniel, Hyde, and Kotelchuck (1977) asserted that poor and ethnically diverse children are more likely to be identified as abused while white and more affluent families are identified as having accidentally inflicted injuries. Hampton and Newberger (1985), in a reanalysis of the national incidence study (NCCAN, 1981), found that class and race were the best predictors of whether an incident was reported by hospitals. Impoverished black families were more likely to be reported than were affluent white families, even if the severity of the incident was comparable. Carr and Gelles (1978) identified a bias toward physician and hospital reports being validated, regardless of the severity of the abuse. O'Toole, Turbett, and Nalepka (1983) found that vignettes were more likely to be identified as abuse if a lower-class caretaker was involved. Again, there are implications for service delivery. Although poor black (and other culturally diverse) families may be treated more punitively, abused affluent white children may fail to receive intervention. Nobody, then, is well served.

The argument about ethnic differences in rates of abuse and neglect cannot, however, be dismissed on the basis of detection and reporting errors and bias. Self-reports on the Conflict Tactics Scales (CTS) indicate that lower socioeconomic status is a risk factor for violent behaviors toward children (Straus, Gelles, & Steinmetz, 1980; Gelles & Straus, 1988). Although violence toward children occurs in all social strata, violent behaviors toward children, particularly severe violence, is more likely in poor families. Gelles (1992) has further refined the analysis to indicate that a subset of the poor are at increased risk of child abuse. Young parents, particularly mothers, with young children living below the poverty line are at the greatest risk of violent behavior toward children. Despite these findings on socioeconomic status, self-report data on the CTS did not find a significant difference between blacks and whites in reported violent acts toward children (Straus et al., 1980). The "other category" (including Native American Indians, Asians, and "other" cultural groups) were most likely to exhibit violent acts toward children.

Because child abuse and neglect is a low-base-rate phenomenon, it is often difficult to assess its prevalence in small populations. Graburn (1987), in studying Inuit peoples, documented severe cases of physical child abuse. However, the rarity of these incidents and their seeming contradiction to his and others' descriptions of nurturant, indulgent, and nonpunitive Inuit parenting made him hesitant to publish these seemingly aberrant cases.

The data available leave many questions unanswered that are critical to a neighborhood-based child protection strategy. Both official reporting data and self-report data indicate that impoverished families are at increased risk of child maltreatment. Cultural and ethnic groups at greatest risk of poverty, then, appear to have increased incidence and prevalence of child maltreatment. Other chapters in this volume (Garbarino & Kostelny, Chapter 7; Lerman, Chapter 8; and Pelton, Chapter 4) provide a more extensive examination of the relationship between socioeconomic status, specifically poverty, and child maltreatment. The purpose of this discussion is to underline that, at present, there is no convincing evidence that disaggregates socioeconomic status and cultural or ethnic identity in rates of reported child abuse and neglect. A critical problem is that the search has nevertheless ensued for cultural factors that are related to maltreatment. This search has been largely speculative and has generated much debate on the relative risk and protective factors that diverse cultures afford.

With rare exception, studies do not link the cultural practice that is thought to lead to higher incidence or prevalence of child maltreatment with these rates in a systematic way. There are some exceptions that consider the relationship between cultural practices and report rates (Dubanoski 1981; Dubanoski & Snyder, 1980; Ritchie & Ritchie, 1981). Dubanoski and Snyder (1980) suggest that Samoan Americans are overreported and Japanese Americans underreported for abuse in Hawaii because of Samoan values on physical punishment and increased aggressiveness. However, actual physical punishment is not measured between the groups, and it is assumed that the value on punishment is linked to increased punishment, which, in turn, is linked to maltreatment. Indeed, other factors could easily be involved. In Hawaii, Japanese Americans are in a much better socioeconomic position, in general, than are Samoan Americans. Further, disruption and change involved in the migration of Samoans may be contributing to their rate of report. Samoan service providers consider physical discipline one of the areas that is likely to be misunderstood by non-Samoans (Gray & Cosgrove, 1985).

In the 1975–1985 national family violence restudy, the rates of severe violence toward black children increased, as did the black–white ratio for severe violence toward children. That black children did not experience the nearly 50% reduction in severe violence found for the population as a whole (Straus & Gelles, 1986) was explained by self-reports on the CTS that blacks were more likely to hit a child with an object (Hampton, Gelles, & Harrop, 1989). While of interest, this finding requires further scrutiny because hitting with an object does not necessarily show a one-to-one correspondence with reported abuse rates. However, a study in Columbus, Ohio, found that black children were overrepresented in child abuse and neglect reports compared with white children. Further, children were more likely to be injured with objects including belts and cords than were white children. While black children constituted 39% of the child abuse reports, they accounted for 91% of the electric cord injuries. Black children over 5 years of age were particularly vulnerable to this pattern of injury.

Ritchie and Ritchie's (1981) discussion of child maltreatment patterns in New Zealand has relevance to the multicultural setting of the United States. Polynesian (specifically Maori) children, who comprise approximately 10% of the child population of New Zealand, constitute over half of the children reported as not being properly supervised. In part, this has to do with cultural conflict in the definition of child maltreatment related to a misunderstanding of the Polynesian practice of sibling caretaking. However, the Ritchies also point out that it is not merely cultural misunderstanding or cultural conflict that accounts for this disparity in reporting statistics. They argue that cultural practices that are valued and adaptive in one setting may indeed be dangerous to children in another. Sibling caretaking in urban environments with substandard housing that catches fire, streets with fast-moving cars, and so on may indeed increase the risk to younger children being cared for by older siblings rather than adults, and therefore justifiably may be treated as neglect even though the behaviors are culturally consistent and nonproblematic in the indigenous setting.

Physical discipline (i.e., spanking), in reality, does not usually find its way into child protection case loads. Nevertheless, debate continues as to whether physical discipline is itself abusive and/or whether it is a powerful contributor to abuse. Acceptance of physical discipline of children among laypersons (Carson, 1986; Gelles & Straus, 1988; Gil, 1970) and physicians (McCormick, 1992) is pervasive. However, cultural differences in the use of physical discipline and force have not been documented. Weller, Romney, and Orr (1987) found that Anglo and Hispanic adolescents did not differ in their judgments about the appropriateness of disciplinary strategies, including physical punishment, nor in the proportion of each group reporting the experience of physical punishment. Billingsley (1969) found that blacks are not more violent toward children than are whites. Blacks and whites do not differ in self-reports of spanking (Stark & McEvoy, 1970).

Parke and Collmer (1975) suggest that physical discipline may be most dangerous among parents who disapprove of its use because it is then used as a measure of last resort when parental anger is highest. They speculate as follows:

> As a result of this cultural shift in attitude [away from the use of physical discipline], the manner in which physical punishment is employed makes the contemporary use of this type of discipline potentially more dangerous than in the past. (p. 27)

Indeed, Kadushin and Martin (1981) have pointed out that while most discipline does not become abuse, most abuse begins with parental intentions (at least retrospectively stated intentions) to discipline.

Sexual Abuse

Incidence and prevalence figures for child sexual abuse pose similar problems for interpretation as statistics concerning physical abuse and neglect. Definitions vary across cultures and across time (Korbin, 1990a; Mrazek, 1981).

Earlier studies of the incidence of child sexual abuse identified ethnically diverse children as the dominant victims of child sexual abuse (DeFrancis, 1969; Peters, 1976). However, these studies were based on clinical samples obtained in medical or social service settings in which poor and ethnically diverse children are likely to be overrepresented.

Survey research on the prevalence of child sexual abuse has not supported the existence of ethnic differences in child sexual abuse. Finkelhor's (1979) study of New England college students utilized a predominantly white middle-class sample, precluding an analysis by culture or ethnicity. However, Finkelhor's (1984) Boston study did not find an association between ethnicity and child sexual abuse. Russell's (1986) prevalence study in San Francisco included four ethnic groups (Latina, Asian, African American, and white American) and found no significant ethnic differences on intrafamilial abuse. Wyatt (1985) studied child sexual abuse prevalence among an equal number of African American and white American women in Los Angeles, specifically sampling for equal representation of both in her research. She found no significant ethnic differences in the prevalence of child sexual abuse. The two national incidence studies (NCCAN, 1981, 1988) also failed to find a relationship between race and sexual abuse.

Finkelhor and Williams's (1988) study of sexual abuse in day care settings found the racial composition of the assaulted children to be in proportion to the racial composition of U.S. children in day care. However, they suggest further research concerning whether children who are racially different within their day care setting are at risk.

Again, the tie between cultural factors and increased or decreased incidence remains unclear. Whereas middle-class child protective services may view co-sleeping as deleterious to children, and as a risk factor for sexual abuse, it is well to remember that most of the world's cultures value and support parents sleeping with infants and small children. Indeed, parent–child co-sleeping is taken for granted in most societies, and its absence is viewed as dangerous to and neglectful of children (Korbin, 1987a). Co-sleeping may be seen as preventing child sexual abuse in some cultures. There is anecdotal evidence that some Native American groups believe that sexual abuse increased when families stopped sleeping together. The dispersal of children to their own rooms provided the conditions of secrecy conducive to abuse that would have been prevented if all adults had been present.

The Relationship of Culture to Child Maltreatment: Risk and Protective Factors

The literature on child maltreatment in single cultural/ethnic groups most often seeks to explain cultural patterns and reasons posed for child maltreatment within those groups (e.g., Daniel 1985; Daniel, Hampton, & Newberger, 1983; Deitrich, 1982; Fischler, 1985; Graburn, 1987; Hampton, 1987; Hauswald, 1987; Holton, 1990; Hong & Hong, 1991; Korbin 1990b; Krantzler, 1987; Larson, Doris, & Alvarez, 1987; Levy, 1964; Protective Services Resource Institute [PSRI], 1977; Reid, 1984; White & Cornely, 1981; Wichlacz, Lane, & Kemp, 1978). This literature most often attempts to identify cultural factors (e.g., childrearing practices, personality profiles, and kinship systems) that might serve as risk-enhancing or risk-reducing factors for child maltreatment.

As discussed in the first section, broad groupings by skin color or descent ignore intracultural differences, are misleading, and fuel racism and stereotypes. At best, such analyses shed some light on macrolevel, or societal level explanations. These analyses, however, leave a residue of argument about whether some groups are under greater stress from poverty or whether these same groups have an increased likelihood of being reported or identified because of their greater contact with public agencies. Such studies also do not address the issue of bias in reporting along the lines of ethnicity, as discussed earlier.

Considering the problems involved in incidence/prevalence studies, it is much more fruitful in examining a potential neighborhood strategy to look at the ways that cultural factors promote or impede child maltreatment rather than to look for differences in rates that are likely to be unreliable and to generate more controversy than insight. The basic question is whether there is something about a culture or something about the circumstances that people find themselves in that leads to abuse. The answer is probably that it is a combination of both. Cultural values may be protective or risk inducing. However, intracultural variability and socioeconomic status cannot be ignored. Efforts directed at the neighborhood level must better understand the etiology of child maltreatment and whether it varies among ethnic groups and neighborhoods.

With respect to a neighborhood-based strategy, Coulton and Pandey (1992) have found that poor neighborhoods are not uniform in their impact on child well-being but differ in the risks to children (assessed by low birthweight or school dropout rates, for example). The concentration of poverty (percentage of the neighborhood residents that are poor) and the persistence of poverty (length of time that the neighborhood has been poor) pose particular risks to children. Additional variables (e.g., housing and crime rates) are being explored for their relationship to rates of child abuse and neglect (Korbin & Coulton, 1991). A preliminary analysis of the data indicates that contiguous census tracts that are presumably at equal risk on the basis of socioeconomic conditions vary substantially in their rates of child abuse and neglect reports.

It is also worthwhile to note the impact of child maltreatment on neighborhood and community mental health status. Community mental health may be adversely affected by the numbers of individuals who experienced childhood abuse and have long-term consequences from that abuse. These individuals, then, have an impact on the mental health status of the community, imposing drains on community resources and posing potential risks for current children (e.g., Scott, 1992).

In the effort to delineate the relationship between culture/ethnicity and child maltreatment it is important not to lose sight of protective factors. Efforts should be directed at naturally occurring strengths as well as weaknesses. For example, in explaining the lack of significant differences between blacks and whites in their self-report survey research, Gelles and Straus (1988) noted that whereas blacks had greater economic problems and scored higher on the incidence of life stresses, they also were more likely to participate in family and community activities, including contact with relatives and reliance on relatives for financial assistance and help with child care. Support from kin, particularly in the arena of child care, can reduce the risk of abuse (Cazenave & Straus, 1979). Stack (1974) has written persuasively about the coping strategies of poor black families who protect children. For example, the strategy of child lending means that if the biological parent(s) is experiencing financial hardship, the child(ren) can go, without stigma or shame, to live with a relative (affinal, consanguineal, or fictive kin) who is not low on food stamps that month. Child protective services tend to look askance at fluid household membership, but this may act to the advantage of some children and families.

Similarly, Dubanoski (1981) found that Hawaiians were overrepresented in Hawaii's child abuse reports. However, Dubanoski also found that child-abusing families were low on 'ohana (extended family) involvement.

In exploring the relationship between culture/ethnicity and child maltreatment, the cultural variable must be "unpacked" (e.g., Tharp, 1991; Whiting, 1976; Weisner, Gallimore, & Jordan, 1988). That is, because culture is not monolithic, it cannot be viewed as having a uniform impact on all members. For example, some aspects of Hawaiian culture may promote good school performance, other aspects may interfere with it, and still other aspects may have no effect at all. Further, while sibling caretaking may promote positive experiences with peer-directed learning, all Hawaiian–Polynesian American children do not participate in sibling caretaking, or do so to different degrees. Similarly, while Stack (1974) describes a functional system of child lending, this may not hold for all inner-city black families.

Social Supports and Embeddedness of Childrearing in a Larger Sociocultural Context

The idea of social networks as a panacea for child maltreatment has been thoughtfully challenged (Thompson, Chapter 3, this volume). Nevertheless, the presence of social networks and social supports to children and families and a positive balance between supports and strains have been posited to be important to child well-being and the prevention of child maltreatment (e.g., Amato, 1990; Garbarino, 1977; Garbarino & Crouter, 1978; Garbarino & Kostelny, 1992; Garbarino & Sherman, 1980; Pilisuk & Parks, 1986; Schorr, 1988; Whittaker & Garbarino, 1983). The cross-cultural literature supports the position that good quality and well-functioning social networks and the embeddedness of childrearing in a larger social context are important protections from child maltreatment (Korbin 1981, 1987b).

Social networks serve multiple protective functions for children: (1) They provide assistance to parents with child care tasks and responsibilities; (2) networks provide options for the temporary and/or permanent redistribution of children; and (3) networks afford the context for collective standards and, therefore, for the scrutiny and enforcement of child care standards. Embeddedness of childrearing in kin and community acts against the social isolation that has been linked with child maltreatment in industrialized nations (Garbarino & Crouter, 1978; Garbarino & Sherman, 1980).

Assistance

Social networks provide options for assistance with child care. This may take the form of alternative caretakers who provide relief from unremitting responsibility for child care. It also may take the form of temporary or permanent fosterage or adoption, which allows redistribution of children who would otherwise be unwanted and vulnerable to maltreatment.

Shared responsibility for children's welfare provides sources of alternative caretakers. Alternative caretakers may be other adults or older household children. If alternative caretakers are older household children, this assistance with caretaking serves the additional function of providing experience in child care that acts against the ignorance of child development and age-inappropriate expectations associated with child maltreatment in industrialized nations.

Redistribution

Social networks with shared responsibility for children and their care also allow redistribution of children, some of whom might be at risk of abuse or neglect with their biological parents. Children who are not wanted by their parents can be absorbed into other households where they are wanted for their economic or emotional contributions. Mechanisms such as child lending, fostering, and informal adoption allow redistribution of children on a temporary or permanent basis.

Informal child lending may ease the stress of children who tax scarce family resources. In some black communities in the United States, children are regularly redistributed among a network of households depending on the need for child helpers and the available resources. If one family is low on its food stamps, for example, the children may go to live for a few weeks with an "aunt" who has a better supply (Stack, 1974).

Among Polynesians, the care of adopted children tends to be warm and loving (Carroll, 1970; Gallimore et al., 1974). *Hanai*, the Hawaiian term for informal adoption, literally means "to feed." Children are frequently adopted because of the emotional value attached to children. Hawaiians believe that "a house without children is a house without life" (Young, 1980, p. 12).

Adopted children are thought to have an advantage because they have two sets of parents, biological and adoptive, who will care about their welfare.

The impact of redistribution of children on maltreatment is inextricably linked to the cultural context. While promoting well-being and even survival for children who might otherwise be subject to abuse or neglect, redistribution does not necessarily ensure an absence of subsequent maltreatment.

Consensus, Scrutiny, and Enforcement

If child care is shared in a community, greater consensus is likely concerning the acceptable boundaries of child socialization methods and goals. Standards are more likely to be enforced and departures more noticeable. If others are regularly involved in child care, intervention across families is less likely to be viewed as unduly intrusive or a strategy of last resort.

While physical discipline, or threats thereof, may be accepted by a community, the presence of networks provides safeguards against excess. If child care tasks and children are shared, rather than considered the property of one or two biological parents, a situation is more likely in which no one needs an invitation to intervene in the case of an overly severe spanking (Olson, 1981). Rural Hawaiian–Polynesian American parents more frequently express concern that hitting a child too often or too hard will cause resentment in the child rather than concern that the child will be physically hurt. Relatives do not hesitate to yell from one house to the next that a spanking has gone on long enough or is too severe for the child's misbehavior. Children are quite open about calling for help more quickly and loudly than a spanking warrants as an effective strategy for disarming an angry parent (Korbin, 1987b, 1990b).

A neighborhood-based, child-centered strategy must include increased willingness of others to intervene on behalf of children. This applies to known and related children as well as to unknown and unrelated children. Intervention can take place on behalf of children in general, such as protecting them from strangers or assisting them when lost. Intervention can take place specifically in response to physical aggression (e.g., spankings) in public (Brown, 1979; Davis, 1991). And, intervention can take place specifically in response to suspected abuse.

For a neighborhood-based child protection strategy to succeed, adults beyond the biological parents must have some investment in children's welfare. Beyond a child's own network of kin, neighbors, and friends, the willingness of nonparental adults, known and unknown to the child, to intervene or act on behalf of children is an important component in neighborhood-based child protection (e.g., Daro, 1991). Anecdotally, people who grew up in small towns and neighborhoods often recall that if they misbehaved or were somewhere they should not be, a neighbor would come outside to let them know that their behavior was being monitored. In our current research on neighborhood factors affecting child abuse and neglect in Cleveland, Ohio, approximately 88% of neighborhood residents ($n = 121$) reported that when they were children, if they misbehaved when their parents were not present, someone else would intervene to make them behave. Only 32% believed that the same would be true today (Korbin & Coulton, 1994.) Among the reasons provided for nonintervention, residents believed that parents would side with the child, or that the parent or child would retaliate against them (Korbin & Coulton, 1994).

The willingness of unknown and/or unrelated others to intervene on behalf of children has not been well studied with respect to child maltreatment. The literature in social psychology on "bystander behavior" (e.g., Dovido, 1984; Baumeister, Chesner, Senders, & Tice, 1988; Tice & Baumeister, 1985) may be relevant to the well-being of children. The literature on bystander behavior seeks to identify situational (e.g., presence of others and appearance of person in need of help) and individual characteristics (e.g., personality factors and leadership position) that promote altruistic or prosocial intervention in public. It is based on simulated circumstances or emergencies where there is little risk to the intervener. While there are limits to the generalizability of this line of research to actual behavior, this kind of intervention could be promoted at the neighborhood level.

The evidence of nonrelated individuals intervening in parental behavior in public is sparse. Although public awareness of child abuse and neglect has increased dramatically, such that almost all adults are aware of the existence of the problem, less than one fifth (17%) of individuals in a random survey indicated that they had acted to make someone stop hitting a child (National Committee for Prevention of Child Abuse, 1990). In the face of a cultural value for minding one's own business and cultural acceptance of physical force directed at children, individuals may be hesitant to intervene in public spankings.

Davis (1991) interviewed 37 individuals (involved in 50 incidents) who initiated an encounter in response to public child punishment. Most of the individuals who intervened were women addressing a punishing mother. Those who intervened received a hostile response from the punishing parent and a mixed reaction from individuals in their own networks. For example, one woman's husband warned her to stay out of the conflict, that she was lucky that the parent did not turn around and hit her. Indeed, "there is a common shift in interactive focus from the wrongful treatment of the child to the deviant involvement of the stranger" (Davis, 1991, p. 242).

Publicity about cases in which neighbors or unrelated others tried to intervene may act to both encourage and discourage such intervention. For example, in the well-known Lisa Steinberg case, neighbors' reports to child protective services did not result in protection for Lisa or prevent her death. In the well-publicized Jeffrey Dahmer case, recordings were played on the radio and television of a woman insisting that the soon-to-be victim looked like a child and pleading with the police to investigate the case and make sure that the boy was safe. Incidents such as these may reinforce a belief that intervention will do little good and that outsiders will not be listened to.

A neighborhood-based strategy that relies on unrelated others must be cognizant of the fact that it runs counter to American values. First, family privacy is a dearly held American value. Neighbors who intervene are sometimes portrayed as snoops or busybodies who peer over their fences or through their blinds (sometimes with binoculars to further make the point). These individuals usually make trouble rather than preventing it or being part of the solution. "Good" neighbors tend to their own business and only intervene in family matters when asked, for example, for a cup of sugar; thus the saying, "Fences good neighbors make."

There is potential, however, for fostering a cooperative neighborhood strategy as indicated by the existence of neighborhood or block parent(s) and neighborhood watch associations. Many informal arrangements exist in neighborhoods, and it is a challenge of a neighborhood-based strategy to identify and capitalize on them. Family privacy may not be threatened when a neighborhood engages itself in a cooperative effort aimed at the well-being of all its children and families and not at identifying and investigating only some.

Second, American values tend toward professionalism in intervention. The tradition of professional law enforcement acts strongly against individual citizen intervention. Vigilantes are strongly discouraged. People who intervene in crimes can be hurt and/or prosecuted if they inflict injury on the perpetrator of the crime. Thus, if neighbors or unknown others are to intervene in child protection, some degree of alteration of basic values will be necessary.

Third, the U.S. tolerance of physical discipline of children and the confusion about where the boundaries ought to be set promote nonintervention in families who are seen punishing their children. Indeed, parents who do not spank their children may be the ones accused of poor parenting. The widespread acceptance of physical punishment of children is reflected in the finding that 70% of family physicians and 59% of pediatricians support the practice (McCormick, 1992).

In a discussion of the positive aspects of network involvement, it must also be mentioned that there may be drawbacks to network involvement (see Thompson, Chapter 3, this volume). First, not all networks are good networks. Proximity of kin does not necessarily mean that those individuals will be helpful or supportive. Further, if individuals in one's network are inadequate parents, this inadequacy may reinforce patterns of abusive or neglectful child treatment in the target parents. Potentially abusive or neglectful parents may take solace or comfort in the idea that they are not "bad" parents but simply behaving like everyone else around them. In a study of fatally abusing mothers, Korbin (1989, 1991) found that networks sometimes reinforced mothers' ideas that they were not abusive parents but within the range of normal.

Along these lines, child abuse and neglect work often engages in a major contradiction. Even though the intergenerational transmission of abusive parenting has been challenged in recent literature (e.g., Kaufman & Zigler, 1987; Widom, 1989), it is still among the most commonly held etiological explanations for child maltreatment. At the same time, family members, including grandparents, are the preferred placements for children who must be removed from parental care. Thus, children are being placed with the very individuals whom the field believes contributed powerfully to the abusive parents' behavior in the first place.

Further, even if informal networks protect children from abuse or neglect in the short run, they may be impeded in the long run. As an example, in Cleveland we are using a case for teaching in which a substance-using young mother repeatedly left her infant unattended in her apartment. An unrelated neighbor, observing this behavior, volunteered to watch the baby when the mother went out. The mother then abandoned the child with the neighbor, who has been caring for the child for 4 years. The boy is bright, healthy, developing well, and regards this neighbor as "mommy." Taken from a viewpoint that only examines whether someone in the informal helping networks will care for the child, it looks as if the neighborhood is functioning well to protect its children. However, nobody has legal custody of the child. Routine health care has been performed because health care providers have assumed the woman bringing the boy to appointments had either a biological or legal relationship with him. However, what happens when the child needs minor surgery requiring a legal consent form or must be registered for school?

Values on Children and Categories of Vulnerable Children

In formulating a neighborhood-based strategy, neither a romantic version of the value of children nor a view that some cultures mistreat their children will be helpful. The cross-cultural literature suggests that child maltreatment is less likely in cultures in which children are highly valued for their economic utility, for perpetuating family lines and the cultural heritage, or as sources of emotional pleasure and satisfaction. Nevertheless, generalized cultural values on children are not sufficient in and of themselves to prevent maltreatment. All cultures espouse a value on children in general and a disvalue on their deliberate harm. However, certain cultural values may place some children at greater risk than others, even in cultures that have a high general value on children. This disvalue or undervalue may be expressed in a range of behaviors. Such children may be subjected to deliberate infanticide, physical abuse and neglect, sexual misuse, psychological maltreatment, or economic exploitation. If, for example, children primarily are valued for their economic contribution, those who fail to be useful may be at increased risk of mal-treatment. If children are valued to perpetuate family lines and cultural tra-ditions, in societies that require males to perform requisite ceremonies, daugh-ters are less valued and at greater risk of maltreatment (Wolf, 1974; Wu, 1981). Further, if children are expected to be sources of psychological and emotional satisfaction, they may fail parental expectations, making them vulnerable to abuse. This has been an important dynamic contributing to child abuse in the United States (Steele, 1980).

The cross-cultural record suggests categories of children who are at greater risk of maltreatment. Some of these categories can be identified through demographic analyses of differential mortality patterns (Johanson, 1984; Scrimshaw, 1978); other categories can be identified only with a thor-ough understanding of the cultural context. All such categories, however, may be exacerbated or mitigated by the cultural context in which they occur. A multicultural neighborhood-based strategy would require an understand-ing of categories of vulnerable children. Examples of categories of under-valued and disvalued children have been discussed elsewhere (e.g., Korbin, 1981, 1987b).

The cross-cultural record strongly suggests that children with diminished social networks are vulnerable to maltreatment. In the work of LeVine and LeVine (1981) in East Africa, children from broken homes or out-of-wedlock births accounted for 2.5% of the population but 25% of malnourished chil-dren. Five of the eight deaths of children under 5 years of age during the 2 years of their study were born of illegitimate unions (LeVine & LeVine, 1981). Fraser and Kilbride (1980) similarly found that children from inter-tribal marriages among the Samia of East Africa were at increased risk of neglect. If the marriage floundered and the children were not well cared for, neither the kin of the mother nor the kin of the father felt that the children necessarily fell under their protection.

Stepchildren are at increased risk of maltreatment in a number of soci-eties. In the United States and European nations, stepchildren are more vul-nerable to abuse (Daly & Wilson, 1985) and sexual molestation (Finkelhor, 1984; Russell, 1984).

A case of neglect in a rural Hawaiian–Polynesian American community underlined the problems of a child who did not have a network of concerned kin. The child was not well liked by his stepfather, and the mother's parents and kin did not live in the community. Unrelated community adults were kind to the child, watched out for him when they could, and fed him when he appeared in their yards. However, he was frequently found wandering about the community well after dark when the rest of the small children had been gathered up and taken home. He frequently complained of stomach-aches and often had a distended belly from gorging himself at the many households in which his requests for food would be met. The child was viewed as neglected by the adults in the community. However, because most were unrelated to the parents, they did not feel that they could actively intervene on behalf of the child. All they could do was feed him and treat him kindly when they stumbled on him. The child's plight was viewed as unacceptable and the parents culpable (Korbin, 1990b).

Although categories of vulnerable children can be delineated cross-culturally, the potential for maltreatment can be mitigated by social networks. Communities vary in the degree of risk for child maltreatment according to the balance of social supports and stresses (Garbarino & Sherman, 1980). When childrearing is a shared concern within a supportive network, the consequences of having an inadequate or aggressive parent are diminished.

With the cultural context carefully considered, a neighborhood-based child protection strategy has the potential to make significant others in protective social networks available for children in their neighborhoods and communities through (1) formal networks (e.g., schools), (2) informal networks (e.g., scouts, Big Brothers, and Big Sisters), (3) mix of formal and informal networks (e.g., churches, religious organizations), and (4) informal networks of kin (i.e., consanguineal, affinal, and fictive).

SOCIOCULTURAL FACTORS AFFECTING THE ACCEPTANCE AND EFFICACY OF CHILD PROTECTIVE SERVICES

The literature in international health and medical anthropology (e.g., Coriel & Mull, 1990; Nichter, 1989; United Nations International Children's Emergency Fund [UNICEF], 1990) is potentially applicable to neighborhood-based child protection services. Efforts in international health programs have shown repeatedly that program acceptance and efficacy depend on congruence with the needs and cultural beliefs of the target community. For example, if diarrheal disease is not perceived to result from contaminated water, then programs to educate mothers to boil water will be unsuccessful. As with international health work centered on smaller living units (e.g., a village), a neighborhood-based child protection strategy will have to assess what the neighborhood residents perceive to be the major problems for child protection. For example, the danger from handguns in the neighborhood may rank higher with residents than a concern about spanking.

Improving acceptance of child protective services cannot be accomplished by addressing cultural values alone. The way that the system addresses clients in general, and culturally diverse clients in particular, must be considered. Cultural values in and of themselves do not impede acceptance of child protective services. However, when combined with mistrust and suspicion of "the system," child protection efforts as currently structured may be compromised. Folk wisdom heard over and over again in clinical settings is that child protective services "takes your kids away" rather than helps families.

Several writers have suggested cultural values that impede use of child protection agencies, such as familialism among the Chinese (Hong & Hong, 1991) or African American values of not "putting your business into the street." Long (1986) provided an example from a Native American community in which an uncle molested his young niece. Even though relatives agreed that the uncle's behavior was wrong and the child victimized, loyalty to the clan remained a critically important variable. Relatives opposed the mother's reporting the abuse to a white agency and relentlessly pressured her not to pursue prosecution of the offending uncle.

Opposition to involvement of child protection agencies, however, does not mean that culturally diverse groups spurn utilizing a wider network for help with family problems and issues, including those related to child maltreatment. For example, in many African American communities, the church is an important vehicle for help with family matters that has been largely unrecognized and underutilized by official social service agencies (e.g., Pinderhughes, 1982). The church is a trusted institution over which members of the community have some control.

In the example of the Native American sexual abuse case discussed above, the mother's refusal to participate in prosecution of the uncle did not mean that she would not act to protect the child. However, protection was accomplished along more culturally congruent lines. The therapist helped the mother and daughter to reintegrate themselves into their support system of maternal relatives and assisted the mother in formulating plans for protecting the daughter in ways that were more culturally acceptable than legal prosecution (e.g., leaving her with other relatives when the uncle was present, particularly if alcohol was being consumed). In maintaining integration in the clan network, the mother may have selected the most effective protective strategy for her child. Reintegration into a network of known individuals who opposed the perpetrator's behavior (even if not willing to extrude the uncle from the group), and who would help to protect the child in the future, was a better bet than trying to punish/prosecute. Prosecution would have excluded the mother and her child from their support network and not necessarily protected the child (particularly because prosecution in child sexual abuse cases is so often unsuccessful).

Further, ethnically diverse groups' hesitancy to utilize child protective services does not necessarily indicate a generalized hesitancy to use helping services. Head Start, for example, has a long tradition of being a helpful institution in the community. Child Protective Services, on the other hand, has been linked with investigations that often result in the removal of children from the home. Thus, in assessing the impact of culture on willingness to use services, the type of service and past experience with that service must be carefully considered. For a neighborhood-based strategy, one important distinction may be more general/generic family services as compared with services specific to child abuse and neglect.

Treatment Modalities and Strategies

In a recent review of the literature on the treatment of culturally diverse children, Tharp (1991) noted that "research on cultural issues in clinical treatment is scant, particularly research addressing such issues with children" (p. 799). Similarly, McGoldrick et al. (1982), in reviewing family therapy, suggested that culturally specific family therapy is underdeveloped.

A neighborhood-based strategy is likely to improve its chances for being effective if it takes the ethnic/cultural backgrounds of residents into account in its interventions. "The hypothesis of cultural compatibility suggests that treatment is more effective when compatible with client culture patterns" (Tharp, 1991, p. 802). Tharp suggests that there are three variants of cultural compatibility in treatment of children. First, there are specific, distinctive, and unique modalities of treatment for different cultures. However, these are rare in the literature. One variant of the culturally specific model is to utilize indigenous treatments and healers. For example, *ho'o'ponopono* is a traditional form of family discussion and conflict resolution among Hawaiians (Shook, 1985) that has been utilized in child abuse intervention. Another variant is to design treatment modalities for specific cultures. Tharp points out that even though the issue of cultural compatibility in treatment is not a new debate, few such treatment modalities have been developed. An example is *cuento* therapy developed for Puerto Rican children, which adapts the traditional use of folktales in child socialization to foster discussion of current difficulties. Bilingual, bicultural therapists were utilized, as were culturally familiar stories and characters. The mother also was involved in the therapy sessions. *Cuento* therapy was reported to reduce children's trait anxiety in comparison to traditional therapy and no intervention and to improve intelligence test scores (Costantino, Malgady, & Rogler, 1986).

Second, there are "two-type" modalities that view the majority culture on one side and all children of color on the other. In this view, ethnically diverse children share common problems (e.g., poverty and oppression), which are at the root of their difficulties. Thus, a single modality addressing these root problems is sufficient and cultural diversity will not be a significant impediment.

Third, there are universalistic strategies that assume that treatment and intervention will work, with perhaps slight variation, for all groups. Tharp (1991) suggests that because universalistic strategies start with the individual, rather than the wider social network, there may be substantial barriers to the success of intervention with children from cultures in which families and social networks are important. He suggests that treatment strategies start with the larger network of individuals involved with a child, a suggestion well suited to a neighborhood strategy. Above all, treatment interventions must be contextualized (Tharp, 1991).

Tharp (1991) suggests that culturally informed therapeutic interventions with children use education as a model. Schools are, by necessity, multicultural and have had to adapt to this reality. Although the educational issues in multicultural education (e.g., bilingual education) can be contentious, and are by no means resolved, the experience of the educational system in educating culturally diverse children provides a body of experience that lends itself to multicultural contexts in other domains, such as child protection.

A major and contentious debate is whether therapists and child protection workers must be matched with clients by ethnicity. Sue (1988) found that "cultural" matching (shared beliefs, behaviors, values based on cultural membership) had a positive impact on therapy, but "ethnic" matching (shared descent but not shared beliefs, behaviors, and values) had no direct impact. Increasing the representation of culturally diverse therapists and service providers will be important in a successful neighborhood-based strategy so that residents will have the option of selecting a service provider or therapist with whom they can best work.

Further, linguistic skills will not necessarily ensure culturally informed, culturally competent child protection. For example, anecdotal information suggests that members of closely knit communities may decline an interpreter in cases of child sexual abuse because they do not want their shame to become widely known (as they assume it will if an interpreter from the community becomes aware of the case). As a second example, some Puerto Ricans in a New York City neighborhood studied by Urciuoli (1990) found the use of the Spanish language by white social service providers to be threatening in that it demeaned them and insinuated that they were ignorant of English. She also suggested that the use of Spanish by outsiders was perceived as an intrusion on the intimacy experienced by those who share the cultural heritage implicated by Spanish language use. Harwood (1981) found that some individuals felt insulted by outsiders' use of Spanish, whereas others preferred communicating in their own language. As with worker and therapist choice, in a culturally informed and culturally competent neighborhood child protection system, individuals should be consulted as to their preferred language for communication.

There is a vast array of unpublished handbooks and guides for working with culturally diverse populations. These publications are often specific to one locality. Although it is difficult to compile this literature on a nationwide basis, such a compilation would be invaluable to a successful neighborhood-based child protection strategy.

It should be stressed, however, that no set of generalizations about any cultural or ethnic population will be sufficient to deal with child maltreatment among culturally diverse populations. As discussed above, the importance of within-culture variability, and the need to "unpack" the cultural variable, precludes the development of a library-like card catalogue of strategies for working with specific cultural groups. Whereas knowledge of general cultural patterns provides an important starting point, a successful neighborhood-based child protection strategy will require each neighborhood to be assessed on its own merits, rather than trying to make it conform to a cultural stereotype.

A CULTURALLY INFORMED, CULTURALLY COMPETENT NEIGHBORHOOD-BASED, CHILD-CENTERED CHILD PROTECTION STRATEGY

Interest in the relationship between culture and child maltreatment has experienced a resurgence. In the mid- to late 1970s in particular, there was a great deal of interest in culture and child maltreatment (e.g., PSRI, 1977). Federal funding was provided for culturally specific resource centers, and issues of culture appeared in national conferences. In the past few years, the issue of culture has emerged again. The National Committee for Prevention of Child Abuse has cultural competence as an top priority. The People of Color Leadership Institute is federally funded. Several innovative programs on cultural competence are being developed and disseminated, some published (e.g., Cross, Bazron, Dennis, & Isaacs, 1989) and some unpublished.

Although most writers acknowledge that the relationship between culture and child maltreatment is poorly understood, culture is widely thought to be of critical importance in understanding child maltreatment as well as developing successful prevention and intervention strategies (e.g., Alfaro, 1981; Beavers, 1986; Cohn, 1982; Cross et al., 1989; Eisenberg, 1981; Garbarino & Ebata, 1983; Gelles, 1987; Green, 1978, 1982; Korbin, 1987b, 1992; Slaughter, 1988).

Flexibility in dealing with cultural issues, a major strength of a neighborhood-based child protection strategy, will also present challenges. Whereas guidelines may exist for some cultural or ethnic populations, stereotypes must be avoided and any search for easy answers is likely to be futile.Prior knowledge of the culture is of immeasurable value but is not sufficient in and of itself to address a problem as complex as child maltreatment. As merely one example, a neighborhood-based child protection strategy in a predominantly African American urban neighborhood would be well advised to begin with the assumption of strong kin and church networks. However, in "unpacking" the concept of culture, it must be remembered that not all individuals in the neighborhood will equally value or participate in kinship networks or church organizations. Of relevance to a child protection strategy, the marginal individuals who do not participate in kin or church networks, or whose networks are deviant or dysfunctional, are most likely to be at risk for abuse and neglect.

Neighborhoods cannot be defined on the basis of socioeconomic status or race alone. All poor neighborhoods are not alike (Coulton & Pandey, 1992). All white neighborhoods are not alike, nor are all black, Hispanic, or Asian neighborhoods. Culture and ethnicity must be self-defined, not defined from the outside.

Individuals, both those who are and those who are not of the same cultural background as the neighborhood being served, should be encouraged and rewarded for spending time in the neighborhood unrelated to child abuse investigation and intervention. This will afford a better understanding of the cultural continuum of behaviors and the point at which deviance in child care is identified.

A neighborhood-based strategy should be flexible enough to subdivide neighborhood designations. Census tracts or city-planning defined neighborhoods may not, in reality, meet residents' delineations of their neighborhoods. Further, rural neighborhoods must not be left out of the child-centered neighborhood-based approach.

Considering the remarkable cultural diversity of the United States, a neighborhood-based child protection system has substantial potential for meeting the dual goals of culturally informed and culturally competent child protection: (1) to respect and encompass cultural diversity and (2) to ensure an equitable standard of care and protection for all children. Neighborhoods, and the individuals who inhabit them, must be empowered to identify and meet their problems and to provide the best possible environment for their children.

ACKNOWLEDGMENT

I would like to express appreciation to the other authors in this volume, to Gary Melton and Frank Barry, and to Byron Gold for their helpful feedback on previous drafts of the paper.

NOTE

1. There is considerable variation on the appropriate terms to use for any cultural group. If terminology varies throughout the chapter, an effort was made to be consistent with literature cited. Further, examples have been used citing particular cultural or ethnic groups. These were intended as examples and not in any way to indicate that problems are unique to the culture or ethnic group used in the example. Descriptions of cultural practices are written in what is termed the "ethnographic present," the time at which such practices were described in the literature. Use of the "ethnographic present" does not necessarily imply that such practices still occur.

REFERENCES

Aber, L., & Zigler, E. (1981). Developmental considerations in the definition of child maltreatment. In R. Rizley & D. Cicchetti (Eds.), *Developmental perspectives on child maltreatment* (pp. 1–29). San Francisco: Jossey-Bass.

Alfaro, J. D. (1981). Child neglect and cultural tradition. *Human Ecology Forum*, 12, 26–30.

Amato, P. R. (1990). Personality and social network involvement as predictors of helping behavior in everyday life. *Social Psychology Quarterly*, 53(1), 31–43.

American Academy of Pediatrics. (1988). Religious exemptions from child abuse statutes. *Pediatrics*, 81(1), 169–171.

Asian tradition at war with American laws. (1988, February 10). *New York Times*, p. 18.

Baumeister, R. F., Chesner, S. P., Senders, P. S., & Tice, D. M. (1988). Who's in charge here? Group leaders do lend help in emergencies. *Personality and Social Psychology Bulletin*, 14(1), 17–22.

Beavers, C. (1986, Fall). A cross-cultural look at child abuse. *Public Welfare*, 44(4), 18–22.

Besharov, D. (1981). Toward better research on child abuse and neglect: Making definitional issues an explicit methodological concern. *Child Abuse and Neglect: The International Journal*, 5(4), 383–390.

Billingsley, A. (1969). Family functioning in the low income Black community. *Social Casework*, 50, 563–572.

Brown, B. W. (1979, January). Parents' discipline of children in public places. *Family Coordinator*, 28, 67–71.

Carr, A., & Gelles, R. J. (1978). *Reporting child maltreatment in Florida: The operation of public child protective service systems* (Report to the National Center on Child Abuse and Neglect). Washington, DC: U.S. Department of Health and Human Services.

Carroll, V. (Ed.). (1970). *Adoption in Eastern Oceania*. Honolulu: University of Hawaii Press.

Carson, B. (1986). *Parents who don't spank: Deviation in the legitimation of physical force*. Unpublished doctoral dissertation, University of New Hampshire.

Cazenave, N., & Straus, M. (1979). Race, class, network embeddedness and family violence. *Journal of Comparative Family Studies*, 10, 281–300.

Cohn, A. H. (1982). Stopping child abuse before it occurs: Different solutions for different population groups. *Child Abuse and Neglect: The International Journal*, 6(4), 473–483.

Coriel, J., & Mull, J. D. (1990). *Anthropology and primary health care*. Boulder, CO: Westview.

Costantino, G., Malgady, R., & Rogler, L. (1986). Cuento therapy: A culturally sensitive modality for Puerto Rican children. *Journal of Consulting and Clinical Psychology*, 54, 639–645.

Coulton, C., & Pandey, S. (1992). Geographic concentration of poverty and risk to children in urban neighborhoods. *American Behavioral Scientist*, 35(3), 238–257.

Cross, T., Bazron, B., Dennis, K., & Isaacs, M. (1989). *Towards a culturally competent system of care: CASSP Technical Assistance Center.* Washington, DC: Georgetown University Child Development Center.

Daly, M., & Wilson, M. (1985). Child abuse and other risks of not living with both parents. *Ethnology and Sociobiology,* 6, 197–210.

Daniel, J. (1985). Cultural and ethnic issues: The black family. In E. Newberger & R. Bourne (Eds.), *Unhappy families. Clinical and research perspectives on family violence* (pp. 145–153). Littleton, MA: PSG.

Daniel, J., Hampton, R., & Newberger, E. (1983). Child abuse and accidents in black families: A controlled comparative study. *American Journal of Orthopsychiatry,* 53(4), 645–653.

Daro, D. (1991). *Public attitudes and behaviors with respect to child abuse and prevention, 1987–1991.* Chicago: National Committee for Prevention of Child Abuse.

Davis, P. W. (1991). Stranger intervention into child punishment in public places. *Social Problems,* 38(2), 227–246.

DeFrancis, V. (1969). *Protecting the child victim of sex crimes committed by adults.* Denver, CO: American Humane Association.

Deitrich, G. (1982). Indian Child Welfare Act: Ideas for implementation. *Child Abuse and Neglect: The International Journal,* 6(2), 125–128.

Dovido, J. (1984). Helping behavior and altruism: An empirical and conceptual overview. In L. Berkowitz (Ed.), *Advances in experimental social psychology* (Vol. 17, pp. 361–427). New York: Academic Press.

Dubanoski, R. (1981). Child maltreatment in European- and Hawaiian-Americans. *Child Abuse and Neglect: The International Journal,* 5(4), 457–466.

Dubanoski, R., & Snyder, K. (1980). Patterns of child abuse and neglect in Japanese- and Samoan-Americans. *Child Abuse and Neglect: The International Journal,* 4(4), 217–225.

Edgerton, R. B. (1976). *Deviance: A cross-cultural perspective.* Menlo Park, CA: Cummings.

Edgerton, R. B. (1985). *Rules, exceptions, and social order.* Berkeley: University of California Press.

Eisenberg, L. (1981). Cross-cultural and historic perspectives on child abuse and neglect. *Child Abuse and Neglect: The International Journal,* 5(3), 299–308.

Feldman, K. W. (1984). Pseudoabusive burns in Asian refugees. *American Journal of Diseases in Children,* 138, 768–769.

Finkelhor, D. (1979). *Sexually victimized children.* New York: Free Press.

Finkelhor, D. (1984). *Child sexual abuse: New theory and research.* New York: Free Press.

Finkelhor, D., & Korbin, J. (1988). Child abuse as an international issue. *Child Abuse and Neglect: The International Journal,* 11(3), 397–407.

Finkelhor, D., & Williams, L. (1988). *Nursery crimes: Sexual abuse in day care.* Newbury Park, CA: Sage.

Fischler, R. S. (1985). Child abuse and neglect in American Indian communities. *Child Abuse and Neglect: The International Journal,* 9(1), 95–106.

Fraser, G., & Kilbride, P. (1980). Child abuse and neglect—Rare, but perhaps increasing, phenomenon among the Samia of Kenya. *Child Abuse and Neglect: The International Journal*, 4(4), 227–232.

Gallimore, R., Boggs, J., & Jordan, C. (1974). *Culture, behavior, and education: A study of Hawaiian-Americans*. Beverly Hills, CA: Sage.

Garbarino, J. (1977). The human ecology of child maltreatment. *Journal of Marriage and the Family*, 39(4), 721–735.

Garbarino, J., & Crouter, A. (1978). Defining the community context for parent–child relations: The correlates of child maltreatment. *Child Development*, 49, 604–616.

Garbarino, J., & Ebata, A. (1983). The significance of cultural and ethnic factors in child maltreatment. *Journal of Marriage and the Family*, 45(4), 773–783.

Garbarino, J., & Kostelny, K. (1992). Child maltreatment as a community problem. *Child Abuse and Neglect: The International Journal*, 16(4):455–464.

Garbarino, J., & Sherman, D. (1980). High risk neighborhoods and high risk families: The human ecology of child maltreatment. *Child Development*, 51, 188–198.

Gelles, R. J. (1982). Toward better research on child abuse and neglect: A response to Besharov. *Child Abuse and Neglect: The International Journal*, 6(4), 485–486.

Gelles, R. J. (1987). What to learn from cross-cultural and historical research on child abuse and neglect: An overview. In R. Gelles & J. Lancaster (Eds.), *Child abuse and neglect: Biosocial dimensions* (pp. 15–30). New York: Aldine De Gruyter.

Gelles, R. J. (1992). Poverty and violence towards children. *American Behavioral Scientist*, 35(3), 258–274.

Gelles, R. J., & Straus, M. A. (1988). *Intimate violence*. New York: Simon & Schuster.

Gil, D. (1970). *Violence against children: Physical child abuse in the United States*. Cambridge, MA: Harvard University Press.

Giovannoni, J., & Becerra, R. (1979). *Defining child abuse*. New York: Free Press.

Giovannoni, J., & Billingsley, A. (1970). Child neglect among the poor: A study of parental adequacy in families of three ethnic groups. *Child Welfare*, 49(4), 196–204.

Graburn, N. (1987). Severe child abuse among the Canadian Inuit. In N. Scheper-Hughes (Ed.), *Child survival: Anthropological perspectives on the treatment and maltreatment of children* (pp. 211–226). Dordrecht, Holland: D. Reidel.

Gray, E., & Cosgrove, J. (1985). Ethnocentric perception of childrearing practices in protective services. *Child Abuse and Neglect: The International Journal*, 9(3), 389–396.

Green, J. W. (1978). The role of cultural anthropology in the education of social service personnel. *Journal of Sociology and Social Welfare*, 5(2), 214–229.

Green, J. W. (1982). *Cultural awareness in the human services*. Englewood Cliffs, NJ: Prentice Hall.

Hampton, R. (Ed.). (1987). *Violence in the Black family: Correlates and consequences*. Lexington, MA: Lexington Books.

Hampton, R. L., Gelles, R. J., & Harrop, J. W. (1989). Is violence in black families increasing? A comparison of 1975 and 1985 national survey rates. *Journal of Marriage and the Family*, 51, 969–980.

Hampton, R. L., & Newberger, E. (1985). Child abuse incidence and reporting by hospitals: Significance of severity, class, and race. *American Journal of Public Health*, 75(1), 45–58.

Harwood, A. (Ed.). (1981). *Ethnicity and medical care*. Cambridge, MA: Harvard University Press.

Hauswald, L. (1987). External pressure/internal change: Child neglect on the Navajo reservation. In N. Scheper-Hughes (Ed.), *Child survival: Anthropological approaches on the treatment and maltreatment of children* (pp. 145–164). Dordrecht, Holland: D. Reidel.

Holton, J. (1990). *Black families and child abuse prevention: An African-American perspective and approach* (Working Paper No. 852). Chicago: National Committee for Prevention of Child Abuse.

Hong, G. K., & Hong, L. K. (1991). Comparative perspectives on child abuse and neglect: Chinese versus Hispanics and whites. *Child Welfare*, 70(4), 463–475.

Horowitz, B., & Wolock, I. (1981). Material deprivation, child maltreatment, and agency interventions among poor families. In L. Pelton (Ed.), *The social context of child abuse and neglect*. New York: Human Sciences Press.

Jason, J., Amereuh, N., Marks, J., & Tyler, C. (1982). Child abuse in Georgia: A method to evaluate risk factors and reporting bias. *American Journal of Public Health*, 72(12), 1353–1358.

Jason, J., Williams, S., Burton, A., & Rochat, R. (1982). Epidemiological differences between sexual and physical abuse. *Journal of the American Medical Association*, 247(24), 3344–3345.

Johansson, S. (1984). Deferred infanticide: Excess female mortality during childhood. In G. Hausfater & S. Hrdy (Eds.), *Infanticide: Comparative and evolutionary perspectives* (pp. 463–486). New York: Aldine.

Kadushin, A., & Martin, J. (1981). *Child abuse: An interactional event*. New York: Columbia University Press.

Kaufman, J., & Zigler, E. (1987) Do abused children become abusive parents? *American Journal of Orthopsychiatry*, 57(2), 186–192.

Kempe, C. H., Silverman, F. N., Droegmueller, W., & Silver, H. K. (1962). The battered child syndrome. *Journal of the American Medical Association*, 181, 17–24.

Korbin, J. (1977). Anthropological contributions to the study of child abuse. *Child Abuse and Neglect: The International Journal*, 1(1), 7–24.

Korbin, J. (1978). *Caretaking patterns in a rural Hawaiian community: Congruence of child and observer reports*. Unpublished doctoral dissertation, University of California, Los Angeles.

Korbin, J. (Ed.). (1981). *Child abuse and neglect: Cross-cultural perspectives*. Berkeley: University of California Press.

Korbin, J. (1987a). Child abuse and neglect: The cultural context. In R. Helfer & R. Kempe (Eds.), *The battered child* (4th ed., pp. 23–41). Chicago: University of Chicago Press.

Korbin, J. (1987b). Child maltreatment in cross-cultural perspective: Vulnerable children and circumstances. In R. Gelles & J. Lancaster (Eds.), *Child abuse and neglect: Biosocial dimensions* (pp. 31–55). New York: Aldine.

Korbin, J. (1989). Fatal maltreatment by mothers: A proposed framework. *Child Abuse and Neglect: The International Journal*, 13, 481–489.

Korbin, J. (1990a). Child sexual abuse: A cross-cultural view. In R. K. Oates (Ed.), *Understanding and managing child sexual abuse* (pp. 42–58). Sydney, Australia: Harcourt Brace, Jovanovich. (Original work published 1987)

Korbin, J. (1990b). Hana'ino: Child maltreatment in a Hawaiian-American community. *Pacific Studies, 13*(3), 6–22.

Korbin, J. (1991, November). *"Good mothers," "babykillers," and fatal child abuse.* Paper presented at the annual meetings of the American Anthropological Association, Chicago.

Korbin, J. (1992). *Cultural competence in child protection.* Unpublished manuscript.

Korbin, J., & Coulton, C. (1991). *Neighborhood impact on child abuse and neglect* (Grant proposal to the National Center on Child Abuse and Neglect). Washington, DC: NCCAN.

Korbin, J., & Coulton, C. (1994). *Neighborhood impact on child abuse and neglect* (Final project report to the National Center on Child Abuse and Neglect). Washington, DC: U. S. Department of Health and Human Services.

Krantzler, N. J. (1987). Traditional medicine as "medical neglect": Dilemmas in the case management of a Samoan teenager with diabetes. In N. Scheper-Hughes (Ed.), *Child survival: Anthropological perspectives on the treatment and maltreatment of children* (pp. 325–338). Dordrecht, Holland: D. Reidel.

Larson, O., Doris, J., & Alvarez, W. (1987). Child maltreatment among East Coast migrant farm workers. *Child Abuse and Neglect: The International Journal, 11*(2), 281–291.

Lauderdale, M., Valiunas, A., & Anderson, R. (1980). Race, ethnicity, and child maltreatment: An empirical analysis. *Child Abuse and Neglect: The International Journal, 4*(3), 163–169.

LeVine, S., & LeVine, R. (1981). Child abuse and neglect in Sub-Saharan Africa. In J. Korbin (Ed.), *Child abuse and neglect: Cross-cultural perspectives* (pp. 35–55). Berkeley: University of California Press.

Levy, J. (1964). The fate of Navajo twins. *American Anthropologist, 66,* 883–887.

Light, R. (1973). Abused and neglected children in America: A study of alternative policies. *Harvard Educational Review, 43,* 556–598.

Long, K. A. (1986). Cultural considerations in the assessment and treatment of intrafamilial abuse. *American Journal of Orthopsychiatry, 56*(1), 131–136.

McCormick, K. (1992). Attitudes of primary care physicians toward corporal punishment. *Journal of American Medical Association, 267*(23), 3161–3165.

McGoldrick, M., Pearce, J. K., & Giordano, J. (Eds.). (1982). *Ethnicity and family therapy.* New York: Guilford Press.

Mendoza, R. (1984). Acculturation and sociocultural variability. In J. L. Martinez (Ed.), *Chicano psychology* (2nd ed., pp. 61–74). New York: Academic Press.

Morris, B. (1979). Value differences in definitions of child abuse and neglect: Jehovah's Witnesses: A case example. *Child Abuse and Neglect: The International Journal, 3*(3/4), 651–655.

Mrazek, P. (1981). Definition and recognition of child abuse: Historical and cultural perspectives. In P. Mrazek & C. H. Kempe (Eds.), *Sexually abused children and their families* (pp. 5–15). New York: Pergamon Press.

National Center on Child Abuse and Neglect. (1981). *Study findings: National study of incidence and severity of child abuse and neglect.* Washington, DC: U.S. Department of Health and Human Services.

National Center on Child Abuse and Neglect. (1988). *Study findings: Study of national incidence and prevalence of child abuse and neglect: 1988*. Washington, DC: U.S. Department of Health and Human Services.

National Committee for Prevention of Child Abuse and Neglect. (1990). *Public attitudes and action regarding child abuse and its prevention, 1990*. Chicago: Author.

Newberger, E., Reed, R., Daniel, J. H., Hyde, J., & Kotelchuck, M. (1977). Pediatric social illness: Towards an etiologic classification. *Pediatrics, 60*, 178–185.

Nichter, M. (1989). *Anthropology and international health: South Asian case studies*. Boston: Kluwer.

Olson, E. (1981). Socioeconomic and psychocultural contexts of child abuse and neglect in Turkey. In J. Korbin (Ed.), *Child abuse and neglect: Cross-cultural perspectives* (pp. 96–119). Berkeley: University of California Press.

O'Toole, R., Turbett, P., & Nalepka, C. (1983). Theories, professional knowledge, and diagnosis of child abuse. In D. Finkelhor, R. Gelles, G. Hotaling, & M. Straus (Eds.), *The dark side of families: Current family violence research*. Beverly Hills, CA: Sage.

Parke, R., & Collmer, C. W. (1975). *Child abuse: An interdisciplinary perspective*. Chicago: University of Chicago Press.

Peters, J. (1976). Children who are victims of sexual assault and the psychology of offenders. *American Journal of Psychotherapy, 30*, 395–421.

Pilisuk, M., & Parks, S. H. (1986). *The healing web: Social networks and human survival*. Hanover, NH: University Press of New England.

Pinderhughes, E. (1982). Afro-American families and the victim system. In M. McGoldrick, J. K. Pearce, & J. Giordano (Eds.), *Ethnicity and family therapy* (pp. 108–122). New York: Guilford Press.

Polansky, N., Chalmers, M., Buttenwieser, E., & Williams, D. (1981). *An anatomy of child neglect*. Chicago: University of Chicago Press.

Protective Services Resource Institute. (1977). Child abuse, neglect and the family within a cultural context [Special issue]. *PSRI Report*.

Reid, S. (1984). Cultural differences and child abuse intervention with undocumented Spanish-speaking families in Los Angeles. *Child Abuse and Neglect: The International Journal, 8*(1), 109–112.

Ritchie, J., & Ritchie, J. (1981). Child rearing and child abuse: The Polynesian context. In J. Korbin (Ed.), *Child abuse and neglect: Cross-cultural perspectives* (pp. 186–294). Berkeley: University of California Press.

Rizley, R., & Cicchetti, D. (Eds.). (1981). *Developmental perspectives on child maltreatment*. San Francisco: Jossey-Bass.

Russell, D. (1984). The prevalence and seriousness of incestuous abuse: Step-fathers versus biological fathers. *Child Abuse and neglect: The International Journal, 7*, 133–146.

Russell, D. E. H. (1986). *The secret trauma: Incest in the lives of girls and women*. New York: Basic Books.

Sandler, A. P., & Haynes, V. (1978). Nonaccidental trauma and medical folk belief: A case of cupping. *Pediatrics, 61*(6), 921–922.

Schorr, L. B., with Schorr, D. (1988). *Within our reach: Breaking the cycle of violence*. London: Doubleday.

Scott, K. (1992). Childhood sexual abuse: Impact on a community's mental health status. *Child Abuse and Neglect: The International Journal, 16*, 285–295.

Scrimshaw, S. (1978). Infant mortality and behavior in the regulation of family size. *Population and Development Review, 4*(3), 383–403.

Shook, E. V. (1985). *Ho'o'ponopono. Contemporary uses of a Hawaiian problem-solving process*. Honolulu: East-West Center.

Singelenberg, R. (1990). The blood transfusion taboo of Jehovah's Witnesses: Origin, development and function of a controversial doctrine. *Social Science and Medicine, 31*(4), 515–523.

Slaughter, D. (1988). Programs for racially and ethnically diverse American families: Some critical issues. In H. B. Weiss & F. H. Jacobs (Eds.), *Evaluating family programs* (pp. 461–476). New York: Aldine.

Snow, L. (1977). Popular medicine in a black neighborhood. In E. Spicer (Ed.), *Ethnic medicine in the Southwest* (pp. 19–95). Tucson: University of Arizona Press.

Stack, C. (1974). *All our kin. Strategies for survival in a black community*. New York: Harper & Row.

Stark, R., & McEvoy, J. (1970, November). Middle class violence. *Psychology Today*, pp. 52–65.

Steele, B. F. (1980). Psychodynamic factors in child abuse. In C. H. Kempe & R. E. Helfer (Eds.), *The battered child* (pp. 48–85). Chicago: University of Chicago Press.

Sternberg, K., & Lamb, M. E. (1991). Can we ignore context in the definition of child maltreatment? *Development and Psychopathology, 3*(1), 87–92.

Straus, M., & Gelles, R. (1986). Societal change and change in family violence from 1975–1985 as revealed by two national surveys. *Journal of Marriage and the Family, 48*, 465–479.

Straus, M., Gelles, R., & Steinmetz, S. (1980). *Behind closed doors: Violence in the American family*. New York: Anchor.

Sue, S. (1988). Psychotherapeutic services for ethnic minorities: Two decades of research findings. *American Psychologist, 43*(4), 301–308.

Tharp, R. G. (1991). Cultural diversity and the treatment of children. *Journal of Consulting and Clinical Psychology, 59*(6), 799–812.

Tice, D. M., & Baumeister, R. F. (1985). Masculinity inhibits helping in emergencies: Personality does predict the bystander effect. *Journal of Personality and Social Psychology, 49*(2), 420–428.

Trotter, R., Ackerman, A., Rodman, D., Martinez, A., & Sorvillo, F. (1983). "Azarcon" and "Greta": Ethnomedical solution to epidemiological mystery. *Medical Anthropology Quarterly, 14*(3), 3, 18.

United Nations International Children's Emergency Fund. (1990). *The state of the world's children, 1990*. New York: Oxford University Press.

U.S. Advisory Board on Child Abuse and Neglect. (1990). *Child abuse and neglect: Critical first steps in response to a national emergency* (Stock No. 017-092-00104-5). Washington, DC: U.S. Government Printing Office.

Urciuoli, B. (1990). The political topography of Spanish and English: the view from a New York Puerto Rican neighborhood. *American Ethnologist, 18*, 295–310.

Wagatsuma, H. (1981). Child abandonment and infanticide: A Japanese case. In J. Korbin (Ed.), *Child abuse and neglect: Cross-cultural perspectives* (pp. 120–138). Berkeley: University of California.

Weisner, T., Gallimore, S., & Jordan, C. (1988). Unpackaging cultural effects on classroom learning: Native Hawaiian peer assistance and child-generated activity. *Anthropology and Education Quarterly, 19,* 327–353.

Weller, S., Romney, A. K., & Orr, D. P. (1987). The myth of a sub-culture of corporal punishment. *Human Organization, 46*(1), 39–47.

White, R. B., & Cornely, D. A. (1981). Navajo child abuse and neglect study: A comparison group examination of abuse and neglect of Navajo children. *Child Abuse and Neglect: The International Journal, 5*(1), 9–17.

Whiting, B. (1976). The problem of the packaged variable. In K. Riegel & J. Meacham (Eds.), *The developing individual in a changing world: Vol. I. Historical and cultural issues.* The Hague, Netherlands: Mouton.

Whittaker, J. K., & Garbarino, J. (1983). *Social support networks: Informal helping in the human services.* New York: Aldine.

Wichlacz, C., Lane, J. M., & Kempe, C. H. (1978). Indian child welfare: A community team approach to protective services. *Child Abuse and Neglect: The International Journal, 2*(10), 29–35.

Widom, C. (1989). Does violence beget violence? A critical examination of the literature. *Psychological Bulletin, 106,* 3–28.

Wolf, A. (1974). Marriage and adoption in Northern Taiwan. In R. Smith (Ed.), *Social organization and the applications of anthropology* (pp. 128–160). Ithaca, NY: Cornell University Press.

Wolock, I. (1982). Community characteristics and staff judgements in child abuse and neglect cases. *Social Work Research and Abstracts, 18,* 9–15.

Wu, D. Y. H. (1981). Child abuse in Taiwan. In J. Korbin (Ed.), *Child abuse and neglect: Cross-cultural perspectives* (pp. 139–165). Berkeley: University of California Press.

Wyatt, G. E. (1985). The sexual abuse of Afro-American and white American women in childhood. *Child Abuse and Neglect: The International Journal, 9,* 507–519.

Yeatman, G. W., Shaw, C., Barlow, M. J., & Bartlett, G. (1976). Psuedobattering in Vietnamese children. *Pediatrics, 58,* 616.

Young, B. (1980). The Hawaiians. In J. McDermott, W. Tseng, & Maretzki, T. (Eds.), *Peoples and cultures of Hawaii: a psychocultural profile* (pp. 5–24). Honolulu: John A. Burns School of Medicine and University of Hawaii Press.

Chapter 6

The Role of Intervention and Treatment Services in the Prevention of Child Abuse and Neglect

David A. Wolfe

Attempts to prevent the abuse of children began soon after attention was drawn to this problem in the early 1960s, and researchers and practitioners have been trying ever since to determine what methods are most effective in this regard. The "treatment" of child abuse is understandably plagued by poor definitions of what (or who) exactly is being treated, what constitutes "success," and how services can be delivered in such a way as to minimize the harm to the child (and his/her family constellation). The complexity of what we have come to consider physical abuse of children poses tremendous challenges to our understanding of this phenomenon and to our choices to intervene and/or prevent its occurrence. It stands to reason, therefore, that little consensus exists as to the formation of policy directions for this problem (e.g., Gerbner, Ross, & Zigler, 1980; Wolfe, 1991).

The treatment of abuse and neglect has been synonymous with the cessation of physical injuries to the child. It has long been reasoned that physical abuse is harmful because the child is at risk for serious physical injuries. Throughout the first decade of child abuse research, the effects of abuse on the child were described in terms of physical injuries and little more. Because the problem landed in the laps of primary medical care facilities, the focus was directed to the physical injuries of the children as well as the presumed underlying psychopathology of the parents. This focus gave the problem visibility and led to a number of positive steps to outline detection and protection services (Daro, 1988). However, recognition of the hidden manner

Portions of this chapter are adapted from the following previously published materials: Wolfe (1987); copyright 1987 by Sage Publications; adapted by permission. Wolfe (1991); copyright 1991 by The Guilford Press; adapted by permission. Wekerle and Wolfe (1993); copyright 1993 by Pergamon Press; adapted by permission.

in which child abuse affects the development of children has emerged gradually (Aber & Cicchetti, 1984). Rather than focusing on physical injuries alone, social scientists have been attempting to document the much more subtle and pervasive psychological injuries that may arise from prolonged maltreatment by caregivers (Garbarino, Guttman, & Seeley, 1986; Shirk, 1988). As well, more attention has been drawn to the factors that often accompany child abusive incidents, with the intention of offsetting the probability of abuse through the reduction of stressful circumstances impinging on families (Belsky & Vondra, 1989; Cicchetti & Rizley, 1981).

Treatment directions for child abuse and neglect have paralleled the predominant theoretical frameworks used to explain this phenomenon over the past three decades. Like most other areas of treatment of psychopathology, the development of treatment strategies for child maltreatment has involved a long process of trial and error in which currently popular ideas are heralded as the "necessary ingredients" for successful treatment outcome, only to be usurped by more popular methods or to fade due to disappointing results. To introduce the theory behind the ideas and procedures described in this chapter, I provide an overview of early conceptualizations of abusive and neglectful behavior. Selected treatment approaches derived from these emerging explanations are briefly described because they formed the basis for important developments in intervention strategies.

EXPLANATIONS FOR PHYSICALLY ABUSIVE BEHAVIOR AND CHILD NEGLECT

Psychopathology of the Parent

Because pediatricians and other medical personnel brought the problem of abuse to worldwide attention, early attempts to explain this phenomenon were couched predominately in terms of the individual psychopathology of the offender. Child abuse was a deviant act; therefore, it was reasoned that the perpetrators of such acts were themselves deviant (Spinetta & Rigler, 1972). The search began for the identification of the psychiatric symptoms or psychopathological processes that were responsible for such inhumane behavior toward one's offspring, and that would respond to psychiatric treatment.

A number of important diagnostic signs of abuse were identified on the basis of this psychopathology viewpoint, as reported in early clinical studies. The most predominant behavioral characteristics of abusive parents included chronic, multisituational aggressive behavior, isolation from family and friends, rigid and domineering interpersonal style, impulsivity, and problems rooted in marital difficulties. At an emotional or cognitive level, such parents were described as being emotionally immature (e.g., expecting the child to "care" for the parent), as showing low frustration tolerance (especially for child-related stress), as having difficulties expressing anger appropriately, as having high expectations for their children (with little regard for the child's needs and abilities), and as possessing deep-seated problems in self-esteem and/or personality adjustment that were related to problems in their family of origin (in particular, their own poor treatment). Neglectful parents, in contrast, have received far less attention than have abusive parents (Drotar, 1992), perhaps because *omissions* of proper caretaking behaviors are more difficult to describe and detect. Based primarily on clinical descriptions (and very few empirical studies) neglectful parents are described as having more pronounced personality disorders (than do comparable nonmaltreating parents), inadequate knowledge of child development and stimulation, and chronic patterns of social isolation and/or deviant subculture identification (Gaines, Sandgrund, Green, & Power, 1978; Wolfe, 1985).

Studies over the past decade confirmed the significance of additional risk factors related to parental adjustment and lifestyle. For example, a national interview study of 1,681 families with a history of child maltreatment revealed that for 10.88% of respondents, alcohol or drug dependence was a major family stress factor (American Association for Protecting Children, 1988). Similarly, Daro and Mitchell (1989) reported extremely high percentages of substance abuse problems among families receiving services from child protection agencies. For example, 68% of the state agencies surveyed across the country reported substance abuse to be the major issue in their case loads. Based on this survey, these researchers estimate that 675,000 children annually are seriously maltreated by substance-abusing caretakers, a figure that seems to be rising at a dramatic rate.

This psychopathology view of abuse and neglect led to early treatment efforts directed primarily at the individual parent. Because it was assumed that child abuse was the result of parental personality disturbance, most treatment focused on parents' insight into their own past experiences, which often included abuse by their own caregivers. In addition, treatment efforts preliminarily explored the use of family visitors or counselors, paraprofessionals who assisted family members to reduce the amount of chaos or stress existing in the family (e.g., Kempe & Helfer, 1972).

The underlying assumption guiding such treatment efforts was that abusive parents behaved aggressively toward their children due to a personality disturbance. With the treatment focus aimed primarily at parental (adult) psychopathology, it is not surprising that the early evaluation studies of such treatment were disappointing in terms of preventing further abuse. For example, in the 1970s the U.S. government evaluated 11 federally funded demonstration programs to determine the effectiveness of traditional methods of lay counseling, parent education, support services, and psychotherapy on the recidivism rates of child abuse. Cohn (1979) reported that 30% of the abusive parents involved in such studies seriously reabused their children during treatment. Similarly, another study involving 328 families (Herrenkohl,

Herrenkohl, Egolf, & Seech, 1979) found that 66.8% of the families involved in their treatment program had incidents of reabuse that were verified. Such failures occurred despite the fact that one quarter of the families received more than 3 years of treatment. Thus, it became clear that traditional approaches of psychotherapy involving personality change in the parent were not addressing the problem appropriately (Azar & Wolfe, 1989).

Influence of Large-Scale Epidemiological Studies

Beginning in the late 1960s, large-scale survey studies expanded our knowledge of the etiology of child maltreatment. Gil (1970), based on nationwide survey data, was among the first to document the role of poverty and family disadvantage on the rates of maltreatment. These findings were followed by investigations into the social isolation and chronic stress of at-risk families, leading Garbarino (1977) to propose that isolation from support systems was a necessary, but not sufficient, condition of child maltreatment. A consensus emerged in which child maltreatment was viewed in relation to economic inequality, because it was reported proportionately more often among economically and socially disadvantaged families (Pelton, 1978). Furthermore, U.S. statistics were collected nationwide (National Center on Child Abuse and Neglect, 1981, 1988) on the sociodemographic characteristics of reported maltreating families, which revealed that, in comparison to all U.S. families with children, maltreated children were twice as likely to live in a single-parent, female-headed household; four times more likely to be supported by public assistance; and likely to be affected by numerous stress factors such as health problems, alcohol abuse, and wife battering (American Humane Association, 1984).

These illustrative data relating situational factors to rates of child maltreatment led to a view of this problem that went beyond the role of the parent alone. Child abuse and neglect began to be defined in relation to its familial and situational context, such as the private and violent nature of family life and the large number of environmental stressors affecting the family. This viewpoint expanded to become an "ecological" model of maltreatment, which espoused the importance of its sociocultural context (e.g., Belsky, 1980; Garbarino, 1977). This perspective argues that as the social structure in which a parent lives becomes less controllable or manageable (or is perceived to be so), the adult may rely more and more on coercion and violence (i.e., abuse) or withdrawal and apathy (i.e., neglect) to control the irritating, daily events that he/she links to such stress.

One of the most significant theoretical and practical contributions to be made by this emerging sociocultural viewpoint is related to pressures to modify the definition and suspected causes of maltreatment. Rather than dichotomizing parents into abusive and nonabusive (or neglectful), this perspective was the first to advance the notion that child maltreatment was more a function of its situational context than it was of an individual's personality weaknesses. That is, abuse and neglect are not isolated social phenomena or a personality defect of the parent per se—rather, they are a "symptom" of a society that condones the use of some violent methods toward family members, that does not provide adequate services and basic needs for all its members, and that chooses to define maltreatment in relative terms rather than in absolute terms. It follows from this viewpoint that inappropriate childrearing practices are not so much a function of individual disturbance as they are of social and cultural forces that establish the parameters of individual behavior (Wolfe, 1987).

Based on these broader explanations, suggestions for improving treatment resources and expanding services to families were offered. Although the ecological viewpoint clarified the causes of child abuse and mobilized some efforts to attack some of its social roots, it was nevertheless difficult to translate some of the causes into treatment or prevention policy. Critics of the status quo definition and policy argued that because child abuse is a symptom of society, society should attack the elements that create such disadvantage rather than attempt to patch together the casualties of such societal ills. The influence of this viewpoint on treatment, therefore, may be described more in terms of its direction for long-term systemic changes in policy rather than in terms of current treatment procedures; however, this remains a highly promising and encouraging trend that may have a major bearing on child abuse prevention in the next generation, as elaborated on later.

Development of Social–Interactional Perspectives

With the emerging knowledge derived from sociodemographic studies, greater dissatisfaction was expressed by professionals regarding definitions that placed a major emphasis on parental deviance and wrongdoing (e.g., Garbarino, 1977; Gelles, 1973; Parke, 1977). This dissatisfaction was due in part to the fact that existing social–legal definitions were aimed primarily at the implicit intent to inflict harm or the incapability of the parent to protect the child from harm. However, research was beginning to suggest that many incidents of physical abuse and neglect, although impulsive acts, were not necessarily maliciously perpetrated by the parent (with the noted exception of sexual abuse, discussed later). Rather, it was becoming apparent that child maltreatment was most likely to emerge among those families who lacked the resources and skills to deal with the everyday discipline and stress-management issues that are a part of childrearing. Thus, social scientists began to place more and more emphasis on social and familial variables that could be susceptible to early intervention and treatment.

As explained by the emerging social–interactional perspective, child abuse and neglect can be viewed as symptoms of an extreme disturbance of childrearing (Burgess, 1979; Starr, 1979) and not necessarily as an individual disorder or psychological disturbance per se. It was further recognized that child abuse is often enmeshed in other serious family problems (such as alcoholism or antisocial behavior), which are all similarly related in some degree to negative developmental outcomes. In light of these developments, the socialization practices that maltreating and other distressed families have in common were pinpointed as areas to receive the majority of attention for defining and treating this problem (e.g., Wolfe, Kaufman, Aragona, & Sandler, 1981).

The social–interactional perspective can be considered to be somewhat of an integration of the concerns expressed by the two previous explanations. That is, this perspective was interested in defining child abuse *in the context of the family, community, and society* (as underscored by the ecological perspective) while stressing the importance of individual factors that play a role in the actual expression of abusive behavior. Most significantly, the parent–child relationship, rather than individual psychopathology or particular stressors, became the target of concern for intervention, due to the belief that this relationship set the stage for the degree of healthy versus abusive interactions. This perspective not only was influenced by clinical studies of other disturbed populations, but also benefited from studies relating to the development of parent–child relationships, early attachment, and the formation of appropriate child care (e.g., Cicchetti & Rizley, 1981). This view was further influenced by the emerging perspective on reciprocal processes of parents and children on each other (Bell & Harper, 1977). The role of normal child behavior thus became a much more important and significant factor to consider in defining and treating child abuse.

Some of the earlier descriptions of maltreating parents as being "disturbed" gave way to new empirical findings that embraced a "person-situation" interaction as the principal factor underlying harmful childrearing practices. In place of personality dimensions, these studies looked specifically at the interactions of family members as well as self-reports of abusive parents' perceptions of their children, physical and emotional symptomatology that may interfere with parenting abilities, and emotional reactivity to stressful childrearing situations. In general, these studies (using comparison groups of physically abusive and nonabusive parents) confirmed the existence of behavioral differences among abusive samples in terms of low frustration tolerance, social isolation, and impaired childrearing skills.

Studies also confirmed several important cognitive differences between maltreating and nonmaltreating parents, including unrealistic expectations of their children, the tendency to view their own child's behavior as being extremely stressful, and their view of themselves as being inadequate or incompetent in the parenting role. Interestingly, with the use of matched comparison samples, these studies also revealed that maltreating families could *not* be readily distinguished from other (matched) families in terms of the type and frequency of child behavior problems, their own negative childhood experiences, and the presence of general symptoms of unhappiness or dis-satisfaction. Thus, it became important to view the psychological character-istics of abusive parents in relation to their role as a parent and the nature of their family and social context (Wolfe, 1987).

Psychological interventions flourished under the social–interactional model, particularly behavioral strategies designed to assist physically abu-sive parents in learning appropriate childrearing methods. The growth of behavioral intervention was due in part to the fact that psychotherapy-based (insight-oriented) methods of treatment for abuse were found to be inadequate or a poor match for this population, as noted previously. In contrast, behav-ioral methods (i.e., behavioral change based on systematic instruction, mod-eling, rehearsal, and feedback) became a good match to abusive families in particular because of the good track record of these procedures for assisting families (nonabusive) with behaviorally disturbed children. Abusive families seemed to respond favorably to such structured teaching methods, in con-trast to efforts aimed at personality change (Ammerman, 1990; Azar & Siegel, 1990). Neglectful parents, however, have seldom been the focus of such inter-vention programs (Lutzker, 1990; see subsequent sections).

Recent efforts are being made to direct the focus of intervention toward the important issues that families face during *each* of the emerging develop-mental stages that the child and parent must endure, rather than attempting to repair the relationship difficulties later on. Such efforts are expanding the focus of intervention to include the early formation of the parent–infant relationship and stimulation of early childhood development, as well as the fundamentals of childrearing skills. Before discussing these emerging ap-proaches, however, a brief review is provided of the most common approach to child abuse intervention—alternative care by the state.

Alternative Care by the State

State intervention was predicated on the assumption that alternative care by the state (i.e., removing children from abusive or dangerous family environ-ments) was a benevolent intervention when families failed or violated stan-dards of care. Alternative care was assumed to remove the child from harm and to provide a stable and therapeutic environment, as well as to provide a brief period for family rehabilitation (Azar & Wolfe, 1989). This view has been challenged more recently by the realization that not all interventions are beneficial and, in fact, can do more harm than good in some cases by introducing further victimization and disruption into the child's life (Melton, 1990; Wolfe & Jaffe, 1990). Thus, much confusion presently exists between the needs and rights of children and families.

This awareness of potential harm to the child has led to an increasing focus on children's rights and some fundamental safeguards regarding their entry into the care of the state and ongoing review of the state's intervention. However, this shift in focus has lost its initial attractiveness because of the awareness that procedural complications may create delays or that a sequence of failed "least intrusive" measures may not be in the child's best interests. The policy issues emanating from this realization point to the need to strike a balance between the two related concerns of children's developmental needs and the state's responsibility to provide them with the least intrusive intervention.

The costs of operating the current North American system of mandated state intervention (without any formal treatment services) are the first issue one faces when describing this approach. Unquestionably, child maltreatment costs the public enormously in terms of alternative placements and protective services. Daro (1988) estimates that *serious* abuse cases (which constitute only 3% of all reports) cost the United States annually at least $20 million in hospital costs and $7 million in rehabilitation costs for the victims. Based on 1983 figures, she notes that the total reported cases cost society a minimum of $460 million in administration and foster care placements. Intensive treatment, if available, can run from $2,860 per family per year (for lay therapy and support services) to over $28,000 per family per year for comprehensive services (including child treatment). Daro points out that if only the severely abused in 1983 had received any of these treatment services for 1 year the costs would have exceeded $662 million. Clearly, many of these dollars are necessary to mount *any* type of widespread attack on abuse and thus costs will always be high. The question that warrants greater consideration, however, is whether these dollars are being spent on the appropriate *type* of service. These shortcomings of apprehension and alternative care were clearly noted by the U.S. Advisory Board on Child Abuse and Neglect (1990):

> The child protection system is a complex web of social service, legal, law enforcement, mental health, health, educational, and volunteer agencies. The many elements of the child protection system increase the complexity of the problem. Families in which maltreatment is suspected or is known to have occurred find themselves the objects of action (or inaction) by numerous public agencies that often are poorly coordinated and may have conflicting purposes. (p. xii)
>
> The most serious shortcoming of the nation's system of intervention on behalf of children is that it depends upon a reporting and response process that has punitive connotations, and involves massive resources dedicated to the investigation of allegations. State and County child welfare programs have not been designed to get immediate help to families based on voluntary requests for assistance. As a result it has become far easier to pick up the telephone to report one's neighbor for child abuse than it is for that neighbor to pick up the telephone to request and receive help before the abuse happens. . . . More resources must be allocated to establishing voluntary, non-punitive access to help. (p. 80)

In conclusion, it would be naive to consider interventions by the state simply as beneficial or damaging. State intervention to remove children from their families is generally accepted in North America as an essential last resort for aiding children in families with major difficulties. Major readjustments to the present system are not impossible, yet such changes will most likely need to be preceded by major revisions of the purpose and intent of state intervention. In keeping with some of the emerging findings on what services work best for disadvantaged families (some of which are reviewed in later sections), child protection agencies may have to be prepared to provide opportunities for the type of training or therapy that this population requires. More and more, courts are indicating that parental rights cannot be terminated when it is shown that agencies did not make appropriate efforts to ensure the provision of therapeutic or remedial services. Unfortunately, in many cases the only intervention is the passage of time, so the requisite skills and modifications needed to return the child to the family are incomplete. Striking a balance between parental rights and children's rights remains a critical challenge for future research and policy development.

Summary and Commentary Regarding Intervention Strategies

Broadly speaking, psychological intervention with reported maltreating parents developed gradually from an individually based pathology model to an all-encompassing ecological model, with an evolving emphasis on the importance of the parent–child relationship and its context. Simultaneously, the orientation toward the treatment issue (i.e., how such behavior is viewed) shifted gradually from a parent-focused, deviance viewpoint more toward one that accounts for the vast number of stress factors that impinge on the developing parent–child relationship. This shift toward a more process-oriented, contextual theory of maltreatment places greater emphasis on the importance of promoting parental competence and reducing the burden of stress on families. As Belsky (1984) explains, parental competence (i.e., sensitivity to the child's developing abilities and communications) is influenced by such factors as (1) parental resources (e.g., education, attitudes about childrearing, and parents' background experiences), (2) the child's characteristics (e.g., temperament, health, and developmental level), and (3) the family context (e.g., the marital relationship, the quality of social networks and supports, and community resources). Available data on maltreating families confirm that the vast majority lack parental competence because of problems associated with all three of these domains.

Although our intervention models have greatly improved and have contributed to encouraging gains in treatment outcomes, the field remains split between promising research findings, on the one hand, and the realities of child protection and welfare, on the other hand. Unfortunately, the dominant theme in most services to maltreating families remains that of protection, not of treatment (Azar & Wolfe, 1989). To assess any gains made over the past two decades in treatment outcome, it is necessary to separate what is truly treatment from what is actually delivered to identified families in practice (Wolfe, 1984). It should also be noted that most intervention tends to occur only after a major identified incident of abuse or neglect, and parents often need a "calling card" of some sort in order to receive appropriate help. That is, current laws and priorities are such that child protection agencies have few resources to assist families who have not, as yet, violated any community standard. The present child welfare system is designed primarily for protection rather than assistance, which leaves inadequate services available to a significant number of parents who are at risk of losing control with their children and who could benefit from early intervention. This requires a retooling of our priorities and procedures within the child welfare system, to encourage parents to seek assistance early on for their important role (Wolfe, 1990).

THE IMPACT OF PHYSICAL ABUSE AND NEGLECT ON CHILDREN'S DEVELOPMENT

Researchers have emphasized that maltreatment should be defined not only in terms of physical injuries to the child but also in terms of its impact on the child's psychological development (Cicchetti & Rizley, 1981; Wolfe, 1987; Zuravin, 1991). Physical and emotional forms of child abuse and neglect, according to the developmental psychopathology explanation, may interfere with long-term development by virtue of the psychological dimensions that are impaired or disrupted by such parental treatment (i.e., socioemotional, behavioral, and social–cognitive dimensions) (Cicchetti, 1989; Wolfe, 1987). This explanation, moreover, corresponds to findings indicating that physically abused children were more likely to be behaviorally or emotionally impaired than were their nonabused counterparts in ways that could not be attributed to physical injuries alone (e.g., Cicchetti & Rizley, 1981). Such children have been reported to be developmentally delayed, behaviorally disordered, and recognizably different from their age peers, although no particular pattern of psychopathology has emerged (Shaw-Lamphear, 1985). Highlights of these recent findings are summarized in the section below.

Maltreated Children's Behavioral, Cognitive, and Emotional Development

Initial studies with children identified as physically abused suggested that such maltreatment was associated with higher rates of acting-out, externalizing disorders (e.g., higher rates of aggression, delinquency, hyperactivity, and similar behaviors) than for nonabused children. This finding has generally held up under more rigorous investigation in recent years, leading to the tentative conclusion that physical maltreatment is associated with (but, of course, may not be the direct cause of) more aggressive, resistant, and avoidant behavior with adults and peers (e.g., see reviews by Ammerman, 1992; Fantuzzo, 1990; Shaw-Lamphear, 1985; Wolfe, 1987). The higher rates of acting-out problems among this population are not surprising in light of the fact that child abuse comprises physically and emotionally aggressive interactions between caregiver and child, which may form the basis for how the child interacts with others (Sroufe & Fleeson, 1986). At the same time, studies have described abused children as being delayed in both language development (e.g., Appelbaum, 1977) and their social competence with peers (e.g., George & Main, 1979). Not surprisingly, such children often report greater feelings of hopelessness, depression, and low self-worth (Fantuzzo, 1990).

Studies of children identified as *neglected* confirm similar disruptions in major areas of socioemotional and behavioral development. Social withdrawal, depression, lower intellectual functioning, and behavior problems have been documented among samples of neglected children (Ammerman, Cassissi, Hersen, & Van Hasselt, 1986), as well as major problems related to the formation of attachment and the mastery of developmental milestones (Egeland & Sroufe, 1981). Although some investigators suspect that children who experience *both* abuse and neglect demonstrate the greatest risk, little systematic research has been conducted in this regard. (According to the American Association for Protecting Children, 1988, multiple forms of maltreatment, such as physical abuse and neglect, are frequently present in a single family; estimates of overlap of abuse and neglect, however, are unreliable; Drotar, 1992).

Despite these overall deficiencies and adjustment problems shown across studies of maltreated children, there has been little confirmation of the initial belief that abuse or neglect leads to *predictable* developmental outcomes for children across their lifespan (Ammerman, 1992; Fantuzzo, 1990; Wolfe, 1987). Rather, findings suggest that child abuse represents the visible aspect of a very major disrupting influence in the child's ongoing development. Such disruptions are of such a pronounced and significant level that the child's behavioral, emotional, and social–cognitive dimensions of development are impaired to varying degrees (Aber & Cicchetti, 1984).

From a developmental perspective, abused children's experiences with their caregivers may have their greatest significance in terms of the formation of positive relationships with others and contentment in their social environment. For example, the formation of attachment is one of the most critical early developmental tasks, which is believed to set the stage for subsequent relationship formation (Sroufe & Fleeson, 1986). In the field of child maltreatment, the attachment concept has been theoretically linked to the perpetuation of maltreatment across generations (Kaufman & Zigler, 1989), the failure of these children to form subsequent relationships with others

(Erickson, Sroufe, & Egeland, 1985), and their vulnerability to additional developmental failures that rely to some extent on early attachment success (Aber & Allen, 1987). Not surprisingly, Cicchetti, Toth, and Bush (1988) report that the vast majority of maltreated infants form insecure attachments with their caregivers (70% to 100% across studies). This poor resolution of attachment may be most significant in terms of influencing a child's relationship formation with peers, future partners, and future offspring.

Such findings regarding the broad and diverse developmental disabilities of abused children point to the importance of studying abuse and neglect in terms of socialization practices rather than in terms of individual acts of commission or omission. Accordingly, the impact of maltreatment on a child's development must be considered in relation to the overall quality of care that the child is exposed to over time. Such a view has important implications for early intervention, as discussed below.

In a recent review of the literature on the effects of maltreatment on children's development, Wolfe, Wekerle, and McGee (1992) noted two themes among the existing findings. The first theme was that developmental problems among maltreated children appeared to be linked most commonly to poor nurturance by their caregivers. Thus, it may be more logical to assume that the deficiencies in development among maltreated children are caused by a poor childrearing environment, in which physical injuries are only one aspect. Ample evidence now exists to indicate that maltreated children are poorly cared for, both emotionally and physically, from an early age, and, thus, it is not surprising to find corresponding problems in attachment and relationship formation.

A second theme to emerge from this literature focused on the child's response or adaptation to his or her environment over time. Studies are confirming that children who are maltreated by parents are more likely than are their nonmaltreated counterparts to show signs of failure in normal adaptation. Thus, how such children learn to respond to their environment is closely related to the level of stimulation and sensitivity provided by their caregivers. Because maltreated children are likely to have had poor opportunities to learn appropriate adaptive skills, their reported level of social competence, self-esteem, and problem-solving abilities are understandably diminished.

Adolescent Maltreatment: A Special Concern

Whereas the psychosocial correlates of maltreatment in younger children have received considerable attention, much less is known of the factors relating to adolescent maltreatment. Because adolescence is a time in which the individual is continuing to develop important emotional, physical, and cognitive abilities, it stands to reason that maltreatment may interfere with the negotiation of these tasks. By the same token, these tasks are considerably different than those of the younger child, leading to the belief that the correlates of maltreatment during adolescence may be expressed somewhat differently (Williamson, Borduin, & Howe, 1991). Moreover, as noted by Garbarino (1992), efforts to understand adolescent maltreatment may serve as a link to constructing a more encompassing, general life-course theory of domestic violence.

The importance of adolescent maltreatment emerges from official and unofficial reports and surveys. Based on the National Incidence Studies, data compiled by the American Humane Association, and related surveys, Garbarino (1992) estimates that the rate of adolescent maltreatment is overrepresentative of the adolescent population (42% of reported cases of maltreatment, compared to 38% of the population under age 18). Significantly, adolescent maltreatment is more often associated with problematic acting-out behavior and/or family dysfunction, which may explain why such cases are seen more often by family service agencies rather than child protection agencies.

The ecological contexts of three forms of adolescent maltreatment were recently explored by Williamson et al. (1991). These researchers discovered that (1) adolescent neglect was associated with extrafamilial problems such as stress, social isolation, and deviant peers; (2) adolescent physical abuse was linked to reports of externalizing behavior problems and rigid family functioning; and (3) adolescent sexual abuse was related to internalizing behaviors and emotional problems of the teen. All three forms of maltreatment, on the other hand, were marked by attentional problems, lower family cohesion, and more daily stress relative to nonmaltreated controls. The results of this study, based on small samples of maltreated teens, provides initial support for distinguishing between different forms of adolescent maltreatment and for underscoring adjustment problems associated with maltreatment during this developmental period. More effort is needed, however, in differentiating between families in which maltreatment was a continuation from childhood patterns and those in which there is escalation of conflict during the transition to adolescence. Presumably, these opposing patterns would respond differentially to prevention and treatment services.

Implications for Prevention and Intervention

An important challenge to our understanding of the effects of maltreatment and our concomitant response lies in our recognition that the effects differ depending on the stage of the child's development and the presence or absence of health-promoting factors (e.g., family stability and alternatives to physical punishment). Such a view provides special attention to developmental limitations and abilities of children who have experienced various forms of maltreatment and is an optimistic framework for establishing early prevention and intervention goals.

If we accept the theoretical and philosophical argument that maltreatment is indirectly responsible for myriad developmental problems, then our understanding of the behavioral and emotional adjustment problems shown by maltreated children rests on an awareness of their developmental deficits (in addition to some direct effects of maltreatment or insensitive parenting). Such a position carries with it important implications for establishing intervention and prevention goals. First, it is important to recognize the developmental differences that may emerge as a function of maltreatment. An individual child's symptoms may be an understandable result of his or her efforts to learn social behaviors without the benefit of sensitive parenting or careful guidance. Accordingly, the identified "referral concern" may shift from one that assesses current problematic behavior alone toward one that identifies the developmental concerns that underlie such expressions. This premise directs intervention to the strengthening of developmentally relevant tasks or skills as well as to specific presenting complaints.

A developmentally guided intervention and prevention strategy works on the principle of providing the least intrusive, earliest assistance possible, instead of relying on aversive contingencies. The focus of intervention can be shifted from identifying misdeeds of the parent more toward promoting an optimal balance between the needs of the child and the abilities of the parent.

Of equal importance is the recognition that intervention and prevention services not only must be planned in relation to issues affecting child development (as is the case in almost all studies to date), but also should include efforts to address the somewhat unique elements of adolescent development. Garbarino (1992) outlines several research-based hypotheses for planning such services with adolescents. For example, female adolescents and those with stepparents are overrepresented in maltreatment reports, whereas socioeconomic status seems to be less of a distinguishing feature. Moreover, adolescent maltreatment is most likely to arise when troubled youth live within a high-risk family. These initial findings point to the need to address features of the family context and sources of family support affecting the parent–adolescent relationship.

An additional, promising direction for adolescent services involves programs specifically geared to the interests and needs of this age group (rather than parent–adolescent conflict per se). Adolescents, both male and female, represent a major high-risk group for sexual abuse and sexual assault victimization and offenses. Moreover, violence toward intimate partners and family members is rooted in sociocultural influences, many of which originate in childhood and adolescence (such as power and status and harsh socialization practices) (Health and Welfare Canada, 1989). For example, child maltreatment is a crucial risk factor associated with later maladjustment in adolescence, particularly in relation to antisocial and violent interpersonal behavior (Dodge, Bates, & Pettit, 1990; Widom, 1989), as well as sexual and nonsexual violence toward women during young adulthood (Fagan & Wexler, 1988).

The developmental course of children from such family environments typically proceeds unabated. They are more likely to associate with delinquent peers and engage in antisocial behaviors (Patterson, DeBaryshe, & Ramsey, 1989), which further serves to impair their ability to master important developmental tasks. Moreover, such associations perpetuate attitudes, motivations, emotions, and beliefs that encourage the likelihood of coercive behavior. This course, combined with added cultural stereotypes for men and women, may lead to both sexual and nonsexual forms of acting out during adolescence and young adulthood in attempts to control and coerce others (Dutton, 1988).

AN INTERVENTION MODEL LINKED TO CRITICAL TRANSITION PERIODS FOR FAMILY MEMBERS

The theoretical viewpoints discussed previously offer explanations as to why a parent might mistreat a child. Although each approach has contributed new knowledge to our understanding of child abuse, further integration of the findings is needed to address the concern of how some parents gradually acquire the preconditions that seem to lead to the rather sudden onset of abusive behavior or the gradual onset of neglect. Rather than focusing on observable factors that are often present once a family has been labeled or reported, this viewpoint looks at the process by which subtle identified contributors to child abuse become transformed over time into a high-risk or abusive situation.

The transitional model of child maltreatment (Wolfe, 1987) was formulated to describe such a course of development in terms that have relevance to prevention and early intervention. The model is based on two presuppositions. First, the development of inappropriate childrearing patterns is presumed to follow a somewhat predictable course in the absence of intervention or major compensatory factors. This course is described in reference to stages, which underscores the contention that abuse and neglect develop from a gradual transformation in the parent–child relationship from mild to very harmful interactions. Accordingly, the initial stage is relatively benign, in comparison to later stages, in that the parent has not as yet behaved in the manner that significantly interferes with the parent–child relationship. However, this viewpoint suggests that failure to deal effectively with the demands of their role early on can readily lead to increased pressure on the parent–child relationship and a concomitant increase in the probability of abusive behavior.

   The second presupposition of this model relates to the importance of psychological processes that are linked to the expression of anger, arousal, and coping reactions in adults. Specifically, these processes include operant and respondent learning principles for the acquisition or maintenance of behavior, cognitive–attributional processes that influence an individual's perception and reaction to stressful events, and emotional conditioning processes that determine the individual's degree of physiological arousal, perceived discomfort, and self-control under stressful circumstances.

   Stage 1 in this model, labeled "reduced tolerance for stress and disinhibition of aggression," begins with the parent's own preparation for this role (in terms of psychological and social resources, attributional style, modeling, and similar learning experiences from childhood) and his/her current style of coping with the daily demands that compete with the parenting role. Parents' responses during Stage 1, when their roles and responsibilities are gradually being acquired, are based largely on their own family of origin and their preparation for this role by their previous child care experiences. For those who are at risk of becoming abusive, training is often inadvertently accomplished over the course of childhood through the modeling of aggressive problem-solving tactics and an external attributional style, rehearsal and reinforcement of aggressive behavior with siblings and peers, and the absence of opportunities to learn prosocial behavior. For those at risk of neglectful parenting style, we often see a family background of deficient maternal–child interaction, lack of maternal availability, and inconsistent parental affect and response to the child.

   Several factors may play a critical role in mediating the expression of aggressive and/or avoidant behavior once the individual becomes a parent. In particular, the degree of control, feedback, and predictability that parents perceive in relation to stressful life events can influence their behavior. For example, if they are able to achieve some success in controlling stressful aspects of their life, they are more likely to adopt a purposeful, planned approach to childrearing. In addition, compensatory factors such as a supportive spouse, socioeconomic stability, success experiences at work or school, and positive social supports, which the individual can draw on for information or assistance (Belsky, 1980; Cicchetti & Rizley, 1981), may buffer some parents from the effects of major stressors during this stage.

   Stage 2 in this model, "poor management of acute crises and provocation," represents the hypothetical point in the development of poor parenting style in which the parent's previous attempts or methods of managing life stress or child behavior begin to fail significantly. The parent often experiences feelings of "losing control," and at this juncture the risk of child abuse (and other forms of poor coping reactions) begins to increase. A parent may "step up" the intensity of power-assertive methods that he/she believes are necessary to reestablish a semblance of control, or, if predisposed to neglect/

avoidance, he/she may develop a diminished pattern of social exchange with the child.

Conditioned emotional responding (i.e., prior reactions of anger and irritation related to the child) may overtake, or impair, the parent's rational behavior at this point. Feelings of extreme agitation and irritation, which may have originated from other sources of anger besides the child (e.g., an employer, a neighbor, or a spouse), are (mis)attributed to the child because the parent has learned (through months or years of interaction with the child) to associate feelings of discomfort or irritation with child provocation (also, the child is often the easiest party to "blame" for such unpleasant feelings of arousal). Consequently, when the child cries or fusses to seek attention, for example, the parent may distort the seriousness or potential harm posed by the situation. This appraisal, in turn, may lead the parent to conclude that excessive countermeasures are justified to gain control of the child's aversive behavior.

Once again, the degree of stress experienced by the parent may be offset by compensatory factors. In particular, improvement in the child's behavior or the involvement of community programs to assist parents in coping with difficult family-related issues holds promise for reducing the acute crisis situation.

Stage 3 in the transitional model of maltreatment, "habitual patterns of arousal and aggression with family members," represents a chronic pattern of irritability, arousal, and/or avoidance of responsibility on the part of the parent. By this time, the parent may maintain that the use of excessive punishment and force is absolutely necessary to control the child's behavior, or, in the case of neglect, the parent may rely on inappropriate avoidance of responsibility. Provocative stimuli, such as child behavior problems, frustration, and emotional arousal, now become commonplace, and the parent's response to such events (such as abusive interchanges or neglectful avoidance) escalate in intensity, duration, and frequency.

At this point, parents often perceive that they are trapped into continuing to use harsh or extreme methods to control their children. Although this perception is somewhat accurate (due to the fact that children can habituate to the higher level of punishment and thus may not respond as well to it), the belief justifies their use of further force/avoidance. The parent is now caught in the vicious cycle of using coercive methods to diminish tension and irritation, and the parent may receive some short-term gain through such methods by the reduction of the child's aversive behavior.

Unfortunately, reversal of this process is difficult by this stage and is aided by few compensatory factors. Although treatment efforts may be directed toward families at this point, the method of interacting with one's children has become so ingrained that it becomes difficult to rely on anything but coercive and avoidant methods. Thus, treatment providers are faced with the dilemma of introducing ways to change well-established patterns of family interaction in such a manner that the parent will recognize that the benefits (e.g., a well-behaved child or more pleasant family interaction) outweigh the cost (e.g., efforts needed to learn different disciplinary methods and pronounced increases in child problem behavior in the short term).

The challenging task for professionals becomes one of interrupting this deterioration and intervening in such a way as to restore the family's ability to cope with external demands and provide for the developmental and socialization needs of their children. According to this view, either the parent–child relationship was never well established or it began to disintegrate during periods of developmental change or family stress. Therefore, an overriding goal of child abuse prevention from the perspective of healthy child development is the establishment of positive socialization practices that are responsive to situational and developmental changes. Such healthy practices buffer the child against other socialization pressures that can be stressful or negative and reduce the need for parents to rely on power-assertive methods to control their children.

INTERVENTION NEEDS AND METHODS FOR IDENTIFIED ABUSIVE AND NEGLECTFUL FAMILIES (STAGES 2 AND 3)

Intervention with abusive and neglecting families differs on a number of levels from more traditional intervention services. First, a greater proportion of these clients are intellectually low functioning, which limits the utility of insight-oriented treatment approaches (Azar & Wolfe, 1989). In addition to such cognitive limitations, maltreating parents often have quite different expectations of what takes place in therapy, which is important for involvement in the therapeutic process. They often approach psychological treatment in much the same way they approach medical treatment, expecting the treatment to eliminate the "problem" they are reporting (Azar & Wolfe, 1989). Finally, we can contrast traditional problems faced in psychotherapy by noting that maltreating parents are not voluntarily seeking assistance. Thus, they may be resistant to the goals of therapy, unfamiliar with the course and nature of psychological treatments, and confused by the explanations and information being provided on their behalf. The result can often lead to a less than desirable outcome on the part of both the client and the therapist. Recognizing these special considerations, I now turn to identifying the major targets of intervention with this population.

Identifying Targets for Tertiary Intervention Efforts

Figure 6.1 summarizes the major intervention targets that emerge from the literature on the multiple causes of child abuse and neglect. These targets

KEY:
• Insufficient Data 🚫 Not Applicable Scale: Better ●◑○◐● Worse

INTERVENTION TARGETS

INTERVENTION STRATEGIES	Family Context			Nature of the Maltreatment				Child Needs					Caregiver Needs					Advantages	Disadvantages	Comments
	Marital Conflict	Chronic SES	Social isolation	Chronic physical abuse	Minor physical abuse	Chronic neglect	Minor neglect	Developmental deficits	Self control & aggression	Problems of older children	Out-of-home placements	Emotional distress	Childrearing skills	Child expectations	Competing lifestyle/habits	Recidivism/Reports	Cost			
Child focused Intervention																				
A. Preschool Programs (n=8)[a]	•	•	•	•	●	•	◑	●	○	•	•		•	•	•	•	N/A	N/A	A,B, D,E	a,b,d
Parent Focused Intervention																				
A. Behavioral/Cognitive-Behavioral (n=10)[b]	○	◑	○	●	◑	○	◑	◑	●	◑	•	◑	●	●	•	●	◑	A-F	b,c,f	1,2
B. Social Network (n=2)[c]	•	•	◑	•	•	◑	◑	N/A	N/A	N/A	•	◑	●	●	•	•	◑	A,E	a-d,e,f,h	3
Comprehensive/Multiservice Programs																				
A. Family Centered Home-Based (n=13)[d]	○	◑	•	•	•	•	•	•	•	•	◑	•	•	•	•	•	●	A-E	a-d,f,g	1,2,4
B. Ecobehavioral (n=10)[e]	○	○	◑	○	○	◑	◑	•	•	•	•	•	•	•	•	◐	●	A-E	a-d,f,g	1,2,4

Key to Advantages:
A. Can be easily interrupted and continued as needed
B. Can be implemented by trained paraprofessionals
C. Can be conducted in either home or clinic setting
D. Perceived by most parents as less threatening or coercive
E. Very flexible in terms of individual needs
F. Typically brief duration (less than one year)
G. Little or no cost

Key to Disadvantages:
a. Limited outcome evaluation studies
b. Limited data on generalization across time, settings, or persons
c. Requires post-graduate degree and/or training
d. Generally takes several months or years to produce change
e. Treatment services are often sporadic or minimal
f. Inconclusive regarding efficacy with male offenders
g. No outcome data available as to effectiveness
h. May be helpful only to a very limited subgroup of parents who can identify their own problems and are motivated to change

Comments:
1. Best suited for families in which knowledge/skills of childrearing are lacking
2. Best suited for parents who prefer specific direction and guidance
3. Best suited for individuals who require basic childrearing information and support
4. Due to multiple needs of the identified population, services per family can become quite extensive and prolonged

Superscripts:
a. Culp et al., 1991; Culp, Richardson, & Heide, 1987; Culp, Heide, & Richardson, 1987; Davis & Fantuzzo, 1989; Fantuzzo, 1990; Fantuzzo et al., 1987; Fantuzzo et al., 1988; Parish et al., 1985.
b. Barth et al., 1983; Crimmins et al., 1984; Dawson et al., 1986; Egan, 1983; Fantuzzo et al., 1986; Nomellini & Katz, 1983; Whiteman et al., 1987; Wolfe et al., 1981; Wolfe et al., 1982; Wolfe & Sandler, 1981.
c. Gaudin et al., 1991; Lovell & Hawkins, 1988.
d. Amundson, 1989; Brunk et al., 1987; Hinckley & Ellis, 1985; Kinney et al., 1977; Frankel, 1988 (citing Janes et al., 1976; Landsman 1983; Leeds, 1984; Lyle & Nelson, 1983; Showell & Hartley, 1983; State of Oregon, 1983; State of Virginia, 1985); Nicol et al., 1988; Wood et al., 1988.
e. Barone, Greene, & Lutzker, 1986; Campbell et al., 1983; Lutzker, 1984; Lutzker & Newman, 1986; Lutzker & Rice, 1984; Lutzker & Rice, 1987; Rosenfeild-Schlichter et al., 1983; Tertinger et al., 1984; Watson-Perczel, 1988; Wesch & Lutzker, 1991.

FIGURE 6.1. Intervention strategies for identified abusive and neglectful families (ratings of relative effectiveness in addressing each intervention target).

242

are then discussed in reference to tertiary intervention programs that have presented evaluation data with samples of maltreating parents.

Problems Related to the Family Context

The literature on abusive and neglectful families has documented the existence of family factors that are direct or indirect causes of child maltreatment. The first factor, marital discord and/or coercive family interactions, is a common feature of such families (Wolfe, 1985). For example, in treatment studies of abusive families, it is common for the woman to be involved in treatment but to receive limited support or commitment from her male partner. A history of violent male partners is also commonplace among such families. (According to a national survey of families, Straus and Gelles, 1990, estimate the comorbidity of marital violence and physical abuse at 40–45%.) Second, the figure contains reference to chronic economic problems and associated socioeconomic stressors, a concern documented by sociological as well as psychological studies. Third, the treatment target described as social isolation is included. Clinical studies have noted the inability of maltreating families to establish meaningful social supports, as well as the preponderance of intervention failures among many maltreating families, suggesting the relevance of this variable in treatment planning.

Nature of the Maltreatment

In determining the relative effectiveness of various tertiary intervention programs, we should consider the type or nature of maltreatment that is being addressed. Whereas some forms of intervention may be successful in eliminating harsh physical punishment, they may be inadequate in addressing the needs of neglecting families. Of equal importance is the discrimination between chronic and multiple forms of maltreatment that pose a considerable challenge to treatment, versus transitory or limited episodes that may respond more readily to assistance. Thus, Figure 6.1 contains reference to the nature of maltreatment by considering four principal categories that correspond to the majority of treatment referrals: (1) chronic patterns of physical and emotional abuse (including the child's exposure to wife assault), (2) transitory/acute patterns of physical/emotional abuse, (3) chronic patterns of neglect, and (4) transitory/acute patterns of neglect.

Child Treatment Needs

Based on the impact of maltreatment on children's psychological development, four prominent intervention considerations are listed in Figure 6.1. Each of these issues warrant some attention in treatment planning for this diverse population: (1) deficits in social sensitivity and relationship development, which includes problems related to poor attachment formation, the development of empathy, and affective expression, as well as cognitive and moral development, which refers to poor social judgment and school performance in particular; (2) problems in self-control and aggression; and (3) behavior problems of older children and adolescents. This latter category was included for the review of intervention efforts because of the importance in discriminating between methods aimed at younger children and those aimed at older children. The vast majority of the programs described below pertain primarily to young children (i.e., under age 8), and thus their effectiveness with families with teens and older children is largely unknown. Suggestions for such programs, however, are contained in the conclusions to this chapter. The fourth category, avoidance of out-of-home placement, was also included due to the number of studies that based their intervention on such outcome and the putative importance of meeting the child's needs within his/her own family context.

Parent/Caregiver Treatment Needs

The majority of intervention studies target the individual needs of the maltreating parent. Figure 6.1 lists four factors corresponding to the principal issues that warrant treatment consideration for the caregiver population. The first of these factors, symptoms of emotional distress, reflects the finding that a significant number of maltreating parents describe themselves as unhappy or distressed (Wolfe, 1985). Although they may not suffer from psychiatric illness, they are more likely to have some limited learning abilities and/or immaturity problems that can contribute to child maltreatment. Emotional arousal and reactivity to child provocation refers to the common finding of problems related to the control of anger and hostility, which contribute to abusive episodes. Similarly, maltreating parents show limited or inappropriate childrearing patterns and skills, the second factor, including inadequate child stimulation, and may be proportionately more negative than positive toward their offspring. The third factor, perceptions and expectations of children, reflects the finding that parental attitudes and beliefs about childrearing are often more rigid and limited. Finally, it is important to consider how negative lifestyle and habits may influence the developing parent–child relationship. For example, treatment programs note problems related to the use of alcohol or drugs, prostitution, and subcultural peer groups among some individuals, which interfere with the delivery of intended services.

Intervention Methods: Tertiary Treatment Programs

Child-Focused Intervention

Although there have been numerous programs created to treat the victims of child abuse and neglect (see Mannarino & Cohen, 1990, for review), many provide only descriptive reports, with no data regarding their effectiveness in meeting the needs of children. Only those studies that have included information on results are presented here; however, even these provide only limited information and are plagued by the same shortcomings that appear throughout the child abuse and neglect literature.

Most studies do not make use of control or comparison groups, and provide only limited information on the subjects treated and the types of maltreatment suffered. Often, follow-up observations are not included or are only brief, making conclusions difficult. In addition, intervention often consists of more than one component, making accurate determinations of benefit difficult. Consequently, data from these programs have to be interpreted with caution and, at best, provide only an indication of the potential of these services to improve the needs of maltreated children.

Preschool-Based Programs

The majority of the services offered to children occur in the context of therapeutic day treatment programs, which provide group activities and peer interaction in combination with various individual therapy components. In a controlled study, Culp, Heide, and Richardson (1987) demonstrated that children who were involved in a therapeutic day treatment program, receiving group and individual treatment as well as services for their parents, showed improvements in areas of development related to fine motor, cognitive, gross motor, social/emotional, and language skills. In a similar but uncontrolled study, Culp, Richardson, and Heide (1987) found gains in development; however, they found that not all children received equal benefit, suggesting that attention to the characteristics of the children and the type of maltreatment may improve the effectiveness of this type of intervention. Culp, Little, Letts, and Lawrence (1991) also found that a comprehensive day treatment program providing similar services to those noted above was effective in improving the self-concept of a group of maltreated children relative to controls, as well as helpful in reestablishing their developmental progress (due to the multifaceted nature of the treatment administered, however, conclusions as to which treatment component was effective cannot be drawn).

Nicol et al. (1988) compared a family-oriented, casework approach to structured play treatment for maltreated children, which revealed more significant reductions in coercive behaviors for the family intervention. Unfortunately, there was a very high rate of attrition for the families involved, such that only about half the families actually completed the treatment program. Although attrition rates are not described for the rest of the studies reviewed, it is obvious that their inclusion would contribute substantially to the accurate interpretation of the program results.

Several intervention studies for victims of abuse were conducted by Fantuzzo and his associates (Fantuzzo, Stovall, Schachtel, Goins, & Hall,

1987; Fantuzzo et al., 1988; Davis & Fantuzzo, 1989). Using adult and con-federate child initiations of play within a playroom setting, these researchers found that the incidence of positive, prosocial responses and initiations im-proved for withdrawn, maltreated children. However, maltreated children who tended to be aggressive showed an increase in negative behaviors in re-sponse to social initiation (Davis & Fantuzzo, 1989). Again, the need for a greater understanding of the interplay between treatment modality and the characteristics of the children being treated is clear.

In sum, the preliminary results of programs designed to treat the vic-tims of abuse and neglect seem favorable in meeting some of their interven-tion needs. Across studies, participants showed improvement in social behavior, cognitive development, self-concept, and reduction in aggressive and coercive behaviors. No mention was made of the applicability of these intervention strategies to older children and adolescents, however, and the information is sketchy at best regarding effectiveness with different forms of maltreatment. Even though these child-focused treatment programs of-ten incorporated parent treatment components, no information was provided as to the effectiveness of these programs in meeting the needs of the parents involved. Similarly, no mention was made of the contribution of these approaches to the improvement of family resources and well-being.

In combination with the methodological concerns noted previously, these considerations underscore that the child-centered intervention programs have provided only limited indications of their usefulness. The potential of these methods, however, merits further investigation because services for child victims have important implications both for the development of the chil-dren involved and for interrupting the intergenerational transmission of child maltreatment.

Parent-Focused Interventions

Behavioral and Cognitive–Behavioral Programs

Behaviorally based treatment services for abusive parents typically involve some form of skills training focusing on child management skills, anger control skills, and/or general stress management (Azar & Wolfe, 1989). Training parents in effective child management skills, by far the most widely explored application of skills training, is based on a practical application of learning principles: educating parents about basic contingency management principles (e.g., reinforcement, punishment, and consistency), modeling for the parents (via films or live demonstrations) new ways of problem solving and increasing child compliance, rehearsing the desired skills in nonthreat-ening situations, with increasingly more and more realistic applications (i.e., practicing in the home with the therapist), and providing feedback (verbal or, in some instances, videotaped) to the parents regarding their performance of these behaviors.

As the application of these principles grew, additional therapeutic techniques (in particular, cognitive restructuring) were added to deal with some of the residual beliefs or emotional responses underlying to some extent the expression of abusive behavior. Self-control and anger-control techniques, derived from studies of nonabusive populations, were explored as a way to reduce abusive parents' heightened arousal level and inadequate coping ability. These techniques most commonly involve several components, including the use of early detection of anger-arousal cues (e.g., physiological and/or cognitive cues), replacing anger-producing thoughts with more appropriate ones, and teaching self-control skills that would lessen the likelihood of emotional outbursts and rage. These latter skills are developed through training in stress reduction, which is often done in conjunction with child management training. Stress reduction generally involves instructing parents in relaxation techniques and cognitive–behavioral methods of reducing stress, followed by rehearsal of new coping strategies during imagined and live interactions with their child.

Programs that utilize cognitive–behavioral intervention methods can be divided into three categories: behavioral programs aimed at improving parenting skills; cognitive programs, which aim to improve parent awareness and coping; or cognitive–behavioral approaches, which attempt to address both parenting skills and coping abilities of abusive parents. Of the studies reviewed herein, five emphasized behavioral interventions, four utilized cognitive approaches, and two used both components in their programs. Two of the programs that utilized both cognitive and behavioral intervention approaches (Egan, 1983; Whiteman, Fanshel, & Grundy, 1987) did so in order to compare the effectiveness of these approaches in treating abusive populations.

Subjects involved in these 11 studies were parents, mostly mothers, who were referred by community agencies dealing with child abuse and who had histories of substantiated maltreatment. Physical abuse was the form of maltreatment most frequently addressed, although cognitive intervention approaches were used to treat neglect in three of the programs and were also used as components of ecobehavioral programs dealing with child neglect issues, as discussed later (e.g., Tertinger, Greene, & Lutzker, 1984; Barone, Greene, & Lutzker, 1986). Parents were taking part in the programs voluntarily, although often in an attempt to preserve or stabilize custody of the children.

Two studies conducted therapy within the families' homes, while the rest used a clinic-based group treatment approach. Homework assignments were often used as part of these programs, and assessment was sometimes conducted by trained observers within the home in order to validate real gains in family effectiveness. Most services were provided in weekly sessions, generally over 6 to 8 weeks.

1. *Success in addressing problems related to the family context.* Although few of the studies directly addressed the problems related to the

family context and resources, there is some evidence of benefit in this regard. Barth, Blythe, Schinke, and Schilling (1983) structured the group treatment sessions in order to maximize the formation of supportive relationships between families. They report that group members socialized outside of the treatment sessions and reported having better feelings about life in general and better relationships with family and friends. Similar findings were noted by Fantuzzo, Wray, Hall, Goins, and Azar (1986) and Brunk, Henggeler, and Whelan (1987) in terms of improvements in the social behavior of the parents in their program. Dawson, de Armas, McGrath, and Kelly (1986), who taught cognitive problem-solving techniques to neglectful parents, report that parents in the treatment condition showed evidence of improved quality of life, including success with finding employment.

In addition, programs that attempted to improve parenting skills also reported success in reducing negative commands and hostile behavior between family members, as well as improving child compliance, thereby reducing the coercive interactions which characterize abusive families. The one study that made mention of marital problems, however, found no significant change (Barth et al., 1983).

2. *Success with different types of maltreatment.* Several cognitive–behavioral programs report consistent positive findings in treating both abuse and neglect, with continued improvement evident at follow-up. Behavioral intervention programs used coaching/modeling of appropriate parenting skills, role playing, reading assignments, and feedback to improve the parenting behaviors of abusive subjects and reported increases in positive parent–child interactions, increased child compliance, and reduced reliance on physical punishment for the parents treated. Reassessment after treatment and at follow-up (generally 1 year) revealed that these improvements were somewhat long lasting and generalized beyond the treatment setting. In addition, and important, further reports or suspicions of abuse did not occur for the families treated in many of the studies (e.g., Wolfe & Sandler, 1981; Wolfe et al., 1981; Wolfe et al., 1982; Crimmins, Bradlyn, St. Lawrence, & Kelly, 1984; Egan, 1983).

Studies of cognitively based interventions, using such techniques as relaxation and self-management skills training, cognitive restructuring, problem solving training, stress and anger management training, and combinations of methods to improve the coping abilities of abusive parents, report similar positive results in reducing the propensity of maltreatment (Nomellini & Katz, 1983; Egan, 1983; Barth et al., 1983; Whiteman et al., 1987). Cognitive intervention techniques also proved effective in teaching judgment and skills to neglectful parents, which presumably may reduce the risk of future incidents (Dawson et al., 1986; Fantuzzo et al., 1986). Studies that combined cognitive and behavioral techniques reported that such an approach may be the most effective method of dealing with maltreatment (Egan, 1983; Whiteman et al., 1987), providing parents with both the tools and the understanding required to properly assess, respond to, and control their children's behavior. However, these findings of cognitive and combined approaches must be approached with caution due to the relative lack of careful follow-up evaluation.

3. *Success in dealing with child intervention needs.* As previously noted, cognitive–behavioral approaches to intervention show promise in addressing the needs of maltreated children directly. Recent studies suggest the merit of these methods for assisting parents as well. For example, gains made in teaching parents appropriate skills and self-control have also been shown to result in collateral decreases in aggressive or negative child behavior and increased mutual expression of positive behavior and emotion between parent and child (e.g., Nomellini & Katz, 1983; Wolfe & Sandler, 1981).

4. *Success in addressing the needs of caregivers.* The evidence favoring successful intervention to meet the needs of caregivers is abundant for the cognitive–behavioral approaches. With the exception of issues related to lifestyle, of which there is little mention, such studies report consistent success in helping maltreating parents improve the conditions that predispose them to abusive and neglectful treatment. Control of emotions and anger is enhanced by cognitive treatment approaches and perceived stress is reduced (Barth et al., 1983; Egan, 1983; Nomellini & Katz, 1983; Whiteman et al., 1987). Parents' judgment, ability to empathize, and realistic perceptions and expectations of children also show improvement (Dawson et al., 1986; Whiteman et al., 1987). Finally, significant and consistent results are reported by all the programs designed to improve the parenting skills of abusive populations. Parents who receive these treatments consistently show improvements in their ability to interact positively with their children and control behavior without overreliance on negative, coercive, physically punitive child management techniques.

Surprisingly, only one study systematically investigated family therapy as a specific means of addressing the identified concerns of abusive families, despite the appeal of this approach. Brunk et al. (1987) randomly assigned 18 abusive and 15 neglectful families to either behavioral parent training or multisystemic family therapy and compared the relative effectiveness of both methods. Families in both conditions revealed decreased psychiatric symptomatology, reduced overall stress, and a reduction in the overall severity of identified problems. Although family therapy was more effective at restructuring parent–child relations, parent training was more effective at reducing identified social problems. The lack of a control group, as well as replications of this approach, make conclusions concerning multisystemic family therapy premature.

5. *Conclusions: Cognitive–behavioral intervention programs.* Several features make cognitive–behavioral intervention approaches attractive in working with parents who may abuse or neglect their children. First, they demonstrate a relatively greater degree of effectiveness in modifying those

parental characteristics that are most relevant to child maltreatment (e.g., parenting skills and perceptions and expectations of children). Several studies, using randomly assigned control groups, also showed reduced recidivism of maltreatment rather than just changes in specific attitudes or behaviors.

Many of the psychological characteristics of abusive caregivers make behavioral skills-based learning approaches quite attractive. Behavioral strategies are concrete and problem focused and, thus, may be more appropriate for assisting the less intellectual client. Interventions based on social learning theory are high in face validity and permit clients to work on the problems that are of most urgency and importance to them. Moreover, because behavioral treatments are often perceived as more "educational" and problem focused in nature, they may be less threatening to such families and make cooperation a bit easier to achieve (Fantuzzo et al., 1986; Azar & Wolfe, 1989; Kaufman & Rudy, 1991).

Despite these strengths, there are some limitations to cognitive–behavioral intervention programs. Most notably, these methods are not clinically effective for assisting those parents who may suffer from long-standing personality or psychiatric disorders, nor are they useful in improving the social or economic conditions of maltreating families. Furthermore, such skills-based educational methods require that parents practice new skills with their children, which poses some degree of resistance or difficulty (i.e., when children are in care). Given that a wide range of different problems often must be addressed with each family, cognitive–behavioral services may offer the greatest benefit in conjunction with other types of services.

Social Network Interventions

This approach to working with maltreating parents is discussed here only briefly because of the limited number of studies that provide evaluative data. The studies described focused their efforts on social support/social network interventions, defined as those strategies that seek to mobilize or modify the support available to targeted populations and/or alter the nature and structure of the social network. Based on the expanding evidence base supporting this approach for families with children at risk for adverse developmental outcomes (e.g., Tracy & Whittaker, 1987), two studies applied this strategy to the treatment of identified abusers.

Gaudin, Wodarski, Arkinson, and Avery (1991) sought to remedy child neglect by strengthening the informal support networks of such parents. Their intervention consisted of personal networking, mutual aid groups, volunteer linking, employing neighborhood helpers, and social skills training. The results, based on 34 experimental and 17 control families, support the value of informal network linkages in improving the adequacy of parenting among this disadvantaged population. For example, almost 60% of the treatment families had their cases closed, and 80% of families who received more than

9 months of treatment improved significantly on measures of parenting adequacy.

In a less elaborate design, Lovell and Hawkins (1988) tested a 26-week group intervention for mothers whose children were attending a therapeutic nursery for abused/neglected children. The goal of the intervention was straightforward—to increase the participants' availability of personal supports. Although the findings showed an increase in the number of identified supports, their network contacts did not provide much assistance/support in childrearing (e.g., on average, 74% of network members never or only rarely provided help with child care responsibilities).

Thus, on the basis of these limited studies, little information is available regarding the efficacy of social network interventions. Interestingly, this approach remains popular with many communities and child welfare agencies (Daro, 1988), perhaps because of the low cost and intangible benefits not measured by these reports. Nevertheless, adequate evaluation of their benefits is needed, especially as the programs pertain to the delivery of multiple services (discussed later).

Comprehensive/Multiservice Programs

Due to the intertwined causes of child abuse (i.e., the interaction of individual, family, marital, community, and sociocultural factors), treatment efforts have also been directed at levels other than (or in addition to) the parent's behavior. Accordingly, some programs have tailored their methods more specifically to the needs of the families they are serving, such as marital, financial, personal, or even employment-related problems. Such comprehensive or multiservice intervention strategies with dysfunctional and maltreating families represent a large and growing segment of current interventions for these diverse populations.

Comprehensive programs attempt to address the multiplicity of needs identified among maltreating families by providing services that are flexible and wide ranging. These services may be selectively chosen from existing methods of individual or group support, skills-based coping and child management techniques, homemaker services, and so forth, in order to tailor the program to the needs of each family. In this manner, they attempt to deal separately or simultaneously with each aspect of a family's particular situation within the context in which the problems occur. The following discussion organizes studies of comprehensive programs according to the two major programmatic efforts that have emerged over the past decade: those following a family-centered home-based orientation, and those with an ecobehavioral orientation.

Family-centered, home-based intervention (FCHBI) services, also known as the "family-preservation movement," arose largely in response to U.S. government initiatives to reduce the rate of child placement outside the home

(Frankel, 1988; Amundson, 1989). Based largely on an ecological model, these programs aim to prevent placement through the provision of a wide range of psychological and concrete services within the natural settings in which the families interact. Such services are generally time limited, team delivered, family oriented, and problem related, aiming to intervene with families in crisis situations, stabilize those situations, and set up support and intervention networks with other individuals and agencies in the community before terminating involvement with the family.

Ecobehavioral intervention programs, which also evolved from ecologically oriented research, assume multiple causation for any particular incident of abuse. Maltreatment occurs within a multifaceted context that extends beyond the parent–child relationship and beyond immediate antecedents and consequences. Abusive or neglectful behaviors are considered in relation to contextual factors, with an emphasis on the reciprocal influences between behavior and environment (Lutzker & Newman, 1986; Kaufman & Rudy, 1991). Treatment may be provided in the family home, or in any environment in which the difficulties arise (e.g., school or day care center). Virtually all research on ecobehavioral intervention centers on Project 12-Ways, a program developed in the early 1980s by Lutzker and associates.

Family-Centered Home-Based Intervention Programs

In accordance with their goal of reducing the number of child placements, FCHBI programs specifically target populations in which it is felt that placement of one or more children will occur, or temporary placement will be prolonged, without intervention. For all but one of the programs reviewed, the avoidance of placement was the primary criterion for selection, also forming the most frequent index of intervention success. Selection of participants in at least one study was also based on the presence of at least one family member who was motivated to keep the family together and on the determination that the home environment posed no danger to the therapist entering it. Thirteen intervention studies fell into this category (several from unpublished sources), as identified in Figure 6.1.

Unfortunately, the type, intensity, and combinations of treatments administered by each of the programs were often not clearly specified. Services listed by these programs include crisis intervention, case management, structural family therapy, supportive counseling, marital therapy, behavior parent training, parent education, behavior modification, assertiveness training, self-control, alcohol referral/treatment, problem solving, job-finding skills, financial and household management, and parent aid services such as homemakers and day care.

Duration of services varied broadly, both between and within the various programs. For those that emphasized brief, intense crisis intervention (six of the programs reviewed), the duration of service varied from 6 to 12 weeks. Further intervention was then continued by a network of other community agencies, with FCHBI personnel remaining on call for support. Six of the remaining programs provided more long-term services, averaging 10–12 months, with one lasting 18 months.

Interpretation of the results of these programs is limited due to several methodological factors. The inclusion of representative control groups and random assignment to the control and experimental groups was often missing. Four of the projects used random assignment to control and experimental groups; one other study utilized a nonrandom comparison. Moreover, data are either not provided or are inadequate regarding descriptions of treatment success in dealing with the various components of the multifaceted abuse problems encountered. Consistent with their concern for the reduction of child placement, results of intervention are frequently restricted to the percentage of placements that occurred during treatment or at follow-up, making it difficult to determine relationships between the type of maltreatment, the specific services provided, and the outcome of the intervention. Finally, interpretation is further clouded by a lack of information on participant attrition. These concerns notwithstanding, the results of FCHBI programs are delineated below, in reference to the identified needs of this population previously noted.

1. *Success in addressing problems related to the family context.* As mentioned earlier, an important component of FCHBI programs is the improvement of family and environmental conditions that contribute to the occurrence and severity of maltreatment. Although FCHBI programs consider the improvement of family functioning to be part of intervention success, there are few specific data presented that address this goal. In general terms, four studies reported modest to significant gains in "family functioning."

The study by Jones et al. (cited in Frankel, 1988) reported an improvement in the "emotional climate of the home" based on caseworker report for 60% of the treated families (in comparison to 36% of the control families). These same researchers also indicated a moderate but significant improvement in marital functioning for these families. Significant improvement in the home environment was also indicated by Nicol et al. (1988), whose study was the only one to examine coercive interactions between family members specifically.

As for family socioeconomic conditions, the few data available indicate no improvement for FCHBI clients, which is somewhat discouraging in light of the repeated finding that poverty and related problems are highly correlated with the failure of these programs to prevent placement (Frankel, 1988). The Second Chance for Families Program (cited in Frankel, 1988) is the only exception, reporting improved income for 52% of its clients, and improvements in housing for two thirds of the experimental group, compared to 8% and 15% for the experimental group. This same study reported improved social contacts, as indicated by relationships with other relatives, for about half of the clients served. Hinckley and Ellis (1985), however, report no improvement in social isolation for their clients, while Amundson (1989) reports an 85% improvement in the use of community resources. Clearly, a need for more specific description of results is evident in order to evaluate intervention success at improving family resources.

2. *Success with different types of maltreatment.* Again, few of the programs provided specific descriptions regarding intervention success according to the nature of the maltreatment involved (see Figure 6.1). It is important to note, however, that the selection procedures for several of the programs are biased against cases involving severe, multiproblem cases of abuse or neglect, because of concerns that the safety of the child must take precedence in such cases.

Amundson (1989) reports a decrease in the use of physical punishment for 95% of the subjects in Family Crisis Care, suggesting that this type of program is successful with minor physical abuse. Although no data are presented, it may be reasonable to assume that FCHBI programs, through the provision of concrete services and services aimed at improving the functioning of caretakers, will also be successful in dealing with less severe forms of neglect.

3. *Success in meeting child intervention needs.* The need of the child to live within a stable home environment and to avoid the disruption and uncertainty associated with outside placement is the primary target of FCHBI programs. However, due to lack of controls in the majority of these studies, placement results must be interpreted cautiously. Although the placement figures quoted in almost all cases are quite favorable, with up to 95% of families remaining intact (Hinckley & Ellis, 1985), those few studies that made use of control groups present figures that are somewhat less supportive. For example, Lyle and Nelson (cited in Frankel, 1988) reported that 67% of the families in the experimental group avoided placement, compared to 45% for the control condition. This relatively low rate for the experimental group occurred despite the fact that the program excluded those cases thought to be at highest risk. Similarly, Frankel (1988) reports that the favorable results initially reported by Jones et al. were found during later replications to be overstated (as stated in their final report). Comparable or lower rates of placement for families in the control group were actually found in the replication samples.

In addition, many of the studies fail to provide information on long-term success, basing their conclusions on placement status at conclusion of service without providing adequate follow-up data. Whether the effectiveness of the programs is maintained after termination of service remains largely a matter of speculation.

Specific data pertaining to the ability of these programs to meet other child intervention needs are largely nonexistent. Jones et al. (1976, cited in Frankel, 1988) report slight to moderate gains for experimental subjects in children's behavior and emotional adjustment, intellectual and school functioning, and social functioning in the community. Improvements in child self-control and aggression may also be inferred from Hinckley and Ellis (1985), who report decreases in physically and verbally violent behavior for all family members. They also report that their program is equally effective with children and adolescents. None of the other studies provided data that directly address the problems of older children in the families treated.

4. *Success in addressing the needs of caregivers.* Although success in adequately meeting the needs of caregivers in often cited as the area of most significant effectiveness for FCHBI programs (Frankel, 1988), once again there are few specific descriptions of the types of problems addressed. Hinckley and Ellis (1985) report a decreased propensity toward violent behavior for the adults in their program. Similarly, Amundson (1989) also reports a substantial decrease in parental use of physical punishment. However, neither of these reports includes suggestions as to the reason for the decrease in violent tendencies, which could be due to decreased emotional arousability, improved parenting skills, or a number of other possible changes. Giblin and Callard (1983, cited in Frankel, 1988) report specific improvement in parental independence and parenting ability for subjects in their program. No other information specific to caregiver needs is described in the studies reviewed.

5. *Costs and recidivism rates.* Intervention during a crisis period may result in a lower financial cost to society than alternatives such as foster care placement, which cost taxpayers $9.1 billion in 1991 (Ames, 1992). Although the determination of cost-effectiveness is as yet preliminary, studies that have addressed this question for FCHBI programs do indicate the potential for significant savings (Kinney, Madsen, Fleming, & Haapala, 1977; Wood, Schroeder, & Barton, 1988; Hinckley & Ellis, 1985). The Homebuilders program (Kinney et al., 1977), for example, presented data several years ago indicating that $5–6 is saved for every dollar invested in the program. In 1985, the cost of such services averaged $2,600 per family (Pransky, 1991); in 1992, this average cost (based on Alabama figures) is still a low $2,800, which compares quite favorably to the $7,400 cost of keeping one child in foster care for 35 months (the state average) (Ames, 1992). Moreover, Homebuilders estimates that 80% of families are still together after one year (Ames, 1992).

Ecobehavioral Intervention Programs

Participants in the ecobehavioral programs reviewed were families who had been identified for abuse or neglect by the Illinois Department of Children and Family Services. A single, unemployed parent with several young children in the home was the most typical participant. Consent of the parent(s) was frequently cited as a condition for selection, although Wesch and Lutzker (1991) indicate that consent may be a reluctantly accepted alternative to child placement.

In keeping with the multifaceted nature of the maltreatment problem assumed by ecological theory, services spanned a broad range and were tailored to meet individual situations. The services described by the researchers included some combination of parent–child training, stress reduction, basic skills training, problem solving, assertiveness training, social support, self-control training, health maintenance and nutrition, leisure skills, home safety, marital therapy, money management, job finding, alcoholism treatment referral, and multiple-setting behavior management (e.g., behavior management in school or day care). Services were provided in the home or in the environment in which problems arose. Precise information on the duration of services is not provided.

Although the information provided regarding the methodology, intervention types, and specific outcomes of intervention for ecobehavioral programs is more specific than the information provided by FCHBI programs, there is still ambiguity in the reports. Once again, numerous intervention tactics are often applied to each specific family situation, but the specific contribution of each intervention component to the success of the program has not been established. The use of control groups or controlled designs is infrequent, making interpretation of the outcomes of these programs limited at present.

1. *Success in addressing problems related to the family context.* There are few specific data regarding improvement in family resources, even though numerous components of the intervention strategy involve attempts to improve the marital, socioeconomic, and social conditions of the families treated. The only report that directly addresses this issue comes from Campbell, O'Brien, Bickett, and Lutzker (1983), based on a Project 12-Ways case study. The data they provide are positive, showing moderate gains in the marital enjoyment of the couple involved, development of a less coercive style of family interaction, and an improvement in the economic situation of the family through the successful application of the job-seeking strategies taught by the program staff. If this case can be considered representative of those served by Project 12-Ways, the program does show significant potential for addressing these aspects of the abusive family situation.

The social isolation of abusive and neglectful families is one problem for which this program seems particularly ineffective. Except for improving the social network of unwed mothers through group interaction, Lutzker (1984) reports that Project 12-Ways has been able to accomplish little in improving the social network of its clients, perhaps due to the extensive geographic area served by the program.

2. *Success with different types of maltreatment.* Project 12-Ways reports success at improving several aspects of family conditions associated with child neglect. Two of the studies (Tertinger et al., 1984; Barone et al., 1986) reported improvements in the safety of the homes of program clients. Similarly, improvements in the cleanliness of both the homes and the children of program clients are reported by Watson-Perczel, Lutzker, Greene, and McGimpsey (1988) and Rosenfield-Schlicter, Sarber, Bueno, Greene, and

Lutzker (1983). More direct evidence of effectiveness in dealing with abuse and neglect comes from reports by Lutzker and Rice (1984, 1987), which indicate program effectiveness in preventing reincidence of abuse and neglect among program participants both during treatment and in follow-up studies. Some suggestion was made, however, that the recidivism rate may increase after discontinuation of treatment, indicating the need for continued contact on a periodic basis between therapists and clients.

3. *Success in meeting child intervention needs.* There are few data specific to the intervention needs of children reported by the ecobehavioral programs reviewed, although intervention does have components aimed at addressing these needs. In a review of the program to date, Lutzker (1990) discussed several case studies that successfully addressed problems related to the child's health and safety. Although the findings are based largely on single case studies, they offer valuable suggestions for dealing with chronic problems associated with neglectful families and about the only evaluation data available specifically on this topic. Using structured behavioral approaches, these case studies revealed important changes in hygiene, nutrition, home safety, and cleanliness of target children.

4. *Success in addressing the needs of caregivers.* Although ecobehavioral programs focus considerable attention on the needs of caregivers, there are few data that refer specifically to this issue. Campbell et al. (1983), in a case study, report success in using relaxation techniques to treat migraine headaches and improve the emotional health of a parent, in addition to improving childrearing skills. Similarly, Lutzker (1990) reviews several additional case studies that successfully modified neglectful parents' affective skills, infant stimulation, and child health care.

5. *Costs and recidivism rates.* Project 12-Ways stands out from other programmatic intervention research in its efforts to document recidivism among participants over a lengthy time span. Using Illinois official reporting sources as their data, Lutzker and Rice (1987) reported a 21.3% recidivism rate for 710 project families, versus 28.5% for comparison families. However, no data regarding cost-effectiveness has been provided for Project 12-Ways.

Conclusions: Comprehensive/Multiservice Intervention Programs

Despite the numerous shortcomings of the studies examined, a few studies (e.g., Kinney et al., 1977; Wesch & Lutzker, 1991) and reviews (Frankel, 1988; Cohn & Daro, 1987) suggested significant advantages inherent in this approach to intervention. Thus, one may conclude that comprehensive programs warrant further study to determine their specific strengths and potential for treatment of abusive populations.

Intervention initiated during crisis situations may benefit from heightened family motivation for change and willingness to try new options ("the teachable moment"). The intensive contact between clients and therapists may allow for more accurate and complete assessment of family situations and may facilitate maximum responsiveness of the treatment program to the changing needs and resources of the families involved. There is an expanded potential for therapist modeling of appropriate behaviors in the environment in which they occur, and intervention can be tailored to build on the strengths of all family members concerned. Finally, initial costs estimates, especially for the home-based programs designed to deter child placements, are very favorable compared to alternative placement costs.

Disadvantages cited for comprehensive intervention programs include the need for extensive training of the therapists involved and a considerable administrative structure; typical limitations faced when working with poor, multiproblem families and severe forms of maltreatment; and a potentially high rate of attrition (Nicol et al., 1988). Most important, because these programs have not received adequate scientific evaluation, the wide-scale effort under way to establish such programs nationwide seems premature.

Summary of Tertiary Interventions

Videka-Sherman (1989) recently conducted a meta-analysis of child abuse and neglect (tertiary) treatment programs. Her review points out some of the common features of these programs and the extent of their effectiveness. From 124 studies involving treatment of child maltreatment, 23% were identified as focusing on physical abuse, 4% neglect, and 23% sexual abuse (the remaining 48% involved mixed samples of maltreatment). After noting that the vast majority of these studies used uncontrolled designs (e.g., 47% were pre–post or one-group ex post facto designs and 29% were single subject), she restricted her analysis to the 25 experimental or quasi-experimental studies that would permit more valid overall conclusions.

Consistent with the present review, the most frequently occurring treatment modality in these 25 studies was some form of treatment of the parent (48%) or the family (35%). The specific strategies included a wide range of (overlapping) approaches, including role modeling and rehearsal (31%), referrals to other social services (35%), child management skills training (31%), teaching about child development (31%), some form of environmental modification or services (34%), shaping new behaviors (28%), use of books or didactic methods (28%), and home visits (48%).

Videka-Sherman (1989) reports that the largest effect sizes were associated with methods based on social learning (average effect size = 1.14, based on 6 studies) and related educational approaches (average effect size = 1.04, based on 5 studies). The relatively few ($n = 4$) psychodynamically based treatment studies produced the lowest average effect size (.47). It is interesting to note that certain intervention components were associated with greater effectiveness across these studies. Specifically, preparing the client in some fashion for the treatment process was associated with higher effect sizes, as were programs that offered specific guidelines to follow. As well, those programs that focused on interpersonal skill enhancement of the parent resulted in better outcomes than did those involved strictly with an intrapersonal or social system emphasis.

This meta-analysis of 25 studies with maltreating parents is suggestive, on the one hand, of important gains that have been made with this population. On the other hand, it points to the caution one must use in drawing conclusions, based on the relative paucity of research. Few studies followed up participants long enough to ensure a low reincidence rate of abuse or its high-risk indicators (e.g., harsh, power-assertive childrearing or use of physical punishment). In view of the concerns noted over a decade ago based on early, uncontrolled clinical trials with abusive families (Cohn, 1979), we still have a considerable way to go toward determining the most effective form of intervention in the long run.

Some of the prominent factors contributing to this lackluster success with tertiary treatment of child maltreatment have to do with the nature of the target population and our general tendency to miss the mark in servicing their needs. First of all, there is a marked tendency for parents to be unwilling to seek help until it is forced on them or the problem becomes major. Their avoidance of services makes sense, however, in light of our current strategy for combating child maltreatment. Currently, our child welfare system functions on the basis of reaction to crises and conflicts, and, consequently, little effort is directed toward the "front end" of the child welfare system. Those families that are most in need often receive very little support and assistance until they commit a major violation of child care practices.

The next section of this chapter looks at the expanding number of programs designed to assist families who may be at risk of maltreatment but have not been identified or have not yet committed such behaviors. By and large, these programs were built on some of the more promising approaches noted in the tertiary intervention literature and then applied to a much broader segment of the parenting population at an earlier point (i.e., Stage 1). Although methodological issues remain with many of these studies as well, several important conclusions may be drawn that have implications for intervention and prevention planning.

INTERVENTION NEEDS AND METHODS FOR NONIDENTIFIED FAMILIES EXHIBITING RISK CHARACTERISTICS (STAGE I)

One may easily argue that all families require some degree of assistance in childrearing today, especially during the child's early years. This view derives from the simple principle that a parent who is well prepared for the life changes associated with childrearing is less likely to succumb to the increasing stress factors that prevail. This viewpoint, moreover, is congruent with the principles of preventive mental health—skills, knowledge, and experiences that boost the individual's coping abilities (e.g., sense of mastery and control over stressful aspects of the individual's role) will increase the individual's resistance to the forces that oppose his/her healthy adjustment (Dohrenwend, 1978). Such parents are said to be socially incompetent, in that they are able to apply interpersonal skills to meet the demands of the situation and provide positive outcomes for all persons involved.

To be socially competent in the parenting role, a person must display interpersonal positiveness such as praising, complimenting, or showing affection; the person must be able to observe the demands of a situation in order to choose the appropriate response; and these manifestations must be rewarding to both interactants (Burgess, 1985). The parent who is socially incompetent, on the other hand, fosters incompetence in the child who, in turn, reacts adversely to the parent. A vicious cycle of rejection, depression, or low self-esteem may result, leading to child maladjustment and parent–child conflict.

Identifying Targets for Early Intervention Efforts

Developmental research informs us that a style of cooperation tends to develop reciprocally among parents and children very early. Parents who are themselves cooperative and attentive to their child's needs and capabilities tend to have children who are similarly cooperative and easier to manage. In sharp contrast, parents who rely on intrusive and power assertive methods of control are more likely to have offspring who reciprocate in kind with annoying and disruptive behavior and who will fail to acquire prosocial behaviors. Thus, it is important to consider the major factors associated with the development of healthy versus high-risk parent–child relationships and to investigate intervention methods that promote such relationships from the earliest point in time. Summarized in this section is a representative list of concerns that may emerge during the prenatal, postnatal, or early childhood periods of parent–infant relationship development. As before, a figure lists the major intervention concerns and available methods for families.

1. *Prenatal factors.* The importance of proper prenatal care in establishing the early beginnings of the parent–child relationship is supported by both medical and psychological research. In terms of intrauterine care, serious disturbances in fetal growth and development, as well as later disturbances of the newborn, can be affected prenatally by maternal nutrition, age, substance abuse, and viral and bacterial infections. Mother's (and perhaps father's) use of drugs, alcohol, and cigarettes has been linked to infant prematurity, low birth weight, slowed development, and the "difficult child

syndrome." These health factors, in addition to genetic endowment, can lead to physical and mental handicaps that impair the mother's and child's later abilities to establish strong ties. Fortunately, there is emerging evidence that many of these problems can be prevented by proper education, medical care, and assistance provided during the prenatal period.

Maternal adjustment and preparation for parenthood are also believed to affect complications during pregnancy, labor, and delivery. This is a grave concern among mothers who experience extreme stress or depression during pregnancy, due either to exogenous conditions (such as relationship conflict or violence or financial instability) or endogenous factors (such as hormonal changes or personality functioning). In addition, how well both parents prepare for their role certainly affects their degree of success with the newborn. Prospective studies (e.g., Brunquell, Crichton, & Egeland, 1981; Egeland, Breitenbucher, & Rosenberg, 1980) have shown that high life stress and change during pregnancy are linked to abuse and related problems, especially among mothers who were anxious, unknowledgeable about children, and ill prepared. Once again, such negative outcomes can be prevented during this period of development. The provision of an adequate support system (e.g., family members and nurse visitors) seems to mitigate the effects of life stress and personal adaptation to a significant degree (as discussed later).

2. *Postnatal/infancy factors.* The formation of healthy infant–caregiver attachment represents a major task during this developmental period, which may have a significant effect on the quality of subsequent patterns of care. Parents who were poorly adjusted or prepared before the child's birth are more likely to have negative outcomes with their child, regardless of the child's birth status (e.g., prematurity and illness). Furthermore, children who receive poor quality of care during early infancy have been found to show interactional patterns of avoidance or anxious attachment to their caregivers, which leads to further developmental decline (Egeland & Sroufe, 1981). In contrast, the parent who is well prepared for the life changes associated with childrearing is less likely to succumb to the increasing stress factors that prevail. Skills, knowledge, experiences, and support that boost the individual's coping abilities will increase their resistance to forces that oppose their healthy adjustment. The same holds true for the infant, whose temperament and responsiveness contributes in important ways to his/her own treatment.

3. *Infancy and early childhood.* During this stage of development, parental resources and responses to the child, as well as the child's opportunity and ability to develop adaptive behavior, appear to be critical determinants of the parent–child relationship. Specific qualities that reflect competence in the parenting role, and thereby enhance the parent–child relationship, include such actions as verbal communication that provides information and stimulation to the infant, physical freedom for the infant to explore his/her environment, responsiveness to the infant's needs in a manner that is consistent

with his/her developmental level, and positive affect that accompanies all supportive verbal and physical interactions (Cicchetti et al., 1988).

In brief, if the parent's responses to the young child are age appropriate, peer supported, and otherwise successful from the perspective of the parent's wishes and the child's needs, the risk of relying on power-assertive control tactics may be reduced and the child's development of adaptive abilities will be enhanced. The value of early assistance and support programs for new families and disadvantaged families is apparent from these findings.

Figure 6.2 lists the major intervention targets that emerge from the literature describing risk factors among dysfunctional families. These targets are then discussed in relation to intervention programs that have been evaluated with samples representing a wide range of risk statuses (e.g., new parents and disadvantaged families). The following summary is representative of the major factors but is not exhaustive.

Problems Related to the Family Context.

The literature reflects the presence of several major risk factors related to family resources and functioning, three of which are summarized here. The first, unstable relationships, reflects the common finding that many young adults are unable to maintain or establish a partnership that is supportive and nonviolent, as reflected by the fact that more than three-quarters of teen parents are single mothers (Canadian Broadcasting Company, 1992). Such families are also plagued by socioeconomic stress, and by social isolation from appropriate supports and resources. For example, they often lack adequate day care, peer groups or close friends, and adequate housing. These factors play an indirect, yet significant, role in the formation and healthy establishment of a positive versus abusive parent–child relationship.

Prenatal/Infant Care

As discussed earlier, the importance of prenatal and postnatal care is paramount in reducing the risk of casualty and establishing a positive developmental outcome. Figure 6.2 lists three factors that should be addressed by intervention programs during this stage: (1) prenatal care, (2) postnatal care, and (3) caregiver sensitivity (including the formation of attachment).

Needs of Toddlers and Young Children

Two primary issues are described as the most viable targets for early intervention concerning the needs of the young child: the successful accomplishment of developmental milestones, such as language and communication, and behavioral competencies, such as positive emotion, normal compliance, and self-control, including developmental immaturity and adjustment.

INTERVENTION TARGETS

| | Family Context | Prenatal/ Infant Care | Toddler/ Child Needs | Caregiver Needs |

INTERVENTION STRATEGIES

Column headers (angled): Unstable Relationships; Socioeconomic Stress; Social isolation; Prenatal Care; Postnatal Care; Caregiver Sensitivity; Developmental Milestones; Behavioral Competencies; Immaturity / Adjustment; Emotional distress; Childrearing skills; Child expectations; Competing lifestyle/habits; Recidivism/Reports; Cost; Advantages; Disadvantages; Comments

Intervention Strategies	Advantages	Disadvantages	Comments
I. Parental Competency Programs (identified Groups)			
A. With Home Visits (n=10)[a]	A,B,D,E	a,b,d,f	1,2,4,5
B. W/O Home Visits (n=3)[b]	A,B,D-F	a,b,d,f	1,2,4,5
II. Parent-Child Support Programs (new parents)			
A. With Home Visits (n=9)[c]	A,B,D,E	a,b,d,f	1,2,4,5
B. With increased Hospital Contact (n=2)[d]	G	a,b,d,	
III. Parent-Child Support			
E. (Teen Parents) (n=6)	A to E F,H	a,b,d	1,2,4,5

Key to Advantages:
A. Can be easily interrupted and continued as needed
B. Can be implemented by trained paraprofessionals
C. Can be conducted in either home or clinic setting
D. Perceived by most parents as less threatening or coercive
E. Very flexible in terms of individual needs
F. Typically brief duration (less than one year)
G. Little or no cost
H. One study supports the use of education classes for teen fathers

Key to Disadvantages:
a. Limited outcome evaluation studies
b. Limited data on generalization across time, settings, or persons
c. Generally takes several months or years to produce change
d. Inconclusive regarding efficacy with male offenders
e. No outcome data available as to effectiveness
f. May be helpful only to a very limited subgroup of parents who can identify their own problems and are motivated to change

Comments:
1. Best suited for families in which knowledge/skills of childrearing are lacking
2. Best suited for parents who prefer specific direction and guidance
3. Best suited for individuals who prefer to explore their own motives and options
4. Due to multiple needs of the identified population, services per family can become quite extensive and prolonged
5. Matching treatment length to each individual's needs may be critical

Superscripts:
a. Andrews et al., 1982; Armstrong & Grailey, 1985; Barrera et al., 1986; Epstein & Weikart, 1979; Gray & Ruttle, 1980; Madden et al., 1984; Slaughter, 1983; Stevenson et al., 1988; Teleen et al., 1989; Travers et al., 1982.
b. Resnick, 1985; Roderiguez & Cortez, 1988; Wolfe et al., 1988.
c. Affleck et al., 1989; Barnard et al., 1985; Gray et al., 1979; Larson, 1980; Olds et al., 1988; Seitz et al., 1985; Siegel et al., 1980; Taylor & Beauchamp, 1988.
d. O'Connor et al., 1980; Siegel et al., 1980.
e. Field et al., 1980; Field et al., 1982; Gutelius et al., 1977; Mitchell & Casto, 1988; Roosa & Vaughn, 1983; Westney et al., 1988.

FIGURE 6.2. Intervention strategies for nonidentified families exhibiting risk characteristics (ratings of relative effectiveness in addressing each intervention target).

Caregiver Needs

The majority of early intervention programming is directed at the adult, as it is during the later stages of maltreatment. Four primary targets are summarized from the literature as being the most important to address during intervention. Because these four are similar to those described in the previous section they are listed here only briefly: (1) emotional distress, (2) limited childrearing skills, (3) inappropriate perceptions and expectations of children, and (4) competing lifestyle/habits.

Intervention Methods:
Secondary Prevention Programs

The view of child maltreatment as a sign of "relational failure" has gained wide acceptance (Cicchetti et al., 1988). Such failure is due to the presence of debilitating factors (poverty, adolescent parenthood, single parenthood, etc.) that place extra burdens on the formative parent–child relationship, as well as the absence of social support and guidance. Accordingly, increasing numbers of researchers and practitioners are focusing on the quality of early interactions between children and parents who may be at risk for child abuse and neglect, with prevention of maltreatment as their goal.

Intervention programs for parents who have not been specifically identified as abusive or neglectful are founded primarily on the premise that promoting a positive and responsive parent–child relationship is both a desirable intervention target as well as a viable child abuse prevention strategy. The rationale for such programs is straightforward: Many families with very young children (under 24 months of age) are not yet experiencing the serious child behavior management problems that bring their counterparts with preschool and school-age children to the attention of child protection agencies. Parent–child interactions are still relatively benign, although subtle indications of future problems may be present. If parents can be assisted in their role at this early stage, the chances of influencing patterns of parenting and promoting healthier parent–infant relationships are improved. Thus, the likelihood of relational failure and signs of child abuse and neglect is diminished.

Young, socially disadvantaged parents are more likely than their older, more advantaged counterparts to lack the skills necessary for effective parenting. They may lack knowledge about infant development and therefore have inappropriate expectations for their infants' behavior in the first 2 years of life. They tend to overestimate the rate of development and often become impatient and intolerant when their infants fail to live up to these expectations (Miller, 1988). When interacting with their infants, such parents display relatively low levels of positive affect and/or tend to display more inappropriate and negative affect, a finding that compares with identified abusive parents (Wolfe, 1985).

For adolescent or immature parents in particular, their own stage of development (e.g., poorly defined personal identities, self-centeredness, and the inability to anticipate the needs of others) can increase their risk of maltreating their children. Thus, programs that help young parents to enjoy their parental role simultaneously serve to promote feelings of self-worth and effectiveness, which in turn enhances behavioral sensitivity (Lamb & Easterbrooks, 1981). The parent's relationship with the child is happier and the increased sense of enjoyment can make the parent more receptive to basic childrearing information.

The following review of intervention programs is organized according to various target populations, rather than particular therapeutic methods per se (as was done in the previous sections). Such a structure reflects the literature in this particular area whereby intervention programs share many of the same "core ingredients" and vary primarily in terms of "with whom" and "when" they focus their efforts at prevention and competency enhancement. Accordingly, the procedures used to achieve their goals often include structured interactions with the child (involving specific stimulation techniques and child management techniques), informal opportunities for parents to learn how to teach and manage their children in a more positive fashion, and the strengthening of personal support networks. Moreover, many of these methods are designed to assist families in a flexible manner that is sensitive to cultural differences and realistic limitations for change.

A common feature in many of the programs described herein is the home-visitor component, in which a professional or trained layperson visits the family home to provide parenting-related instruction and to act as a liaison with other community and health care systems. Thus, chiefly through education and support, these programs strive to enhance adult competency to help parents gain control over their lives (Pransky, 1991). Family support programs may be directed at various types of parents who are at risk for becoming abusive. The following review breaks these groups into three (overlapping) populations: parental competency programs for identified target groups (such as physician referrals), parent–child support programs for new parents, and parent–child support programs for teen parents. One important subpopulation included in this approach is adolescents who are pregnant or with young children, because they are considered to possess both specific and general risk indicators.

Parental Competency Programs for Select Target Groups

Support programs intended for an identified group of parents and/or children who are considered to be at some risk of maltreatment usually state procedural specifications for determining individuals in the population who warrant preventive services. Thirteen intervention studies over the past decade fell into this category. These studies are identified in Figure 6.2. Almost all these studies selected participants according to single or multiple socio-demographic variables that have been associated with verified maltreatment in the literature (e.g., low income and at least one young child in the home); four studies also used a cutoff score on some measure of abuse potential.

Of the 13 studies, 10 chose a home-visitor approach to intervention. These visits were provided by a nurse or trained visitor, occurred on a weekly to monthly basis, and ranged in duration from 3 months to 3 years, with the majority from 1 to 3 years. For studies specifically targeting child developmental delay prevention, the focus of visits was to encourage the parent-as-teacher approach, emphasizing knowledge of child development and child cognitive stimulation. For studies targeting abuse prevention, home visits and supplemental group instruction and support focused on child management issues. The remaining 3 studies utilized a variety of group approaches emphasizing either a parent training curriculum or a personal development/life skills strategy.

Success at Addressing the Needs of Toddlers and Young Children

As noted previously, the primary needs of children at this stage focus on accomplishing developmental milestones and strengthening behavioral competencies. In terms of gains in developmental milestones, the majority of studies reported modest positive cognitive gains for program children over no treatment controls at posttest. These studies tended to use multisite treatment groups and had robust treatment delivery. For example, Andrews et al. (1982) reported consistent positive results across sites at posttest indicating the efficacy of both home-visitor and group approaches. These were maintained at a 1-year follow-up conducted in the group intervention sites (although based on fewer subjects). Also, Barrera, Rosenbaum, and Cunningham (1986) found that child management visits were as effective as child cognitive stimulation visits, compared to no-treatment controls.

Studies that failed to obtain these posttest results either used limited samples (Gray & Ruttle, 1980) or noted problems in the delivery of development-focused services (Travers, Nauta, & Irwin, 1982). Although Madden, O'Hara, and Levenstein, (1984) found positive posttest results for the cohort whose treatment delivery was well monitored, maintenance at follow-up was not found. They speculate that a number of factors, including compensatory activities of controls, may have diluted the experimental-control distinction over time.

In terms of child behavioral competency, positive results were found in several studies utilizing direct observation of longer durations and with larger samples (e.g., Andrews et al., 1982; Slaughter, 1983). The maintenance of these effects remain unclear, however, because only one study reported follow-up interactional data (Epstein & Weikart, 1979). Behavior rating scales yielded less positive results, with only one study (Wolfe, Edwards, Manion,

& Koverola, 1988), finding group differences favoring program children on maternal ratings of child behavior at posttest and at 3-month follow-up.

These findings suggest modest short-term child cognitive benefit for programs that provide instruction in child development and child management. The superiority of either home- or group-based intervention was not demonstrated. Less consistent results for the maintenance of both cognitive and behavioral gains, due primarily to a lack of follow-up studies, limits conclusions regarding the long-term efficacy of parental competency programs with respect to the prevention of child developmental and behavioral impairment.

Success at Addressing the Needs of Caregivers

Needs of the caregiver at this stage, as described in the previous section, include emotional reactivity to child-related stress, limited childrearing skills, inappropriate perceptions and expectations of children, and competing lifestyle habits. To evaluate their ability to meet these diversified needs, the 13 studies measured a variety of adult adjustment variables that were the direct or indirect targets of change in their programs. It should be noted, however, that almost all studies involved mothers only, and therefore conclusions are specific to women who participated.

In terms of personal adjustment, program mothers reported greater improvements in life satisfaction (Andrews et al., 1982), financial independence and/or resource use (Andrews et al., 1982; Roderiguez & Cortez, 1988; Travers et al., 1982), more modern social values and ego development (Slaughter, 1983), and better overall adjustment (Stevenson, Bailey, & Simpson, 1988; Travers et al., 1982) than did controls. In contrast, of the four studies examining depression and self-esteem, only Wolfe et al. (1988) found greater reductions in depression scores for parent training mothers than controls (at posttest only).

The majority of studies found positive results favoring program mothers on measures of childrearing skills. Compared to controls, program mothers had better scores in teaching and interacting (Andrews et al., 1982; Gray & Ruttle, 1980; Madden et al., 1984; Slaughter, 1983; Travers et al., 1982), responsivity (Barrera et al., 1986), and use of negative language and control techniques (Andrews et al., 1982). These effects were maintained at 1 to 2 years follow-up (Andrews et al., 1982; Gray & Ruttle, 1980; Madden et al., 1984), although Epstein and Weikart (1979) found no group differences at 5 years postprogram. Studies that found no group differences in observed childrearing skills had small samples (e.g., Resnick, 1985; Wolfe, 1988).

Three studies that measured parental perceptions and expectations of children found program mothers to show greater gains in positive attitudes than did controls (Resnick, 1985; Roderiguez & Cortez, 1988; Slaughter, 1983). Moreover, all five studies that rated the home environment (i.e., lifestyle issues and the presence of appropriate child stimulation materials) found program mothers had better scores at posttest relative to their initial levels and/or to controls. There was some evidence of maintenance of such effects at 3 years postprogram (e.g., Armstrong & Frailey, 1985).

Additional positive results were found in terms of managing contextual and child-related stress. Armstrong (1981), for example, reported fewer psychosocial stressors for home-visited mothers at posttest and at 3-year follow-up (Armstrong & Frailey, 1985), and Teleen, Herzog, and Kilbane, (1989) found that program mothers reported less child-related stress as compared to controls. Program mothers also reported greater support and less social isolation than did controls in this latter study, with those in the self-help support group showing greater improvement than those in the parent training group.

Finally, program participants had fewer abuse reports at posttest and 3-year follow-up than did post hoc controls (Armstrong, 1981; Armstrong & Frailey, 1985). Teleen et al. (1989) found no abuse reports for treatment subjects during intervention. Similarly, program participation was associated with lower child abuse potential scores (Wolfe et al., 1988) and less self-reported use of physical/severe punishment (Roderiguez & Cortez, 1988; Stevenson et al., 1988).

These results of changes in parental attitudes and in self-reported and observed behavior related to the childrearing role (e.g., stimulating home environment and better teaching approaches) reveal favorable gains for program participants in the short term and suggest longer-term benefits as well. Because these gains were found in both home-visit and group approaches, as well as child management and cognitive stimulation, conclusions regarding treatment type and treatment efficacy remain more global than specific.

Conclusions: Parental Competency Programs for Select Target Groups

While acknowledging the limitations of these studies, in general the findings support the short-term efficacy of family support with identified target groups. Taking child and parental outcome results together, no approach to service delivery with these families emerges as preferred. The pattern that does emerge is that fairly intensive group and home visit interventions providing parental support and instruction in child management and/or child cognitive stimulation exert their main benefits in the domains of parental attitudes and behavior and overall maternal adjustment. Positive child cognitive results seem to emerge in studies involving large samples and consistent delivery of child development-focused interventions, although these seem to be short term in nature. Similarly, positive child behavioral gains are found in studies with larger samples and sounder assessment methods.

From a prevention perspective, these results are encouraging because theorists have emphasized parental characteristics and the interactional quality between parent and child as important determinants of parental behavior (e.g., Belsky, 1984; Wolfe, 1987). While positive gains were found for *indirect* measures of abuse and neglect prevention (e.g., parenting attitudes and behavior), few investigations attempted to measure abuse prevention directly (e.g., agency reports), thereby highlighting the need to include both types of measures. Also, given the increased cost of home visitation, the comparability of home versus group parenting education approaches merits further study.

Parent–Child Support Programs for New Parents

Another early intervention/prevention strategy that has received considerable attention over the past decade emphasizes the importance of establishing positive early beginnings for new, inexperienced parents and their infants. Most commonly, such programs aim their interventions either during pregnancy or during the period following birth. Although these populations may be considered at risk of abuse or neglect by virtue of the fact that they are new parents, many researchers also used additional risk factors to define their populations, such as socioeconomic disadvantage.

Ten studies were identified that focused their education and training efforts mostly on new parents during the perinatal and postnatal periods (see Figure 6.2). Although several studies selected participants based on additional "stress factors" (e.g., social disadvantage), the primary selection criterion was new parenthood. Based on attachment theory as well as on a prevention philosophy, these efforts were designed to assist new parents in their challenging role in order to strengthen the parent–infant relationship from the beginning. Most of these studies involved medical professionals and/or hospital services to implement the expanded services provided to participants in the experimental conditions. All studies utilized a home-visitor approach except for O'Connor, Vietze, Sherrod, Sandler, and Altemeier (1980), which studied the impact of increased mother–infant in-hospital contact following delivery. Visits began on a weekly basis with reduced frequency over time and ranged in duration from 1 month to more than 30 months. The majority of studies provided 1 to 3 years of home visits, with 3 studies offering less than 4 months of service (Affleck, Tennen, Rowe, & Roscher, 1989; Taylor & Beauchamp, 1988; Siegel, Bauman, Schaefer, Saunders, & Ingram, 1980).

The nature of the home visits in these studies of new and expectant parents differed from the previous studies described in that most were begun either prenatally (generally the third trimester) or in the early postpartum period. A further contrast relates to the focus on parental guidance and support in these latter studies. That is, a consultation model in which parenting issues were explored in more of a supportive and unstructured way was followed, rather than a didactic parenting education or infant-focused curriculum. However, this is not to imply that this model is somehow haphazard; in general, guidelines regarding content were specified. Detailed curricula were used in two studies; Olds, Henderson, Chamberlain, and Tatelbaum (1986) focused on instruction in child development and management and Booth, Mitchell, Bernard, and Spieker (1989) provided counseling in maternal social and parenting skills.

Success at Addressing the Needs of Toddlers and Young Children

Although improvements in child development per se were not the main target of these studies, positive results were found by investigators who specifically targeted child stimulation either through day care (Seitz, Rosenbaum, & Apfel, 1985) or home-visitor instruction (Olds et al., 1986). For example, Seitz et al. (1985) noted positive findings favoring program children at posttest and 5-year follow-up, although these were not maintained at 10 years postprogram. Olds et al. (1986) found positive results only for the most at-risk group, and a trend toward better scores for program children of high risk, home-visited mothers as compared to controls at 1 year of program and at posttest was reported (these researchers viewed these cognitive gains to be clinically significant) (Olds & Kitzman, 1990). These findings, limited by the small number of investigations, preliminarily suggest that modest child cognitive benefits may be derived from home-visit intervention and that these gains are likely to be short rather than long term.

In terms of changes in child behavioral competencies, consistent positive results favoring program participants were reported in studies using larger samples and longer interventions. For example, Olds et al. (1986) found home-visited mothers rated their children as having more positive temperaments than did controls. On interview items, trends favoring home-visited, high risk mothers suggested these children were viewed as less problematic than were controls. Seitz et al. (1985) reported that program mothers rated their children more positively than did controls, but for male children only. In contrast, home visitation was not found to predict subsequent child behavior in two studies that utilized a fairly brief home-visitation intervention (Affleck et al., 1989; Siegel et al., 1980). Finally, home-visit and early-contact interventions were linked with gains in child health in three of five studies reporting on this concern (Larson, 1980; O'Connor et al., 1980; Olds et al., 1986).

Taken together, the extent of child positive outcome for home-visit and early-contact interventions is only modest. However, it should be noted that the prime target of these interventions is not child focused, and that those programs that follow a detailed curriculum of child development and management (e.g., Olds et al., 1986) or provided child care (Seitz et al., 1985) reported the most positive results. Because few studies simultaneously measured a variety of child outcomes, these issues await further study.

Success at Addressing the Needs of Caregivers

In terms of maturity and personal adjustment concerns, home-visited mothers reported greater educational attainment, financial status, and smaller family size in a study by Seitz et al. (1985). In two studies, maternal positive mood, greater perceived control, and better social skills were predicted by home-visitation interaction with subject characteristics. That is, Affleck et al. (1989) reported that with increasing need for support, the effect of home visitation on perceived control/coping was more positive; similarly, the effect of home visits was more beneficial as infant risk status increased. Booth et al. (1989) similarly reported that home visits were most beneficial in terms of attainment of treatment goals and improved mother–child interactions for mothers beginning treatment with low levels of social skills. These latter studies suggest that home visitation yields more positive maternal adjustment with those most at risk or in need of treatment (i.e., severe neonatal status, low support, or low social skills).

Adult childrearing skills as measured by observer ratings of the home environment and mother–child interactions showed the most positive results on such aspects as provision of appropriate play materials, greater level of interaction, and less power assertiveness for the home-visited than for control mothers (Affleck et al., 1989; Booth et al., 1989; Larson, 1980; Olds et al., 1986; Taylor & Beauchamp, 1988). Again greater benefits for subjects at higher risk were noted (Affleck et al., 1989; Booth et al., 1989; Olds et al., 1986); however, Taylor and Beauchamp's (1988) results also suggest that brief home visitation is most beneficial to low-risk mothers. The only study that failed to find consistent positive results had interventions that were brief and failed to specify content clearly (Siegel et al., 1980). In terms of child abuse reports, intensive home visitation was most beneficial with mothers displaying more risk factors (Olds et al., 1986). Finally, the only study that measured parenting attitudes and knowledge of child development found that home-visited mothers evinced more positive attitudes and greater knowledge than did controls, and these were maintained at 2 months post-program (Taylor & Beauchamp, 1988).

These results of changes in parental behavior show that the more intensive home-visit interventions (1–3 years) yielded the greatest gains in maternal adjustment and behavior, especially among those parents who possessed more risk factors. Brief home interventions (under 1 month) seem to be efficacious with parents possessing few risk factors, such as first-time parenthood (Taylor & Beauchamp, 1988). However, very brief interventions, such as increased in-hospital contact, show minimal gains in parental outcome (O'Connor et al., 1980; Siegel et al., 1980). Because few studies conducted follow-up assessments of these parental measures, the maintenance of these short-term benefits once again remain at issue.

Conclusions: Parent–Child Support Programs for New Parents

Taking child and parental outcome results together, they echo the findings reported previously with identified at-risk parents. That is, greater gains were shown in measures of parental rather than child adjustment, and the efficacy of fairly intensive home visitation (1–3 years) is supported. The finding that positive results were reported for home visits following both a consultation model and a more formal curriculum suggests that parenting information and support garnered from either approach is beneficial. Brief home visits and/or home visits conducted in the absence of clearly specified program objectives and content did not seem to work as well.

The present findings indicating greater gains for subjects possessing more initial risk factors and receiving fairly intensive interventions argue for the matching of treatment length to the need of each participant. This is supported in the first instance by the positive results of brief home visitations for low-risk subjects (i.e., new parents who were 18 years of age and older and not excluded on the basis of any demographic factor, such as education level, income, or marital status) reported by Taylor and Beauchamp (1988). These findings, although preliminary, support the utility of a community-wide prevention approach in which such services are offered routinely as part of prenatal and postpartum care.

In the second instance, the importance of matching treatment length to subject need or risk is supported by the findings indicating that high-risk parents benefit more from intensive, long-term involvement. Brief interventions of early and extended contact appear insufficient for producing lasting beneficial effects among identified risk populations. Further, Olds and Kitzman (1990) argue that with higher-risk subjects, establishing a therapeutic alliance is a crucial factor in influencing outcome. Consequently, more intensive efforts may be needed to ensure the development of a stable and enduring helper-family bond, because these families may be more socially isolated and mistrustful of service providers.

Parent–Child Support Programs for Teen Parents

Adolescents having children has become an increasing concern due to the rising number of teen births and the number of teens retaining custody of their child. This growing population of teen parents is considered to be at risk for child maltreatment due to the presumed stress of being both an adolescent and a parent (rather than age per se). The relationship between teen parenting and child maltreatment can be understood by taking into account conditions that often coincide with teen parenthood, such as living in poverty, lacking education, and having a single-parent home. Consequently, problems associated with inadequate parenting have been noted with higher frequency among teenage parents. For example, teen mothers (under age 17) are more likely than older mothers to have children with lower birthweights (Alan Guttmacher Institute, 1981). Teen parents also are more likely to show suboptimal childrearing attitudes and expectations (Field, Widmayer, Stringer, & Ignatoff, 1980), tend to be more socially isolated than more mature parents (Rogeness, Ritchey, Alex, Zuelzer, & Morris, 1981), and are less likely to be self-supportive (Group for the Advancement of Psychiatry, 1986).

Another potential risk factor is the preponderance of early sexual victimization among teen parents. In a statewide survey of 445 teen mothers in Illinois, investigators found that 61% had a history of their own sexual victimization (Gershenson et al., 1989). Similarly, a survey of pregnant and parenting teens in Washington state reported that the majority of respondents indicated previous rape and/or molestation (Boyer, LaFazia, & Fine, 1989). Compared to nonabused respondents, sexually abused teen mothers had greater drug and alcohol use at first pregnancy and were more likely to have been in physically violent relationships with men.

Given these potential risk factors, support programs for teen mothers have received increasing attention. The major goal of these programs is to provide teen parents with basic knowledge of child care and child development. Supplemental goals may also include social support, job training, and/or child management and stimulation programs. Six studies are reviewed in this section (see Figure 6.2). Only one study (Westney, Cole, & Munford, 1988) employed expectant fathers rather than mothers as subjects.

Three of the six studies utilized a home-visitor approach (Gutelius, Kirsch, MacDonald, Brooks, & McErlean, 1977; Field et al., 1980; Field, Widmayer, Greenberg, & Stoller, 1982), with Gutelius et al. (1977) providing multiple treatment services including supportive group and pediatric care components. The visits were begun prenatally in the latter study, and ranged in duration from 4 to 8 months to 3 years postpartum across studies. In the study by Gutelius, nurse visitors followed a less structured, more problem-focused format to provide parental guidance, support, and instruction in child cognitive stimulation. A more structured format aimed at enhancing childrearing practices and knowledge of child development was followed in the Field studies. A structured educational curriculum was combined with an on-site nursery (Roosa & Vaughn, 1983) and with maternal health care, personal development, and support (Mitchell & Casto, 1988). Services spanned from 1 month to 2 years.

Success at Addressing the Needs of Toddlers and Young Children

Group differences on child development measures favoring children of program mothers were reported in the three studies that utilized home visitation. These differences were maintained at follow-up in one study (Field et al., 1982) and were found to decrease over time in another (Gutelius et al., 1977). There was also some evidence that a practicum component may be more effective than home visitation alone (Field et al., 1982). The two group intervention studies that found no group differences both had methodological weaknesses such as delayed posttest (Roosa & Vaughn, 1983), early program evaluation (Mitchell & Casto, 1988), and small samples (Roosa & Vaughn, 1983; Mitchell & Casto, 1988). These results suggest that home visitations that include instruction in child cognitive stimulation yield modest short-term cognitive benefits for infants.

In terms of child behavioral competence, positive results favoring program participants were reported in both studies using direct observation of child behavior (Field et al., 1980, 1982), indicating that children of home-visited mothers were more interactive and positive than were children of control mothers. Further, home-visited mothers rated their children as having better temperaments than did controls, with some indication that an additional practicum component is superior to home visitation alone (Field et al., 1982). These preliminary results suggest that moderately intensive home visits that specifically address child development and interactional skills yield positive gains in observed and maternal ratings of child behavior.

Success at Addressing the Needs of Caregivers

Compared to controls, home-visited mothers reported greater educational attainment (Field et al., 1982; Roosa & Vaughn, 1983) and fewer repeat pregnancies (Field et al., 1982), with some evidence for the importance of a practicum component (Field et al., 1982). No group differences were reported in maternal anxiety or in self-esteem and locus of control in these studies.

In terms of parental expectations for children, home-visited mothers and those enrolled in an alternative school reported more positive attitudes and more realistic developmental expectations than did controls (Field et al., 1980). Fathers receiving prenatal classes also had greater gains in knowledge of child development than did controls (Westney et al., 1988). With respect to childrearing skills, home-visited mothers reported more positive parenting practices and received more positive interactional ratings than did controls across the three studies.

Taken together, these preliminary studies suggest that fairly intensive home visitation (4 months to 3 years) yields gains in maternal attitudes, knowledge, and self-reported and observed childrearing behavior. Not surprisingly, group education curricula seem to be most effective at producing gains in knowledge or attitudes, whereas home visits were best for producing changes in childrearing skills among teen parents.

Conclusions: Parent–Child Support Programs for Teen Parents

Despite the small number of studies and methodological weaknesses, results with adolescent parents serve to reinforce the conclusions drawn from the previous sections on procedurally defined at-risk parents and new and expectant parents. Specifically, relatively intensive home-visit interventions with at-risk mothers yield modest short-term child cognitive gains and greater gains in child behavior and parental outcome measures. The findings reported by Field et al. (1982) suggest that a supervised interactional component that improves parenting and socioeconomic status may be particularly useful with low-income adolescent parents. An important contribution of these studies is the finding that brief, education-oriented group classes are useful for enhancing parenting-related knowledge with expectant fathers (Westney et al., 1988). Further, their finding that fathers (across both the experimental and control groups) who had greater total knowledge scores were more likely to report supportive behaviors toward the mother suggests that enlisting the father not only may improve his parenting skills, but may potentially improve maternal skills through increased support.

The comparative effectiveness of group versus home-visit interventions remains at issue because no study directly contrasted these approaches. Moreover, the true preventive potential of these interventions remains unknown until child abuse reports or child health variables (e.g., emergency admissions, and number of accidents) are collected in future studies. Because a number of parenting programs with teen mothers are approaching the evaluation stage (Miller, 1988), these next years will offer an important opportunity to judge the preventive impact of support programs with this population.

Summary of Secondary Intervention Programs

Family support studies ranging in definition of at-risk parents have found short-term positive outcomes, particularly for parental outcome measures and for those mothers deemed at greatest risk (e.g., poor, single, or young). While positive gains have been found in terms of indirect measures of parental behavior (knowledge and attitudes), several studies have also found improvements in observed parental behavior and, to a lesser extent, indicators of maltreatment (child abuse reports). Also, these studies show that family support programs improve general maternal functioning rather than specific dimensions of personal adjustment.

There is initial, yet persuasive, evidence to suggest that multilevel programs (i.e., offering additional services as parents require them over a longer period of time) are worth the additional effort and expense, compared to less intensive services for higher-risk families. Further support comes from an analysis of participants in the Resource Mother program, which provided pre- and postnatal care to disadvantaged teens (Unger & Wandersman, 1988). This study found that the earlier in pregnancy the teens were recruited, the more likely it was that they would continue participation once their child was born. One could speculate that greater involvement in intervention may lead to greater identification with and ownership of the growth process set in motion by preventive efforts.

Overall, those programs that span from 1 to 3 years and provide a personalized approach (e.g., home visits) stand out as most successful in achieving the desired outcomes and most successful with higher-risk individuals, a conclusion shared by Roberts, Wasik, Casto, and Ramey (1991) in their review of informal and formal home-visitor programs. This apparent intervention-population matching may be best understood by considering the often isolated, unskilled, and impoverished characteristics of these mothers. That is, their need for support, parenting instruction, and resource linkage seems to be fulfilled by the more personalized, outreach nature of the home-visitor approach.

EMERGING DIRECTIONS FOR CHILD SEXUAL ABUSE INTERVENTION

Intervention with Victims or Potential Victims

There is a rapidly expanding body of literature investigating the wide-ranging effects of child sexual abuse and suspected risk factors associated with this phenomenon. Both Canada and the United States have experienced a surge in sexual abuse investigations conducted by state and provincial child protection agencies, as evidenced by more than a fivefold increase in official reports of sexual abuse in both countries during the late 1970s and early 1980s (American Humane Association, 1984; Committee on Sexual Offenses Against Children and Youth, 1984). Random surveys of adults provide prevalence estimates suggesting that approximately 28% of women and 16% of men were victims of sexual abuse before the age of 16 (based on the general definition of abuse as any unwanted childhood sexual experiences, ranging from fondling to sexual intercourse, perpetrated by an adult who is more than 5 years older than the child) (Finkelhor, 1990). Many of these victims may require short- or long-term intervention by health service providers, due to the suspected pervasive impact that sexual abuse experiences have on the child's developing personality and interpersonal behavior.

These staggering prevalence estimates of child sexual abuse were accompanied by investigations into the short- and long-term impact of such abuse on the child's development and psychological functioning. Recent reviews of both controlled and uncontrolled studies indicated that a significant portion of the victim population shows initial adjustment problems in the months following disclosure or discovery of the abuse, such as anger, fear, anxiety, depression, somatic complaints, or sexually inappropriate behavior (Finkelhor, 1990; Gomes-Schwartz, Horowitz, & Cardarelli, 1990; Hansen, 1990; Wolfe & Wolfe, 1988). Similarly, long-term behavioral patterns indicative of poor adult adjustment were identified, such as depression, self-destructive behavior, feelings of isolation and stigma, poor self-esteem, problems forming relationships, substance abuse, and sexual maladjustment (Finkelhor, 1990; Gold, 1986; Harter, Alexander, & Neimeyer, 1988).

Particular characteristics of sexual abuse warrant consideration in seeking an understanding of the wide range of problems shown among these children. Unlike other forms of child maltreatment discussed earlier, incestuous sexual abuse is less related to caregivers' attempts to control or manage child- or family-related stress. Rather, it represents a most distinct form of maltreatment that involves both betrayal of trust and physical violation, accompanied by some degree of coercion or deceit (Haugaard & Reppucci, 1988). Private and specific fears related to aspects of the abuse may develop, which the child is often unable to discuss due to the fear itself, as well as developmental limitations in expression (Foa & Kozak, 1986). Abrupt or gradual changes in the child's psychological well-being and behavior may occur, but others (including professionals) may not identify these changes as being a function of sexual abuse (Friedrich, Urquiza, & Beilke, 1986; Gomes-Schwartz et al., 1990).

These emerging findings suggest that children's adjustment following sexual abuse disclosure can be described in part as a specific reaction to the nature of their trauma. Persons and places that previously signaled safety or support have become associated with danger and fear. The child's world becomes less predictable and controllable, and the child may search for an explanation for these events. Guilt and self-blame have been identified as common outcomes of this process (Silver, Boon, & Stones, 1983). In relation to child sexual abuse, therefore, the combination of the unpredictability of the abuse and the child's perception that he/she did not exercise enough control to stop the abuse (i.e., guilt and self-blame) may create psychological problems that warrant intervention. The two most prominent interventions for child sexual abuse victims, legal-based services and psychologically based treatments, are reviewed here.

Legal-Based Interventions to Prepare Children for the Role of Witness

The last decade saw an increasing number of clinicians and researchers expressing concern about the negative emotional effects evident in sexually abused children who have to testify about their experiences in court (e.g., Berliner & Barbieri, 1984; Jaffe, Wilson, & Sas, 1987; Wolfe, Sas, & Wilson, 1987). Empirical studies, moreover, confirm many of these concerns, revealing that the overall court process can lead to secondary victimization of children (Runyan, Everson, Edelson, Hunter, & Coulson, 1988; Goodman et al., 1989). For example, Whitcomb et al. (1991) reported that abused children were highly distressed at the time of their initial interview, regardless of whether the offender was intra- or extrafamilial. Based on a multisite sample of 256 children, these researchers also found that older children were more likely to experience harsh cross-examination. Thus, the harshness of the testifying experiences in combination with emotional sequelae related to the abuse itself can result in a high level of stress for children and affect their ability to provide competent and compelling evidence in a court of law.

Increased recognition of the difficulties children experience in a courtroom setting, in particular their fear of the accused and confusion about the process, led many states and provinces to implement new evidentiary procedures. Most notably, these changes include the use of closed-circuit television to physically remove the child from the courtroom, videotaping of children's disclosure and investigative interviews, and the use of a screen to block the child's direct view of the accused in court. The impact of these changes is currently being evaluated, particularly in terms of how they may attenuate the child victim's level of stress and long-term adjustment problems.

A recent, innovative program to assist children in preparing for court testimony about their abuse was reported by Sas, Austin, Wolfe, and Hurley (1991). These investigators first identified the nine most frequently occurring stressors as (1) delays, (2) public exposure (i.e., having to recount embarrassing and frightening experiences in a public courtroom), (3) facing the accused, (4) understanding complex procedures, (5) change of prosecuting attorneys (and the common lack of a comfortable, familiar relationship with counsel), (6) cross-examination (a quote from a recent article typifies the opportunistic attitudes promoted by some defense counsel toward cross-examination of child witnesses: "You have to go in there as defense counsel and whack the complainant hard at the preliminary. . . get all the medical evidence, get Children's Aid Society records—you've got to attack the complainant with all you've got so that he or she will say I'm not coming back in front of 12 good citizens to repeat this bullshit story that I've just told the judge," Schmitz, 1988, p. 6). (7) exclusion of witnesses (i.e., being "alone" in the courtroom), (8) apprehension and placement outside of the home, and (9) lack of preparation for the role of witness.

To assist children in coping with these system stressors, Sas et al. (1991) developed a court preparation protocol with the goal of (1) demystifying the court process through education and (2) reducing the fear and anxiety of testifying by teaching stress management techniques. Using a random assignment of 120 participants either to this program or to existing services (i.e., a tour of the courtroom and a verbal explanation of court procedures), these investigators found that children who received court preparation as described above (4–6 individual sessions, on average) improved in their knowledge of court, reduced their fears related to court, and were more appropriate in their courtroom behavior than were controls. The presence of additional supports (e.g., mother's support of the child's disclosure), as well as stressors (e.g., delays) also played a role in mediating the overall impact of this educational program, although overall the results support the view that adequate preparation is beneficial to children's accurate testimony and subsequent adjustment.

Psychological and Educational Programs

Therapeutic programs for sexually abused children and family members have expanded rapidly over the last decade, as have school-based prevention programs. Treatment has been extended to victims, parents, siblings, and offenders, and involves many different modalities (e.g., behavioral, psychodynamic, and family therapy). The goals of treatment vary considerably given the diversity of this population and the preliminary nature of current investigations (Kolko, 1987), but most programs emphasize group/individual support for the victim and nonoffending parents, management of anxiety and fear symptoms, and/or empowerment strategies (e.g., Deblinger, McLeer, & Henry, 1990; Giarretto, 1982). Presently, scientific evidence regarding the benefit or impact of such programs is limited, primarily due to methodological concerns that have not been overcome (e.g., use of control groups and proper measures of outcome).

Prevention programs, on the other hand, are directed at the general population of school-age children. Most programs emphasize gains in knowledge about potential abuse situations, "touch" discrimination, and behavioral strategies to avoid/escape abusive situations. As a whole, evaluations provide some limited support for the efficacy of sexual abuse prevention programs (Reppucci & Haugaard, 1989). The most common and consistent finding is a statistically significant, yet often slight, increase in knowledge about sexual abuse following a prevention program (Conte, Rosen, Saperstein, & Shermack, 1985; Harvey, Forehand, Brown, & Holmes, 1988; Saslawsky & Wurtele, 1986). However, no evidence exists that links such changes in knowledge to changes in behavior. In the few studies that examined differences between school-age and preschool children, the younger children learned less (Borkin & Frank, 1986; Conte et al., 1985). This finding raises questions regarding whether programs that are useful for school-age children are appropriate for younger children.

Most evaluations of sexual abuse prevention programs have basic design problems. Although a few studies used matched, nonexperimental control groups (Harvey et al., 1988; Saslawsky & Wurtele, 1986; Wolfe, McPherson, Blount, & Wolfe, 1986; Wurtele, Kast, Miller-Perrin, & Kondrick, 1989), many did not. Other design flaws included small sample sizes, lack of attention to the reliability and validity of the measuring instruments, no pretesting to establish a baseline of knowledge, and short-term follow-up assessments (i.e., less than 2 months).

More thorough evaluations of ongoing prevention programs are necessary in order to determine both their effectiveness and their potential for injury. As mentioned by Reppucci and Haugaard (1989) and Melton (1992), the programs may have two types of adverse reactions: (1) They may harm a child's positive relationships with meaningful people in his or her life or cause the child undue worry or fear at least in the short run, and (2) they may actually place some children at a greater risk for sexual abuse if parents, teachers, and others who work with children abdicate their responsibility as guardians against abuse to these programs. The complexity of the process that a child must go through to repel or report abuse, the variety of abusive situations that a child may encounter, and the short duration of most prevention programs virtually ensure that a child cannot be assumed to be protected simply because of participation in a program. Adults must be encouraged to continue and to increase their protective efforts rather than be reassured that children are learning to be self-protective.

Intervention with Offenders

Various theories have been proposed to explain why some adults, almost exclusively males, engage in sexual activity with children (e.g., biological/organic, psychodynamic, family systems, and cognitive–behavioral theories). Certain psychologically based approaches to treatment are emerging as having a significant impact on the recidivism of known child molesters. A brief discussion of behavioral treatment is presented because this method shows the most promise in community-based programs aimed at reducing the risk of child sexual abuse.

The most widely used and successful form of treatment reported in the literature is some form of aversion therapy. A study by Barbaree and Marshall (1988) best exemplifies this approach. These researchers treated nonincarcerated child molesters with electrical aversion, masturbatory reconditioning, self-administration of smelling salts contingent upon deviant thoughts or urges, and skills training. Based on a follow-up period ranging from 1 to 11 years, they found a recidivism rate of 13.2% for treated men ($n = 68$), compared to 34.5% for the untreated group ($n = 58$). Two factors predicted higher recidivism: younger age (less than 40) and genital contact with the victim.

Becker and Hunter (1992) recently reviewed the major therapeutic approaches to the treatment of child molesters, and they conclude that most studies, especially those with a cognitive–behavioral focus, indicate low recidivism rates for child molesters (i.e., "Data indicate that [treatment works] for some in the short-run and for others in the long-run," p. 89). Marshall, Jones, Ward, Johnston, and Barbaree (1991), in their recent review of the treatment literature with sex offenders, similarly conclude that comprehensive cognitive–behavioral programs are the most effective, especially for child molesters, incest offenders, and exhibitionists. However, considerable methodological advancement must be applied to this area to establish the parameters of what form of treatment works for whom. Issues regarding the identification of high-risk or accomplished child molesters who would benefit from this form of intervention are complex, yet the emerging literature is encouraging in terms of desired change for those individuals who are identified.

CONCLUSIONS AND RECOMMENDATIONS

Research and Methodology: Gaps and Recommendations

Theoretical and Conceptual Advances

A conceptual model to guide intervention and outcome evaluation necessitates the identification of the common antecedents of the categorical problem behaviors (abuse, neglect, etc.). This identification procedure may be informed by empirical findings, clinical observations, and theoretical applications. Thus, if it is proposed that parents maltreat their children due to the direct effects of poor knowledge and skill in childrearing, as well as improper support and assistance, the strategy for prevention should address these specific needs. Intervention and measurement should be directly connected to the hypothesized causal model. An important addition to presumed direct effects is the identification of mediators of the relationships between antecedents and abuse. Intervention that targets both indirect and direct influences would be expected to be more efficacious than those addressing either alone.

Recommendation. There is a critical need for prevention programs to be driven by an underlying conceptualization of the processes involved in child abuse and neglect.

Research Design and Program Evaluation

Although research designs have improved significantly since the first reviews of intervention studies by Isaacs (1982) and Plotkin, Azar, Twentyman, and Peri (1981), recent studies still contain methodological inadequacies common to the field of child maltreatment that must be taken into account in interpreting their findings (Mash & Wolfe, 1991). For example, research designs are often inadequate to draw firm conclusions, because most studies are naturalistic correlational field research that does not permit true experimentation. Many studies involve subject samples that in all likelihood contain mixed forms of maltreatment (e.g., physical, sexual, and psychological abuse), which confounds the findings that may relate to physical abuse alone. In addition, child abuse researchers face a major challenge in attempting to control for related factors that may have direct or indirect effects on children's adjustment, such as marital discord, socioeconomic disadvantage, poor social supports, and so on. Finally, it is worthwhile to note that the newly emerging prevention-focused programs (designed for families who have not yet been identified as abusive or neglecting), although promising, have yet to demonstrate actual prevention if one limits such criteria simply to the occurrence of an incident. On the other hand, the burgeoning evidence that such programs enhance parental effectiveness and child competence argues for the preference of such outcome variables over the unreliable and somewhat arbitrary official reports of maltreatment.

More specifically, intervention studies often pose a number of restrictions that make interpretation difficult. Fink and McCloskey (1990), for example, reviewed 13 major evaluations of child abuse and neglect prevention programs published between 1978 and 1988 (i.e., those types of programs that have the greatest likelihood of influencing policy decisions). They found that only half of these evaluations used control groups, and virtually all the researchers failed to define abuse more specifically, beyond simple report information. This finding is reflected in the wider range of intervention studies as well. In a recent review of child abuse prevention programs, Wekerle and Wolfe (1993) found that interpretation of findings is commonly hampered by lack of adequate sample size, limited follow-up evaluation, insufficient measurement of behavior change, lack of random assignment, and failure to involve a no-treatment control group. These limitations clearly pose major obstacles to formulating unambiguous social policy recommendations.

There is a critical need for appreciable follow-up periods so that maintenance of gains and "sleeper" effects (i.e., those emerging after program completion) may be assessed. Other design issues include the need to conduct more controlled evaluations through randomization procedures and to incorporate greater sensitivity into program design in an effort to maximize the likelihood of finding true effects. Such efforts as calculating necessary conditions (e.g., number of subjects) to meet adequate levels of statistical power, monitoring the consistency, content, and quality of service delivery, and utilizing more psychometrically sound and multimethod measurement procedures would facilitate accurate evaluation of program effects. Although it is recognized that some treatment target areas may not have sufficient evaluation devices currently available, greater utilization of existing knowledge bases is in order.

Prospective designs have resulted in major advances in our understanding of risk factors affecting the developmental course of maltreated children (e.g., Starr, MacLean, & Keating, 1991; Egeland, 1991; Herrenkohl, Herrenkohl, Egolf, & Seech, 1991; Vietze, O'Connor, Sherrod, & Altemeier, 1991). Longitudinal designs carry several major advantages, including precision in timing and measurement, heterogeneity of outcome (i.e., study of both "successes" and "failures"), and an analysis of the causal chain among complex social variables (Black, 1991). However, these advantages come at the cost of extensive data collection, subject attrition, interference from life changes and events, and measurement problems associated with developmental changes. Innovative research designs (other than experimental, prospective designs) with longitudinal components also merit careful consideration. For example, Willett, Ayoub, and Robinson (1991) recently reported on the use of growth modeling to examine change in the functioning of at-risk parents as a function of intervention. This methodology takes advantage of the richness of longitudinal data to estimate changes over time more accurately than traditional two-wave, pre–post designs.

Recommendation. The importance of testing promising intervention models through the use of prospective designs is underscored.

Recommendation. Prevention programs aimed at child maltreatment, in particular home-visitation programs, have matured to the point where specificity issues should be addressed as part of the outcome. In addition to asking whether prevention programs work, the question of which programs work for whom and under what circumstances must be addressed. Consequently, greater attention must be given to the pretreatment assessment of subjects so that an adequate array of individual difference and contextual variables would be available to help categorize who benefited, deteriorated, or was unaffected by treatment.

Selection of Participants

Currently, a major roadblock to the implementation of effective early intervention and prevention programming is the lack of information pertaining specifically to the nature of the population. Although there was some evidence supporting each of the interventions reviewed, little specificity is provided that allows one to match intervention type to individual needs of persons or families. The comprehensive/multiservice programs come closest in this regard, yet conclusions cannot be drawn until more complete evaluation is available.

The decision as to who should receive preventive services is often a difficult and ambiguous one. Concerns for the efficient use of funds have often popularized a narrow definition of the target population to include only those individuals having specific "risk indicators." Although understandable, this practice raises some precautions regarding the identification and participation of individuals determined to be at risk. The problem of determining risk status is complicated by the absence of clearcut guidelines for identification procedures, the lack of complete knowledge concerning risk factors, and the relatively low incidence of child maltreatment in the general population. Thus, if identification procedures are faulty, those identified as at risk may be subjected to a variety of adverse consequences (e.g., derogatory labels, self-fulfilling prophecy, and invasion of privacy). Consequently, to the extent that risk indicators are used, it has been recommended that intervention remain on a voluntary basis (Wald & Cohen, 1988).

Recommendation. An alternative approach to targeting subjects with specific risk indicators, in which general indicators (e.g., first-time parenthood) serve as entry criteria for prevention programs should be explored. An advantage of targeting new parents is that habitual, negative patterns of parent–child interaction have not been established (although dysfunctional parenting tendencies may be present), and prevention programs are not stigmatized by an "at-risk" label.

Participation of Fathers and Male Partners

Almost without exception, the studies reviewed herein include only female participants. No matter what conclusions one draws from these studies, it is necessary to keep in mind that the results apply primarily to women. Regrettably, many of the factors identified by the ecological model of child maltreatment implicitly or explicitly highlight the importance of the man's role in either contributing to or preventing such events. At this time, however, there is little information with which to design and implement services to families that will best meet the needs of men who are at risk of becoming violent toward children or partners. This finding of underrepresentation of fathers compared to mothers is consistent with the literature on developmental psychopathology in general. Despite the growing knowledge that fathers play a significant role in the development of child and adolescent problems and in the etiology of physical and sexual abuse (Phares & Compas, 1992), intervention programs have generally not included men in their programs.

Recommendation. There exists an urgent need to recognize and address the male role in the occurrence and the prevention of child maltreatment. Program additions and modifications that encourage male participation and improve family functioning hold promise for expanding the impact of early intervention services.

Program Development and Social Policy: Gaps and Recommendations

The Importance of Matching Services to the Needs of Parents, Children, and Families: What Works for Whom?

A major finding to emerge from this review is that no particular method of intervention is likely to lead to desirable outcomes for even a majority of families, especially by the time child maltreatment has been identified. From a cost–benefit perspective, the cost of remediating serious childrearing concerns is prohibitive.

These costs may be reduced by placing greater emphasis on preparing parents for their childrearing role well in advance of the emergence of problems and having a wider range of appropriate services available. Such a model requires staff who are trained to assist with families at a level that is most beneficial rather than attempting to detect and intervene after the fact. Staff would have to be sensitive to individual, community, and cultural preferences, as well as to socioeconomic limitations, that constitute the majority of disadvantaged families and be willing to tolerate such differences for the purpose of establishing a basis for improving the parent–child relationship. This approach requires more investment in family development at an earlier point but holds considerable promise in reducing the costs and failures of the current reactive system.

On what basis should early intervention services be provided and matched to families? An issue that emerged clearly from this review was the need to match interventions to the needs of each family as best as possible. Although this seems obvious, the literature shows repeated attempts to design and implement a particular strategy to any given sample of maltreating parents with little regard to the needs of each participant (especially cultural and ethnic minorities; see below). Whereas some parents require information and assistance in basic childrearing, many others require social support, child care respite, and/or personal counseling. Yet, the interventions persist in attempting to "fit" the patient to the "cure," rather than the reverse. Although the expanding multiservice programs are promising in this regard, they lack thorough evaluation and follow-up and tend to have weak or inadequate research designs.

Willett et al. (1991), for example, found a sizable group of at-risk families that showed no change at all in family functioning over time, even after lengthy intervention involving parenting skills and community supports. These researchers speculate that intervention may be maintaining family functioning at its initial level and preventing decline (no untreated control group was used in this study, however). Families who respond well to structured intervention may actually be leaving the programs after a relatively brief period of time; thus, families who remain in treatment are more likely to show "zero growth" and take up the majority of resources just to maintain their entry level of functioning. This conjecture, if correct, has important implications for the delivery of services to families in need, due to limited resources and the importance of reaching families as early as possible.

Moreover, few programs have been directed at the developmental needs of abused and neglected children. Rather, treatment has been predominately aimed at adults. Although our understanding of the developmental impact of these problems has grown, efforts to remediate and/or prevent such problems have been slow to develop. Neglected children, in particular, suffer major psychological consequences that have been inadequately addressed by current approaches.

Many of the conclusions from this review mimic those mentioned by Cohn and Daro (1987), and, unfortunately, the evidentiary base has not improved dramatically. Those authors concluded, on the basis of 89 federally funded child abuse and neglect projects conducted between 1974 to 1982, that the most effective interventions were (1) group approaches, (2) use of nonprofessional lay helpers, (3) parent education and support groups, and (4) skills training to supplement professional help. They added that programs that relied on traditional parent-focused therapy or brief interventions were least successful, and that multiservice interventions are essential for successful intervention with abuse and neglect.

Additions to the earlier conclusions by Cohn and Daro (1987), based on the conclusions in this chapter, are listed below.

Recommendation. The current review supports the utility and cost–benefit of (1) home visits, especially those begun prior to the onset of maltreatment; (2) specific skills training that addresses parental misperceptions and false expectations of young children; (3) specific skills training that promotes alternatives to physical punishment and the use of more prosocial, developmentally relevant activities for the parent to engage in with his/her child; (4) parental competency programs broadly aimed at nonidentified individuals, a strategy that reduces concerns due to labeling and detection; and (5) preschool-based programs for child victims, which emphasize developmental gains and prosocial peer interactions. These findings highlighted the theme of matching relevant services to the changing needs of families.

Recommendation. Major efforts should be launched to determine the impact on child maltreatment of an incentive-based program of child development screening and child development prescriptions and resources offered to the general public from conception through 5 years of age. This program could be offered through the local school system and serve as a bridge to similar services in the schools when school age is reached (this model is compatible with and could be a core element of the "neighborhood-based services" model recommended by the U.S. Advisory Board on Child Abuse and Neglect).

Recommendation. Program development should focus on providing child development and parenting information that is easily understood, practical, and accessible to all present and potential parenting populations.

Recommendation. Early-intervention programs to assist child victims of abuse and neglect should be expanded. In conjunction with efforts to assist the parents in their caregiving role, such programs offer additional developmental stimulation and peer contact for children.

Marital/Partnership Issues and Children Who Witness Wife Assault

The findings from this review point to some important areas of intervention that have been identified but rarely addressed. Based on the most popular ecological view of the causes of child maltreatment, a number of treatment targets were identified at the family, child, and parent level (community and cultural issues were beyond the scope of this review). Many of the methods noted earlier showed some success in addressing issues associated with the parent–child relationship (which is, of course, a central concern); however, the findings point to a lack of information concerning issues related to family functioning.

The relationship between marital/partnership problems and the risk of maltreatment has been noted by clinical researchers but rarely studied systematically. Again, this absence may be due to the lack of male involvement, or it could possibly reflect an unintentional, yet disconcerting, overemphasis on the woman's responsibility/blame for child maltreatment. Empirical studies have generally supported the organizational view, which posits that for both men and women, abusive backgrounds make one more likely to become subsequently involved in coercive relationships with peers, intimate partners, and children (e.g., Malamuth, Sockloskie, Koss, & Tanaka, 1991). Specifically, witnessing violence between parents (Jaffe, Wolfe, & Wilson, 1990), being the victim of physical and/or sexual child abuse (Fagan & Wexler, 1988; Wolfe, 1987), or experiencing pronounced psychological abuse or emotional neglect from caregivers (McGee & Wolfe, 1991) is at the foundation of the development of adversarial, hostile biases and behavior concerning male–female, parent–child, and similar intimate relationships.

Recommendation. Programs that address male violence against female partners, as well as those that address marital disharmony, need to be considered necessary components of intervention and prevention for identified high-risk families.

Effective Ways to Address Corollary Family Problems

To date, the potentiating effects of socioeconomic stress, family disadvantage, and substance abuse on abuse and neglect have not received adequate attention. Although most researchers acknowledge the presence and impact of these contextual factors, few approaches actually were designed to address these problems in a systematic manner. The comprehensive and social network programs are, again, promising in this regard but have as yet provided limited evaluation data. Similarly, the influence of the parent's competing (negative) lifestyle and habits, which is often cited as a major concomitant factor among maltreating families, was addressed only serendipitously rather than systematically. Like the male offenders, perhaps such individuals rarely participate in treatment outcome studies.

Recommendation. Expand service delivery to include multiservice capabilities to address the negative influence of major contextual stress factors on effective family functioning. Subsidized day care and housing, respite programs, homemaker services, and so on show promise in this regard but require systematic implementation and evaluation.

Programs to Address the Needs of Ethnic Minorities

Attention must be directed to societal influences that play a role in child abuse and neglect, especially in circumstances in which families are exposed to major effects of poverty, health risks, and environmental conflict (Sipes, 1992). Research needs to identify the special risks and strengths of diverse cultural and ethnic groups and to be sensitive to ethnic and cultural issues in the planning of services (Fantuzzo, 1990). Such a cross-cultural perspective to child abuse and neglect intervention and prevention would redirect the focus away from individuals and families and explore societal and cultural conditions that attenuate or exacerbate these problems (Sipes, 1992).

Recommendation. Although there is a general lack of research with maltreated children from ethnic and minority communities, adequate information exists to recommend the implementation and evaluation of culturally relevant intervention and prevention methods.

Programs Aimed at Adolescents

Youth represent a sizable proportion of child maltreatment reports, yet, they typically receive less than adequate assistance. From an intervention perspective, there is reason to support the extension of programs that have shown effectiveness with clinically referred youth to an at-risk youth population. The most effective programs for parent–adolescent conflict, which have been in existence for several years, involve several components, such as effective communication, parent training, contingency management, and family therapy (see, e.g., Forehand, Thomas, Wierson, Brody, & Fauber, 1990; Foster & Robin, 1988). Although such methods may not be capable of overcoming long-standing parent–adolescent conflict and abuse, they may be effective in addressing the emerging issues that accompany adolescent development, especially for families with a limited history of protective service involvement.

Prevention services for youth populations could integrate educational concepts (e.g., attitudes and knowledge issues affecting healthy vs. violent relationships) with practical skills aimed at noncontrolling conflict resolution. Such efforts have been undertaken recently by school boards (e.g., Jaffe, Sudermann, & Reitzel, 1992) and by protective service agencies (Wolfe, 1992), following from the belief that this age group offers a unique window of opportunity to challenge existing beliefs and attitudes concerning the use of power and aggression toward others.

Recommendation. Educationally focused prevention programs targeted to low- and high-risk adolescents merit development and evaluation in schools, communities, and service agencies on such topics as control and power in relationships, sexual and physical violence, and family and child-rearing values.

The Need for a Multiservice, Public Health Model of Ongoing Support for Families

Given its prevalence, child maltreatment can be compared to other major threats to public health, such as AIDS, childhood diseases, poverty, and home safety. Therefore, it makes sense in the long run to address the causes of this problem from a public health vantage point rather than tertiary intervention. Evidence for the effectiveness of such a model can be found in reports from Scandinavian countries. Sweden, Finland, and Denmark all have nationwide programs that resemble the family support programs being explored in the United States. In addition, these countries have the benefits of universal insurance, free tuition for academic and vocational training, paid educational leave to upgrade skills, yearly cash allowances for each child under age 16 and for nonworking mothers for 6 months during pregnancy, maternal child health services, subsidized primary health care, and other benefits. Pransky (1991) summarizes the results of these benefits:

- Some 95% of pregnant mothers start prenatal care before the end of the fourth month, compared to less than 85% in the United States.
- Fewer than 4% of mothers are under the age of 20 at the time of their first birth, compared with 10% in the United States.
- Infant mortality rates and births of low-birth-weight babies are among the lowest in the world.
- Infant death from respiratory disease is at the rate of 22–67 per 100,000 (compared with 107/100,000 in the United States).
- Prevalence of mild mental retardation is 8–10 times lower than in the United States.
- Rates of child abuse are about 8 times lower than in the United States.

Expenditures for health care as a percentage of gross national product (GNP) in these countries are less as well (7–10% vs. 11% in the United States). The percentage of GNP spent on social services, however, is much greater (25–35% vs. 18% in the United States). We should keep these comparative expense figures in mind when considering the costs of the current U.S. approach to childrearing and family concerns. For example, on a national basis it cost approximately $19 billion in 1987 to assist families that were started by teenagers, nearly 66% of daughters of single women later go on welfare, and the costs of providing high-quality prenatal care are almost double for high-risk infants, on average, than are the costs for normal, low-risk infants ($706 vs. $476, respectively) (Child Welfare League of America, 1989).

As noted by Pransky (1991), such family support programs as those in place in Scandinavian countries have considerable social and political appeal: "strengthening and promoting well-functioning, independent, self-supporting families that produce children who, in turn, will become independent, self-supporting adults" (p. 59).

Recommendation. A public health approach to the prevention of child abuse and neglect is a promising strategy that merits serious consideration. Such a strategy would not undermine existing efforts at treatment and early intervention but, rather, would be designed to approach the widespread problem of child maltreatment from a broader, more fundamental vantage point.

Special Issues Concerning Child Sexual Abuse

Treatment and prevention activities directed at the underestimated problem of child sexual abuse have emerged rapidly over the past decade. Although there are beneficial therapeutic programs both for child victims and for offenders, it is still too early to draw conclusions regarding their overall impact. However, legal-based services to assist children in preparing to testify in court merit careful evaluation and dissemination, as do group and individual programs for children that address their anxiety, fears, and symptoms of posttraumatic stress which may emerge in the aftermath of disclosing sexual abuse. Perhaps because child abuse prevention programs have emerged so rapidly, there is insufficient data at present to either promote or deter such efforts. The initial findings presented here point to the considerable gap in knowledge related to determining which methods work to teach what types of skills to which children. Because these gaps must be addressed before conclusions can be drawn about such prevention efforts, the following recommendations point to several of the more basic issues facing research and program development.

Therapeutic and Educational Programs

Recommendation. Prevention programs need to expand beyond the focus on potential victims (i.e., children). Kolko (1987) recommends that programs be directed toward three primary groups: children, parents, and school/community agency staff. There is a conspicuous absence of programs that target other adults who come into contact with children, with either a detection or primary prevention goal in mind, yet these adults are the most likely candidates to whom children will report abuse.

Recommendation. Several areas of program curriculum development and clarification for child sexual abuse prevention merit improvement and expansion if such child-focused programs are to expand. Program content should extend beyond a discussion of the touch continuum to include related topics of importance (e.g., personal safety, assertiveness, and problem solving) (Kolko, 1987). Moreover, affiliated staff should be trained to continue providing opportunities for students to discuss the issues brought forth during training.

Recommendation. Child sexual abuse prevention must turn its attention to some of the underlying social and cultural issues that are suspected to be at the root of such exploitation and abuse. To date, little research has been conducted on the motivating factors involved in child sexual abuse. Because almost all of the offenders are male, a long-term strategy should be developed that addresses some of the suspected roots of such behavior from a socialization perspective. More responsibility for prevention should be directed at socialization agents (e.g., schools, parents, and clubs) in an effort to heighten society's awareness of the problem and to attack the roots of sexism that exist at all levels.

Recommendation. Legal-based services for child victims, such as the availability of nonstandard evidentiary procedures (e.g., screen and video-taped testimony), and the use of educational/therapeutic services to prepare children for the stress of testifying in court warrant investigation as to their possible role in decreasing the long-range negative impact of sexual abuse and its disclosure.

Recommendation. Treatment services for child victims and for sex offenders have shown promise in assisting victims and in reducing recidivism. Well-designed investigations should be launched on a wide-scale basis to determine the most effective forms of intervention for offenders and victims.

REFERENCES

Aber, J. L., & Allen, J. P. (1987). Effects of maltreatment on young children's socioemotional development: An attachment theory perspective. *Developmental Psychology, 23,* 406–414.

Aber, J. L., & Cicchetti, D. (1984). The socio-emotional development of maltreated children: An empirical and theoretical analysis. In H. Fitzgerald, B. Lester, & M. Yogman (Eds.), *Theory and research in behavioral pediatrics* (Vol. 2, pp. 147–205). New York: Plenum Press.

Affleck, G., Tennen, H., Rowe, J., Roscher, B., & Walker, L. (1989). Effects of formal support on mothers' adaptation to the hospital-to-home transition of high-risk infants: The benefits and costs of helping. *Child Development, 60,* 488–501.

Alan Guttmacher Institute. (1981). *Teenage pregnancy: The problem that hasn't gone away.* New York: Author.

American Association for Protecting Children. (1988). *Highlights of official child neglect and abuse reporting, 1986.* Denver, CO: American Humane Association.

American Humane Association. (1984). *Trends in child abuse and neglect: A national perspective.* Denver, CO: Author.

Ames, K. (1992, June 22). Fostering the family: An intensive effort to keep kids with parents. *Newsweek,* pp. 64, 67.

Ammerman, R. T. (1990). Etiological models of child maltreatment: A behavioral perspective. *Behavior Modification, 14,* 230–254.

Ammerman, R. T. (1992). The role of the child in physical abuse: A reappraisal. *Violence and Victims, 6,* 87–101.

Ammerman, R., Cassissi, J. E., Hersen, M., & Van Hasselt, V. R. (1986). Consequences of physical abuse and neglect in children. *Clinical Psychology Review, 6,* 291–310.

Amundson, M. J. (1989). Family crisis care: A home-based intervention program for child abuse. *Issues in Mental Health Nursing, 10,* 285–296.

Andrews, S. R., Blumenthal, J. B., Johnson, D. L., Kahn, A. J., Ferguson, C. J., Lasater, T. M., Malone, P. E., & Wallace, D. B. (1982). The skills of mothering: A study of parent child development centers. *Monographs of the Society for Research in Child Development, 47*(6, Serial No. 198).

Appelbaum, A. S. (1977). Developmental retardation in infants as a concomitant of physical child abuse. *Journal of Abnormal Child Psychology, 5,* 417–423.

Armstrong, K. A. (1981). A treatment and education program for parents and children who are at-risk of abuse and neglect. *Child Abuse and Neglect, 5,* 167–175.

Armstrong, K. A., & Frailey, Y. L. (1985). What happens to families after they leave the program? *Children Today, 14,* 17–20.

Azar, S. T., & Siegel, B. R. (1990). Behavioral treatment of child abuse: A developmental perspective. *Behavior Modification, 14,* 279–300.

Azar, S. T., & Wolfe, D. A. (1989). Child abuse and neglect. In E. J. Mash & R. A. Barkley (Eds.), *Treatment of childhood disorders* (pp. 451–493). New York: Guilford Press.

Barbaree, H. E., & Marshall, W. L. (1988). Deviant sexual arousal, offense history, and demographic variables as predictors of reoffense among child molesters. *Behavioral Sciences and the Law, 6,* 267–280.

Barnard, K. E., Magyary, D., Summer, G., Booth, C. L., Mitchell, S. K., & Spieker, S. (1988). Prevention of parenting alternatives for women with low social support. *Psychiatry, 51,* 248–253.

Barone, U. J., Greene, B. F., & Lutzker, J. R. (1986). Home safety with families being treated for child abuse and neglect. *Behavior Modification, 10,* 93–114.

Barrera, M. E., Rosenbaum, P. L., & Cunningham, C. E. (1986). Early home intervention with low-birth-weight infants and their parents. *Child Development, 57,* 20–33.

Barth, R. P., Blythe, B. J., Schinke, S. P., & Schilling, R. F. II. (1983). Self-control training with maltreating parents. *Child Welfare, 62,* 313–324.

Becker, J. V., & Hunter, J. A. Jr. (1992). Evaluation of treatment outcome for adult perpetrators of child sexual abuse. *Criminal Justice and Behaviour, 19,* 74–92.

Bell, R. Q., & Harper, L. (1977). *Child effects on adults.* Hillsdale, NJ: Erlbaum.

Belsky, J. (1980). Child maltreatment: An ecological integration. *American Psychologist, 35,* 320–335.

Belsky, J. (1984). The determinants of parenting: A process model. *Child Development, 55,* 83–96.

Belsky, J., & Vondra, J. (1989). Lessons from child abuse: The determinants of parenting. In D. Cicchetti & V. Carlson (Eds.), *Child maltreatment: Theory and research on the causes and consequences of child abuse and neglect* (pp. 153–202). New York: Cambridge University Press.

Berliner, L., & Barbieri, M. K. (1984). The testimony of the child victim of sexual assault. *Journal of Social Issues, 40,* 125–137.

Black, M. (1991). Longitudinal studies in child maltreatment: Methodological considerations. In R. H. Starr & D. A. Wolfe (Eds.), *The effects of child abuse and neglect: Issues and research* (pp. 129–143). New York: Guilford Press.

Booth, C. L., Mitchell, S. K., Barnard, K. E., & Spieker, S. J. (1989). Development of maternal social skills in multiproblem families: Effects on the mother–child relationship. *Developmental Psychology, 25,* 403–412.

Borkin, J., & Frank, L. (1986). Sexual abuse prevention for preschoolers: A pilot program. *Child Welfare, 6,* 75–83.

Boyer, D., LaFazia, M. A., & Fine, D. (1989). *Pilot study on teen parent victimization. Preliminary report.* Seattle, WA: Washington Alliance Concerned with School Age Parents.

Brunk, M., Henggeler, S. W., & Whelan, J. P. (1987). Comparison of multisystemic therapy and parent training in the brief treatment of child abuse and neglect. *Journal of Consulting and Clinical Psychology, 55*, 171–178.

Brunquell, D., Crichton, L., & Egeland, B. (1981). Maternal personality and attitude in disturbances of childrearing. *American Journal of Orthopsychiatry, 51*, 680–691.

Burgess, L. (1979). Child abuse: A social interactional analysis. In B. B. Lahey & A. E. Kazdin (Eds.), *Advances in clinical child psychology* (Vol. 2, pp. 142–172). New York: Plenum Press.

Burgess, R. L. (1985). Social incompetence as a precipitant to and consequences of child maltreatment. *Victimology: An International Journal, 10*, 72–86.

Campbell, R. V., O'Brien, S., Bickett, A. D., & Lutzker, J. R. (1983). In-home parent training, treatment of migraine headaches, and marital counseling as an ecobehavioral approach to prevent child abuse. *Journal of Behavior Therapy and Experimental Psychiatry, 14*, 147–154.

Canadian Broadcasting Company. (1992, March 12). *Special report on youth from DeGrassi High*. Toronto: Author.

Child Welfare League of America. (1989). *Children's legislative agenda*. Washington, DC: Author.

Cicchetti, D. (1989). How research on child maltreatment has informed the study of child development: Perspectives from developmental psychopatholgoy. In D. Cicchetti & V. Carlson (Eds.), *Child maltreatment: Theory and research on the causes and consequences of child abuse and neglect* (pp. 377–431). New York: Cambridge University Press.

Cicchetti, D., & Rizley, R. (1981). Developmental perspectives on the etiology, intergenerational transmission, and sequelae of child maltreatment. In D. Cicchetti & D. Rizley (Eds.), *New directions for child development: Developmental perspectives on child maltreatment* (pp. 31–55). San Francisco: Jossey-Bass.

Cicchetti, D., Toth, S., & Bush, M. (1988). Developmental psycho-pathology and incompetence in childhood: Suggestions for intervention. In B. B. Lahey & A. E. Kazdin (Eds.), *Advances in clinical child psychology* (Vol. 11, pp. 1–77). New York: Plenum Press.

Cohn, A. H. (1979). Essential elements of successful child abuse and neglect treatment. *Child Abuse and Neglect, 3*, 491–496.

Cohn, A. H., & Daro, D. (1987). Is treatment too late: What ten years of evaluative research tell us. *Child Abuse and Neglect, 11*, 433–442.

Committee on Sexual Offenses Against Children and Youth. (1984). *Sexual offenses against children in Canada: Summary*. Ottawa: Author.

Conte, J. R., Rosen, C., Saperstein, L., & Shermack, R. (1985). An evaluation of a program to prevent the sexual victimization of young children. *Child Abuse and Neglect, 9*, 319–328.

Crimmins, D. B., Bradlyn, A. S., St. Lawrence, J. S., & Kelly, J. A. (1984). In-clinic training to improve the parent–child interaction skills of a neglectful mother. *Child Abuse and Neglect, 8*, 533–539.

Culp, R. E., Heide, J., & Richardson, M. T. (1987). Maltreated children's developmental scores: Treatment versus nontreatment. *Child Abuse and Neglect, 11*, 29–34.

Culp, R. E., Little, V., Letts, D., & Lawrence, H. (1991). Maltreated children's self-concept: Effects of a comprehensive treatment program. *American Journal of Orthopsychiatry, 61*, 114–121.

Culp, R. E., Richardson, M. T., & Heide, J. S. (1987). Differential developmental progress of maltreated children in day treatment. *Social Work*, 497–499.

Daro, D. (1988). *Confronting child abuse: Research for effective program design.* New York: Free Press.

Daro, D., & Mitchell, L. (1989). *Child abuse fatalities continue to rise: Results of the 1988 annual fifty state survey (Fact Sheet #14).* Chicago: National Committee for Prevention of Child Abuse.

Davis, S. P., & Fantuzzo, J. W. (1989). The effects of adult and peer social initiations on the social behavior of withdrawn and aggressive maltreated preschool children. *Journal of Family Violence, 4*, 227–248.

Dawson, B., de Armas, A., McGrath, M. L., & Kelly, J. A. (1986). Cognitive problem-solving training to improve the child care judgment of child neglectful parents. *Journal of Family Violence, 1*, 209–221.

Deblinger, E., McLeer, S. V., & Henry, D. (1990). Cognitive behavioral treatment for sexually abused children suffering post-traumatic stress: Preliminary findings. *Journal of the American Academy of Child and Adolescent Psychiatry, 29*, 747–752.

Dodge, K. A., Bates, J. E., & Pettit, G. (1990). Mechanisms in the cycle of violence. *Science, 250*, 1678–1683.

Dohrenwend, B. (1978). Social stress and community psychology. *American Journal of Community Psychology, 6*, 1–14.

Drotar, D. (1992). Prevention of neglect and nonorganic failure to thrive. In D.J. Willis, E.W. Holden, & M. Rosenberg (Eds.), *Prevention of child maltreatment: Developmental and ecological perspectives* (pp. 115–149). New York: Wiley.

Dutton, D. G. (1988). *The domestic assault of women: Psychological and criminal justice perspectives.* Boston: Allyn & Bacon.

Egan, K. (1983). Stress management with abusive parents. *Journal of Clinical Child Psychology, 12*, 292–299.

Egeland, B. (1991). A longitudinal study of high-risk families: Issues and findings. In R. H. Starr & D. A. Wolfe (Eds.), *The effects of child abuse and neglect: Issues and research* (pp. 33–56). New York: Guilford Press.

Egeland, B., Breitenbucher, M., & Rosenberg, D. (1980). Prospective study of the significance of life stress in the etiology of child abuse. *Journal of Consulting and Clinical Psychology, 48*, 195–205.

Egeland, B., & Sroufe, A. (1981). Attachment and early maltreatment. *Child Development, 52*, 44–52.

Epstein, A. S., & Weikart, D. P. (1979). The Ypsilanti-Carnegie infant education project. *Monographs of the High/Scope Educational Research Foundation* (No. 6). Ypsilanti, MI: High/Scope Press.

Erickson, M. F., Sroufe, L. A., & Egeland, B. (1985). The relationship between quality of attachment and relationship problems in preschool in a high-risk sample. In I. Bretherton & E. Waters (Eds.), *Monographs of the Society for Research in Child Development, 50*(1–2), 147–166.

Fagan, J., & Wexler, S. (1988). Explanations of sexual assault among violent delinquents. *Journal of Adolescent Research, 3*, 363–385.

Fantuzzo, J. W. (1990). Behavioral treatment of the victims of child abuse and neglect. *Behavior Modification, 14,* 316–339.

Fantuzzo, J. W., Jurecic, L., Stovall, A., Hightower, A. D., Goins, C., & Schachtel, D. (1988). Effects of adult and peer social initiations on the social behavior of withdrawn, maltreated preschool children. *Journal of Consulting and Clinical Psychology, 56,* 34–39.

Fantuzzo, J. W., Stovall, A., Schachtel, D., Goins, C., & Hall, R. (1987). The effects of peer social initiations on the social behavior of withdrawn maltreated preschool children. *Journal of Behavior Therapy and Experimental Psychiatry, 4,* 357–363.

Fantuzzo, J. W., Wray, L., Hall, R., Goins, C., Azar, S. T. (1986). Parent and social skills training for mentally retarded parents identified as child maltreaters. *American Journal of Mental Deficiency, 91,* 135–140.

Field, T. M., Widmayer, S. M., Greenberg, R., & Stoller, S. (1982). Effects of parent training on teenage mothers and their infants. *Pediatrics, 69,* 703–707.

Field, T. M., Widmayer, S. M., Stringer, S., & Ignatoff, E. (1980). Teenage, lower-class, black mothers and their preterm infants: An intervention and developmental follow-up. *Child Development, 51,* 426–436.

Fink, A., & McCloskey, L. (1990). Moving child abuse and neglect prevention programs forward: Improving program evaluations. *Child Abuse and Neglect, 14,* 187–206.

Finkelhor, D. (1990). Early and long-term effects of child sexual abuse: An update. *Professional Psychology: Research and Practice, 21,* 325–330.

Foa, E. B., & Kozak, M. J. (1986). Emotional processing of fear: Exposure to corrective information. *Psychological Bulletin, 99,* 20–35.

Forehand, R., Thomas, A. M., Wierson, M., Brody, G., & Fauber, R. (1990). Role of maternal functioning and parenting skills in adolescent functioning following parental divorce. *Journal of Abnormal Psychology, 99,* 278–283.

Foster, S. L., & Robin, A. L. (1988). Family conflict and communication in adolescents. In E. J. Mash & L. G. Terdal (Eds.), *Behavioral assessment of childhood disorders* (2nd ed., pp. 717–775). New York: Guilford Press.

Frankel, H. (1988). Family-centered home-based services in child protection: A review of the research. *Social Service Review, 61,* 137–157.

Friedrich, W. N., Urquiza, A. J., & Beilke, R. L. (1986). Behavior problems in sexually abused young children. *Journal of Pediatric Psychology, 11,* 47–57.

Gaines, R., Sandgrund, A., Green, A. H., & Power, E. (1978). Etiological factors in child maltreatment: A multivariate study of abusing, neglecting, and normal mothers. *Journal of Abnormal Psychology, 87,* 531–541.

Garbarino, J. (1977). The human ecology of child maltreatment: A conceptual model for research. *Journal of Marriage and the Family, 39,* 721–735.

Garbarino, J. (1992). Preventing adolescent maltreatment. In D. J. Willis, E. W. Holden, & M. Rosenberg (Eds.), *Prevention of child maltreatment: Developmental and ecological perspectives* (pp. 94–114). New York: Wiley.

Garbarino, J., Guttman, E., & Seeley, J. (1986). *The psychologically battered child.* San Francisco: Jossey-Bass.

Gaudin, J. M., Jr., Wodarski, J. S., Arkinson, M. K., & Avery, L. S. (1991). Remedying child neglect: Effectiveness of social network interventions. *Journal of Applied Social Sciences, 15,* 97–123.

Gelles, R. J. (1973). Child abuse as a psychopathology: A sociological critique and reformulation. *American Journal of Orthopsychiatry, 43,* 611–621.

George, C., & Main, M. (1979). Social interactions of young abused children: Approach, avoidance, and aggression. *Child Develpoment, 50,* 306–318.

Gerbner, G., Ross, C. J., & Zigler, E. (Eds.). (1980). *Child abuse: An agenda for action.* New York: Oxford University Press.

Gershenson, H. P., Musick, J. S., Ruch-Ross, H. S., Magee, V., Rubino, K. K., & Rosenberg, D. (1989). The prevalence of coercive sexual experience among teenager mothers. *Journal of Interpersonal Violence, 4,* 204–219.

Giarretto, H. (1982). A comprehensive child sexual abuse treatment program. *Child Abuse and Neglect, 6,* 263–278.

Gil, D. G. (1970). *Violence against children: Physical child abuse in the United States.* Cambridge, MA: Harvard University Press.

Gold, E. R. (1986). Long-term effects of sexual victimization in childhood: An attributional approach. *Journal of Consulting and Clinical Psychology, 54,* 471–475.

Gomes-Schwartz, B., Horowitz, J. M., & Cardarelli, A. P. (1990). *Child sexual abuse: The initial effects.* Newbury Park, CA: Sage.

Goodman, G. S., Taub, E. P., Jones, D. P. H., England, P., Port, L. K., Rudy, L., & Prado, L. (1989). *Emotional effects of criminal court testimony on child sexual abuse victims* (Final report. Grant No. 85-IJ-CX-0020). Washington, DC: National Institute of Justice.

Gray, J. D., Cutler, C. A., Dean, J. G., & Kempe, C. H. (1979). Prediction and prevention of child abuse and neglect. *Journal of Social Issues, 35,* 127–139.

Gray, S. W., & Ruttle, K. (1980). The family-oriented home visiting program: A longitudinal study. *Genetic Psychology Monographs, 102,* 299–316.

Group for the Advancement of Psychiatry. (1986). *Teenage pregnancy: Impact on adolescent development.* New York: Bruner/Mazel.

Gutelius, M. F., Kirsch, A. D., MacDonald, S., Brooks, M. R., & McErlean, T. (1977). Controlled study of child health supervision: Behavioral results. *Pediatrics, 60,* 294–304.

Hansen, R. K. (1990). The psychological impact of sexual assault on women and children: A review. *Annals of Sex Research, 3,* 187–232.

Harter, S., Alexander, P. C., & Neimeyer, R. A. (1988). Long-term effects of incestuous child abuse in college women: Social adjustment, social cognition, and family characteristics. *Journal of Consulting and Clinical Psychology, 56,* 5–8.

Harvey, P., Forehand, R., Brown, C., & Holmes, T. (1988). The prevention of sexual abuse: Examination of the effectiveness of a program with kindergarten-age children. *Behavior Therapy, 19,* 429–435.

Haugaard, J. J., & Reppuci, N. D. (1988). *The sexual abuse of children.* San Francisco: Jossey-Bass.

Health and Welfare Canada. (1989). *Family violence: A review of theoretical and clinical literature* (Cat. No. H21-103/1989E). Ottawa: Minister of Support Services Canada.

Herrenkohl, R. C., Herrenkohl, E. C., Egolf, B. P., & Seech, M. (1979). The repetition of child abuse: How frequently does it occur? *Child Abuse and Neglect, 3,* 67–72.

Herrenkohl, R. C., Herrenkohl, E. C., Egolf, B. P., & Wu, P. (1991). The developmental consequences of child abuse: The Lehigh longitudinal study. In R. H. Starr & D. A. Wolfe (Eds.), *The effects of child abuse and neglect: Issues and research* (pp. 57–81). New York: Guilford Press.

Hinckley, E. C., & Ellis, W. F. (1985). An effective alternative to residential placement: Home-based services. *Journal of Consulting and Clinical Psychology, 14,* 209–213.

Isaacs, C. D. (1982). Treatment of child abuse: A review of the behavioral interventions. *Journal of Applied Behavior Analysis, 15,* 273–294.

Jaffe, P. G., Sudermann, M., & Reiztel, D. (1992). An evaluation of a secondary school programme on violence in intimate relationships. *Violence and Victims, 7,* 129–146.

Jaffe, P., Wilson, S., & Sas, L. (1987). Court testimony of child sexual abuse victims: Emerging issues in clinical assessments. *Canadian Psychology, 28,* 291–295.

Jaffe, P., Wolfe, D. A., & Wilson, S. (1990). *Children of battered women.* Newbury Park, CA: Sage.

Kaufman, K. L., & Rudy, L. (1991). Future directions in the treatment of physical child abuse. *Criminal Justice and Behavior, 18,* 82–97.

Kaufman, J., & Zigler, E. (1989). The intergenerational transmission of child abuse and the prospect of predicting future abusers. In D. Cicchetti & V. Carlson (Eds.), *Child maltreatment: Research and theory on the causes and consequences of child abuse and neglect* (pp. 129–150). New York: Cambridge University Press.

Kempe, C. H., & Helfer, R. E. (1972). *Helping the battered child and his family.* Philadelphia: Lippincott.

Kinney, J. M., Madsen, B., Fleming, T., & Haapala, D. A. (1977). Homebuilders: Keeping families together. *Journal of Consulting and Clinical Psychology, 45,* 667–673.

Kolko, D. J. (1987). Treatment of child sexual abuse: Programs, progress, and prospects. *Journal of Family Violence, 2,* 303–318.

Lamb, M., & Easterbrooks, M. A. (1981). Individual differences in parental sensitivity: Origins, components, and consequences. In M. E. Lamb & K. R. Sherrod (Eds.), *Infant social cognition: Theoretical and empirical considerations* (pp. 127–154). Hillsdale, NJ: Erlbaum.

Larson, C. P. (1980). Efficacy of parenatal and postpartum home visits on child health and development. *Pediatrics, 66,* 191–197.

Lovell, M. L., & Hawkins, J. D. (1988). An evaluation of a group intervention to increase the personal social networks of abusive mothers. *Children and Youth Services Review, 10,* 175–188.

Lutzker, J. R. (1984). Project 12-Ways: Treating child abuse and neglect from an eco-behavioral perspective. In R. F. Dangel & R. A. Polster (Eds.), *Parent training: Formulations of research and practice* (pp. 260–291). New York: Guilford Press.

Lutzker, J. (1990). Behavioral treatment of child neglect. *Behavior Modification, 14,* 301–315.

Lutzker, J. R., & Newman, M. R. (1986). Child abuse and neglect: Community problem, community solutions. *Education and Treatment of Children, 9,* 344–354.

Lutzker, J. R., & Rice, J. M. (1984). Project 12-Ways: Measuring outcome of a large in-home service for treatment and prevention of child abuse and neglect. *Child Abuse and Neglect, 8*, 519–524.

Lutzker, J. R., & Rice, J. M. (1987). Using recidivism data to evaluate Project 12-Ways: An ecobehavioral approach to the treatment and prevention of child abuse and neglect. *Journal of Family Violence, 2*, 283–290.

Madden, J., O'Hara, J., & Levenstein, P. (1984). Home again: Effects of the mother–child home program on mother and child. *Child Development, 55*, 363–647.

Malamuth, N. M., Sockloskie, R. J., Koss, M. P., & Tanaka, J. S. (1991). Characteristics of aggressors against women: Testing a model using a national sample of college students. *Journal of Consulting and Clinical Psychology, 59*, 670–681.

Mannarino, A. P., & Cohen, J. A. (1990). Treating the abused child. In R. T. Ammerman & M. Hersen (Eds.), *Children at risk: An evaluation of factors contributing to child abuse and neglect* (pp. 249–268). New York: Plenum Press.

Marshall, W. L., Jones, R., Ward, T., Johnston, P., & Barbaree, H. E. (1991). Treatment outcome with sex offenders. *Clinical Psychology Review, 11*, 465–485.

Mash, E. J., & Wolfe, D. A. (1991). Methodological issues in research on physical child abuse. *Criminal Justice and Behavior, 18*, 8–29.

McGee, R., & Wolfe, D. A. (1991). Psychological maltreatment: Towards an operational definition. *Development and Psychopathology, 3*, 3–18.

Melton, G. B. (1990). Child protection: Making a bad situation worse? *Contemporary Psychology, 35*, 213–214.

Melton, G. B. (1992). The improbability of prevention of sexual abuse. In D. J. Willis, E. W. Holden, and M. Rosenberg (Eds.), *Prevention of child maltreatment: Developmental and ecological perspectives* (pp. 168–189). New York: Wiley.

Miller, S. H. (1988). The Child Welfare League of America's Adolescent Parents Project. In H. B. Weiss & F. H. Jacobs (Eds.), *Evaluating family programs* (pp. 371–388). New York: Aldine de Gruyter.

Mitchell, H., & Casto, G. (1988). Team education for adolescent mothers. In alternative futures for rural special education. *Proceedings of the annual ACRES (American Council on Rural Special Education), National Rural Special Education Conference.*

National Center on Child Abuse and Neglect. (1981). *Study findings: National study of the incidence and severity of child abuse and neglect.* Washington, DC: U.S. Government Printing Office.

National Center on Child Abuse and Neglect. (1988). *Study findings: Study of the national incidence of and prevalence of child abuse and neglect.* Washington, DC: U.S. Government Printing Office.

Nicol, A. R., Smith, J., Kay, B., Hall, D., Barlow, J., & Williams, B. (1988). A focused casework approach to the treatment of child abuse: A controlled comparison. *Journal of Child Psychology and Psychiatry, 29*, 703–711.

Nomellini, S., & Katz, R. C. (1983). Effects of anger control training on abusive parents. *Cognitive Therapy and Research, 7*, 57–68.

O'Connor, S., Vietze, P. M., Sherrod, K. B., Sandler, H. M., & Altemeier, W. A., III. (1980). Reduced incidence of parenting inadequacy following rooming-in. *Pediatrics, 66*, 176–182.

Olds, D. L., & Kitzman, H. (1990). Can home visitation improve the health of women and children at environmental risk? *Pediatrics, 86,* 108–116.

Olds, D. L., Henderson, C. R. Jr., Chamberlain, R., & Tatelbaum, R. (1986). Preventing child abuse and neglect: A randomized trial of nurse home visitation. *Pediatrics, 78,* 65–78.

Olds, D. L., Henderson, C. R., Jr., Tatelbaum, R., & Chamberlain, R. (1988). Improving the life-course development of socially disadvantaged mothers: A randomized trial of nurse home visitation. *American Journal of Public Health, 78,* 1436–1445.

Parish, R. A., Myers, P. A., Brandner, A., & Templin, K. H. (1985). Developmental milestones in abused children and their improvement with a family-oriented approach to the treatment of child abuse. *Child Abuse and Neglect, 9,* 246–250.

Parke, R. D. (1977). Socialization into child abuse: A social interactional perspective. In J. L. Tapp & F. J. Levine (Eds.), *Law, justice, and the individual in society: Psychological and legal issues* (pp. 183–199). New York: Holt, Rinehart, & Winston.

Patterson, G. R., DeBaryshe, B. D., & Ramsey, E. (1989). A developmental perspective on antisocial behavior. *American Psychologist, 44,* 329–335.

Pelton, L. H. (1978). Child abuse and neglect: The myth of classlessness. *American Journal of Orthopsychiatry, 48,* 608–317.

Phares, V., & Compas, B. E. (1992). The role of fathers in child and adolescent psychopathology: Make room for daddy. *Psychological Bulletin, 111,* 387–412.

Plotkin, R. C., Azar, S., Twentyman, C. T., & Perri, M. G. (1981). A critical evaluation of the research methodology employed in the investigation of causative factors in child abuse and neglect. *Child Abuse and Neglect, 5,* 449–455.

Pransky, J. (1991). *Prevention: The critical need.* Springfield, MO: Burrell Foundation.

Reppucci, N. D., & Haugaard, J. J. (1989). Prevention of child sexual abuse: Myth or reality. *American Psychologist, 44,* 1266–1275.

Resnick, G. (1985). Enhancing parental competence for high risk mothers: An evaluation of prevention effects. *Child Abuse and Neglect, 9,* 479–489.

Roberts, R. N., Wasik, B. H., Casto, G., & Ramey, C. T. (1991). Family support in the home: Programs, policy, and social change. *American Psychologist, 46,* 131–137.

Roderiguez, G. G., & Cortez, C. P. (1988). The evaluation experience of the Avance parent–child education program. In H. B. Weiss & F. H. Jacobs (Eds.), *Evaluating family programs* (pp. 287–302). New York: Aldine de Gruyter.

Rogeness, G. A., Ritchey, S., Alex, P. L., Zuelzer, M., & Morris, R. (1981). Family patterns and parenting attitudes in teenage parents. *Journal of Community Psychology, 9,* 239–245.

Roosa, M., & Vaughan, L. (1983). Teen mothers enrolled in an alternative parenting program. *Urban Education, 18,* 348–360.

Rosenfield-Schlichter, M. D., Sarber, R. R., Bueno, G., Greene, B. F., & Lutzker, J. R. (1983). Maintaining accountability for an ecobehavioral treatment of one aspect of child neglect: Personal cleanliness. *Education and Treatment of Children, 6,* 153–164.

Runyan, D. K., Everson, M. D., Edelson, G. A., Hunter, W. M., & Coulter, M. L.

(1988). Impact of legal intervention on sexually abused children. *Journal of Pediatrics, 113*, 647–653.

Sas, L., Austin, G., Wolfe, D., & Hurley, P. (1991). *Reducing the system-induced trauma for child sexual abuse victims through court preparation, assessment, and follow-up* (Project #4555-1-125). Ottawa: National Welfare Grants Division, Health and Welfare Canada. (Available from the authors, London Family Court Clinic, 254 Pall Mall Street, Suite 200, London, Canada, N6A 5P6)

Saslawsky, D. A., & Wurtele, S. K. (1986). Educating children about sexual abuse: Implications for pediatric intervention and possible prevention. *Journal of Pediatric Psychology, 11*, 235–245.

Schmitz, C. (1988, May 27). Whack sexual assault complainant at preliminary hearing. *Lawyer's Weekly*, pp. 22–23.

Seitz, V., Rosenbaum, L. K., & Apfel, N. H. (1985). Effects of family support intervention: A ten-year follow-up. *Child Development, 56*, 376–391.

Shaw-Lamphear, V. S. (1985). The impact of maltreatment on children's psychosocial adjustment: A review of the research. *Child Abuse and Neglect, 9*, 251–263.

Shirk, S. R. (1988). The interpersonal legacy of physical abuse of children. In M. Straus (Ed.), *Abuse and victimization across the lifespan* (pp. 57–81). Baltimore: Johns Hopkins University Press.

Siegel, E., Bauman, K. E., Schaefer, E. S., Saunders, M. M., & Ingram, D. D. (1980). Hospital and home support during infancy: Impact on maternal attachment, child abuse and neglect and health care utilization. *Pediatrics, 66*, 183–190.

Silver, R. L., Boon, C., & Stones, M. H. (1983). Searching for meaning in misfortune: Making sense of incest. *Journal of Social Issues, 39*, 81–102.

Sipes, D.S.B. (1992). *Review of the literature on cultural considerations in treatment of abused and neglected ethnic minority children*. Paper presented to the Working Group on Treatment of Child Abuse and Neglect, American Psychological Association, Washington, DC.

Slaughter, D. T. (1983). Early intervention and its effects on maternal and child development. *Monographs of the Society for Research in Child Development, 48* (4, Serial No. 202).

Spinetta, J. J., & Rigler, D. (1972). The child abusing parent: A psychological review. *Psychological Bulletin, 77*, 296–304.

Sroufe, L. A., & Fleeson, J. (1986). Attachment and the construction of relationships. In W. W. Hartup & Z. Rubin (Eds.), *Relationships and development* (pp. 51–71). Hillsdale, NJ: Erlbaum.

Starr, R. H. Jr. (1979). Child abuse. *American Psychologist, 34*, 872–878.

Starr, R., MacLean, D. J., & Keating, D. P. (1991). Life-span developmental outcomes of child maltreatment. In R. H. Starr & D. A. Wolfe (Eds.), *The effects of child abuse and neglect: Issues and research* (pp. 1–32). New York: Guilford Press.

Stevenson, J., Bailey, V., & Simpson, J. (1988). Feasible intervention in families with parenting difficulties: A primary preventive perspective on child abuse. In K. Browne, C. Davies, & P. Stratton (Eds.), *Early prediction and prevention of child abuse* (pp. 121–138). Chichester, England: Wiley.

Straus, M. A., & Gelles, R. (1990). *Physical violence in American families: Risk factors and adaptations to violence in 8,145 families*. New Brunswick, NJ: Transaction.

Taylor, D. K., & Beauchamp, C. (1988). Hospital-based primary prevention strategy in child abuse: A multi-level needs assessment. *Child Abuse and Neglect*, 12, 343–354.

Teleen, S., Herzog, B. S., & Kilbane, T. L. (1989). Impact of a family support program on mothers' social support and parenting stress. *American Journal of Orthopsychiatry*, 59, 410–419.

Tertinger, D. A., Greene, B. F., & Lutzker, J. R. (1984). Home safety: Development and validation of one component of an ecobehavioral treatment program for abused and neglected children. *Journal of Applied Behavior Analysis*, 17, 159–177.

Tracy, E. M., & Whittaker, J. K. (1987). The evidence base for social support interventions in child and family practice: Emerging issues for research and practice. *Children and Youth Services Review*, 9, 249–270.

Travers, J., Nauta, M. J., & Irwin, N. (1982). *The effects of a social program: Final report of the Child and Family Resources Program's Infant Toddler Component* (AAI No. 82-31). Cambridge, MA: ABT.

Unger, D. G., & Wandersman, L. P. (1988). A support program for adolescent mothers: Predictors of participation. In D. R. Powell (Ed.), *Parent education as early childhood intervention: Emerging directions in theory, research, and practice* (pp. 105–130). Norwood, NJ: Ablex.

U.S. Advisory Board on Child Abuse and Neglect. (1990). *Child abuse and neglect: Critical first steps in response to a national emergency* (Stock No. 017-092-00104-5). Washington, DC: U.S. Government Printing Office.

Videka-Sherman, L. (1989, October). *Therapeutic issues for physical and emotional child abuse and neglect: Implications for longitudinal research*. Paper presented at a research forum entitled "Issues in the longitudinal study of child maltreatment," The Institute for the Prevention of Child Abuse, Toronto, Canada.

Vietze, P. M., O'Connor, S., Sherrod, K. B., Altemeier, W. A. (1991). The early screening project. In R. H. Starr & D. A. Wolfe (Eds.), *The effects of child abuse and neglect: Issues and research* (pp. 82–99). New York: Guilford Press.

Wald, M. S., & Cohen, S. (1988). Preventing child abuse: What will it take? In D. J. Besharov (Ed.), *Protecting children from abuse and neglect* (pp. 295–319). Springfield, Illinois: C. C. Thomas.

Watson-Perczel, M., Lutzker, J. R., Greene, B. F., & McGimpsey, B. J. (1988). Assessment and modification of home cleanliness among families adjudicated or child neglect. *Behavior Modification*, 12, 57–81.

Wekerle, C., & Wolfe, D. A. (1993). Prevention of child physical abuse and neglect: Promising new directions. *Clinical Psychology Review*, 13, 501–540.

Wesch, D., & Lutzker, J. R. (1991). A comprehensive 5-year evaluation of Project 12-Ways: An ecobehavioral program for treating and preventing child abuse and neglect. *Journal of Family Violence*, 6, 17–35.

Westney, O., Cole, O. J., & Munford, T. (1988). The effects of prenatal education intervention on unwed prospective adolescent fathers. *Journal of Adolescent Health Care*, 9, 214–218.

Whitcomb, D., Runyan, D. K., DeVos, E., Hunter, W. M., Cross, T. P., Everson, M. D., Peeler, N. A., Porter, C. Q., Toth, P. A., & Cropper, C. (1991). *Child victim as witness research and development program* (Report prepared under Grant No. 87-MC-CX-0026). Washington, DC: Office of Juvenile Justice and

Delinquency Prevention, Office of Justice Programs, U.S. Department of Justice.

Whiteman, M., Fanshel, D., & Grundy, J. F. (1987). Cognitive-behavioral interventions aimed at anger of parents at risk of child abuse. *Social Work, 32,* 469–474.

Widom, C. S. (1989). Does violence beget violence? A critical examination of the literature. *Psychological Bulletin, 106,* 3–28.

Willett, J. B., Ayoub, C. C., & Robinson, D. (1991). Using growth modeling to examine systematic differences in growth: An example of chance in the functioning of families at risk of maladaptive parenting, child abuse, or neglect. *Journal of Consulting and Clinical Psychology, 59,* 38–47.

Williamson, J. M., Borduin, C. M., & Howe, B. A. (1991). The ecology of adolescent maltreatment: A multilevel examination of adolescent physical abuse, sexual abuse, and neglect. *Journal of Consulting and Clinical Psychology, 59,* 449–457.

Wolfe, D. A. (1984). Treatment of abusive parents: A reply to the special issue. *Journal of Clinical Child Psychology, 13,* 192–194.

Wolfe, D. A. (1985). Child abusive parents: An empirical review and analysis. *Psychological Bulletin, 97,* 462–482.

Wolfe, D. A. (1987). *Child abuse: Implications for child development and psychopathology.* Newbury Park, CA: Sage.

Wolfe, D. A. (1988). Child abuse and neglect. In E. J. Mash & L. G. Terdal (Eds.), *Behavioral assessment of childhood disorders* (2nd ed., pp. 627–669). New York: Guilford Press.

Wolfe, D. A. (1990). Preventing child abuse means enhancing family functioning. *Canada's Mental Health, 38,* 27–29.

Wolfe, D. A. (1991). *Preventing physical and emotional abuse of children.* New York: Guilford Press.

Wolfe, D. A., Edwards, B., Manion, I., & Koverola, C. (1988). Early intervention for parents at risk of child abuse and neglect: A preliminary investigation. *Journal of Consulting and Clinical Psychology, 56,* 40–47.

Wolfe, D. A., & Jaffe, P. (1990). The psychosocial needs of children in care. In L. C. Johnson & D. Barnhorst (Eds.), *Children, families, and public policy in the 1990's* (pp. 231–246). Toronto: Thompson Educational Publishing.

Wolfe, D. A., Kaufman, K., Aragona, J., & Sandler, J. (1981). *The child management program for abusive parents: Procedures for developing a child abuse intervention program.* Ocoee, Florida: Anna Publishing.

Wolfe, D. A., McPherson, T., Blount, R., & Wolfe, V. (1986). Evaluation of a brief intervention for educating school children in awareness of physical and sexual abuse. *Child Abuse and Neglect, 10,* 85–92.

Wolfe, D. A., St. Lawrence, J. S., Graves, K., Brehony, K., Bradlyn, A. S., & Kelly, J. A. (1982). Intensive behavioral parent training for a child abusive mother. *Behavior Therapy, 13,* 438–451.

Wolfe, D. A., & Sandler, J. (1981). Training abusive parents in effective child management. *Behavior Modification, 5,* 320–335.

Wolfe, D. A., Wekerle, C., & McGee, R. (1992). Developmental disparities of abused children: Directions for prevention. In R. DeV. Peters, R. J. McMahon, &

V. L. Quinsey (Eds.), *Aggression and violence throughout the lifespan*. Newbury Park, CA: Sage.

Wolfe, V. V., Sas, L., & Wilson, S. (1987). Some issues in preparing sexually abused children for courtroom testimony. *Behavior Therapist*, *10*, 107–113.

Wolfe, V. V., & Wolfe, D. A. (1988). Sexual abuse of children. In E. J. Mash & L. G. Terdal (Eds.), *Behavioral assessment of childhood disorders* (2nd ed., pp. 670–714). New York: Guilford Press.

Wood, S., Schroeder, C., & Barton, K. (1988). In-home treatment of abusive families: Cost and placement at one year. *Psychotherapy*, *25*, 409–414.

Wurtele, S., Kast, L., Miller-Perrin, C., & Kondrick, P. (1989). Comparison of programs for teaching personal safety skills to preschoolers. *Journal of Consulting and Clinical Psychology*, *57*, 505–511.

Zuravin, S. J. (1991). Suggestions for operationally defining child physical abuse and physical neglect. In R. H. Starr & D. A. Wolfe (Eds.), *The effects of child abuse and neglect: Issues and research* (pp. 100–128). New York: Guilford Press.

Chapter 7

Neighborhood-Based Programs

James Garbarino
Kathleen Kostelny

In its search for innovative ways to respond to the national emergency facing protective services and the prevention of child maltreatment, the U.S. Advisory Board on Child Abuse and Neglect has thrown its support to "neighborhood-based programs" (U.S. Advisory Board on Child Abuse and Neglect [the Board], 1991). Such programs include "neighbor helping neighbor," with service delivery in the home or the adjacent community and related efforts to identify, generate, and maintain enduring social structures at the local level that meet the needs of families in positive ways and prevent child maltreatment. Such a neighborhood-based approach will both improve the viability of a neighborhood and provide needed services to individual families (Barry, 1991).

From this broad commitment, we will address a number of specific topics. First among these are the meaning of "neighborhood" (including both the historical context and the geographic dimension) as well as the concepts of neighboring and neighborhood-based programming. Next, neighborhood-based research on child maltreatment is reviewed, addressing issues of the relationship of community violence to child maltreatment and its implications for delivering social services to families. Included is consideration of ameliorating factors in reducing stress, promoting resiliency, and enhancing participation in the social network for children and families. Neighborhood-based programs—both those aimed at child abuse prevention and other neighborhood intervention programs—are also examined. In addition, some general principles derived from existing programs and research, focusing on creating resiliency through family and community support, are presented. Finally, the research and demonstration needs of neighborhood-based programs are discussed.

NEIGHBORHOODS AND NEIGHBORING

The concept of neighborhood has a history as a focal point for research, theory, policy, and practice in the United States (Hawley, 1950; Warren, 1978). The Board (1991) uses the following definition of neighborhood: "a small geographic unit consensually identified as a single community (includes rural and urban settings)" (p. 55).

The issue of size is problematic for rural areas, of course, once we move beyond small towns and villages to farms, ranches, and isolated dwellings. Nonetheless, the Board's approach is in keeping with most such efforts, which contain an attempt to limit geographic borders—most notably in terms of the walking distance of a young child (cf. Bryant, 1985 discussing "the neighborhood walk methodology"). Coupled with this spatial dimension is some effort to respect history (the evolution of residential patterns) and psyche (some sense of shared identity among the residents, as in a common inclination to "name" the neighborhood).

Such efforts have led to three elements in the definition of neighborhoods: a social component, a cognitive component, and an affective component (Unger & Wandersman, 1985). Thus, we see definitions of neighborhood (and neighboring) in terms of interaction patterns, a common understanding of boundaries and identity, and a set of shared feelings of belonging.

The social component of neighborhoods includes both informal social supports (emotional, instrumental, and informational) and social networks (links to other people). This social component is central in offering support and in providing resources for coping with stressors at both an individual and a neighborhood level.

However, some observers have noted a shift in the function of neighborhoods. With advances in communication, technology, and transportation, neighborhoods have lost some of the important functions that they once had. Now, many activities and relationships take place outside a person's neighborhood. Such a view makes it necessary to consider "communities without propinquity," that is, communities not limited by their geographical boundaries (Wellman, 1979). However, while people may belong to a variety of communities depending on their interests, people will belong to only one neighborhood based on where they live. Thus, a neighborhood is a geographic area where people feel physically, although not necessarily socially, close to each other (Barry, 1991).

The cognitive component of a neighborhood refers to the thoughts or ideas that individuals have about their neighborhood's social and physical environment. This cognitive component can be used both to understand the neighborhood and to develop ways of dealing effectively with neighborhood issues. One aspect of neighborhood cognition involves a mental mapping process resulting from repeated experiences in the neighborhood, thus allowing individuals to better manage their neighborhood. For example, cognitive mapping in dangerous neighborhoods would determine where people felt safe to walk or where they could socially interact with others without fearing harm.

A neighborhood also has an affective dimension, including a sense of mutual help, a sense of community, and an attachment to place. The sense of mutual help involves the belief that assistance is available when needed, even though neighbors are not frequently contacted. Indeed, when there is heavy actual use of neighborhood resources it may well lead to a reduction in neighboring due to overload. Thus, neighborhood support is best understood in terms of confidence rather than utilization.

A sense of community encompasses feelings of membership and belongingness and shared socioemotional ties with others in the neighborhood. Attachment to place develops through an analysis by individuals in their neighborhood where the costs and benefits of living in their neighborhood are compared with other neighborhoods.

Although most of the conceptual rhetoric surrounding "neighborhood" focuses on urban settings, many observers seek some way to incorporate rural settings (Fitchen, 1981). However, in rural areas, providing community-based programs is often problematic for several reasons. First, because rural communities are spread out, families often have difficulty getting to the programs. Second, there is the tendency to duplicate urban program models to rural communities, thereby disregarding the needs and characteristics of the rural population and disempowering the rural residents if these programs come under external control (Myers-Walls, 1992). Going still further, we must recognize that different ecologies generate different patterns of neighborhoods (e.g., the rural area of the American West vs. Appalachia; the organizational pattern of "old" urban neighborhoods in New England vs. the diffused patterns of Sun Belt cities).

NEIGHBORHOOD-BASED PROGRAMMING

However we define neighborhood, we must struggle to understand the potential and actual impact of "neighborhood-based programming" in supporting families and protecting children (Garbarino, Stocking, & Associates, 1980). The defining characteristics of a neighborhood-based approach are premised on the notion that deliberately engineered social support, provided during a formative period in child and family development, can buffer the child and family from some of the psychological and social effects of poverty, promote personal development and psychological well-being, and stimulate healthy patterns of interaction both within the family and between the family and the broader environment (Weiss & Halpern, 1991). In starker terms, it may be argued that deliberately engineered social support can be potent enough to alter parenting capacities and styles acquired and reinforced through a lifetime of experience in a particular familial and social world.

The role of social support systems in preventing child maltreatment is the linking of social nurturance and social control (Garbarino, 1987). Such support systems give feedback to individuals, validating their accomplishments, but also guiding and correcting them when their behavior falls short of the group norm (Caplan & Killilea, 1976).

Two corollary premises are embedded in a personal-change strategy. The first is that the support provided can be internalized in some manner, and thus have an effect beyond the period during which it is provided. The second is that support provided can strengthen childrearing enough to have a meaningful effect on child health and development (Weiss & Halpern, 1991).

These concerns reverberate through all analyses of family support in the form of two recurrent questions: Can family support be a "treatment" or must it be a condition of life? Can family support succeed amidst conditions of high risk? Both call our attention to the limiting factors on neighborhood support: whether it is possible to "synthesize" neighborhood and whether neighborhood-based programming is feasible among the neediest families.

Beyond these fundamental issues of efficacy stand a number of issues concerning process. For example, to what extent can and should social support programs for families be staffed at least in part by indigenous volunteers and/or paraprofessionals? To what extent can and should efforts be aimed at assisting neighbors in helping each other? In short, to what extent is neighborhood-based programming for families inextricably tied to issues of empowerment?

Historical Perspective

One of the origins of the social support "movement" lies in the settlement houses that were created as part of liberal reform movements in the 19th century—(e.g., Hull House in Chicago) (Halpern, 1990b). These settlement houses sought to provide a neighborhood focus and to serve a wide range of needs—ameliorative, preventive, and enabling. Staff lived in the settlement house, and the overall theme was one of establishing a center for promoting the culture, values, and resources of middle-class America among the poor and immigrant populations.

A second origin of the social support approach lies in the early concept of the visiting nurse. By sending nurses into the community, and by defining their role as "holistic," the visiting nurse programs of the 19th and early 20th centuries complemented the settlement house by incorporating the concept of "friendly visitors" and "mutual help" into day-to-day practice. Visiting nurses clearly bear a direct conceptual (and often historical) relationship to contemporary approaches to family social support, where "community nursing" figures prominently (Froland, Pancoast, Chapman, & Kimboko, 1981; Kagan, Powell, Weissbourd, & Zigler, 1987).

From the 1930s through the 1950s, other neighborhood-based strategies emerged. One of these, the Chicago Areas Project, targeted reducing juvenile delinquency and general community breakdown by identifying natural community leaders who could mobilize other community members. Another neighborhood approach, developed by Saul Alinsky in his community-organizing work, was more militant. This approach deliberately engendered conflict to emphasize the power and control of institutions outside the community, with the goal of bringing the community together against these outside institutions (Alinsky, 1970).

From the 1950s through the 1980s, the Gray Areas program of the Ford Foundation was the prototype for many neighborhood-based initiatives (Halpern, 1991). Like earlier initiatives, this approach had its foundation in the idea that mainstream institutions and disenfranchised residents of poor neighborhoods had similar goals but were frustrated by not knowing how to achieve them either independently or together.

Community Progress Inc. was one of the most widely known Gray Areas programs. Based in New Haven, Connecticut, it was developed by a tightly knit group of young, reform-minded professionals. They deliberately excluded the leadership of large, established agencies such as schools, social services, and health departments. However, one drawback to their approach was that while they were committed to neighborhood members providing services, they did not encourage neighborhood members to participate in the planning process.

Current approaches include a wide and proliferating variety of programs and organizations designed to establish social support in the environment of families. These efforts are often called family support and education programs (e.g., the Family Focus program developed by Weissbourd & Kagan, 1994), social support networks (Belle, 1989), parent education projects (e.g., the New Parents as Teachers Program, Pfannesntiel & Seltzer, 1989), or home health visitor programs (e.g., the Elmira, New York, project; Olds, Henderson, Tatelbaum, & Chamberlain, 1986; Olds & Henderson, 1990).

In the political and cultural climate prevailing in the United States since the 1970s, such efforts have great appeal. They reflect private and local initiative. They play to themes of voluntarism ("one thousand points of light") that have received prominent political sponsorship. They echo recurrent themes of "empowerment" and "ownership" that are offered as a complement, or even a substitute, for increased public investment and control in local affairs, as articulated, for example, by Robert Woodson of the Washington-based Enterprise Institute.

Such an approach deemphasizes "treatment" and the role of therapeutic professionals. The resulting models are "community based." Yet, this widespread rhetorical appeal leaves some important questions unanswered (and often even unasked).

Intuitive Appeal versus Rigorous Grounding in Theory and Research

Do existing program evaluations strongly confirm the validity of the assumptions underlying community-based family support and education programs, or has their intuitive appeal in the current political and cultural climate sustained them in the absence of conclusive empirical evidence? If forced to answer this question, we must acknowledge that family support programs rest primarily on a foundation of faith. Few studies exist to address the validity of these approaches, particularly with high-risk families in high-risk communities.

Matching Services and Needs

What is the "market" for neighborhood support efforts? Weissbourd and Kagan (1994) present the assumptions of Family Focus thus: A third of the families are functioning well without us; a third need and can profit from us; a third are too troubled to make good use of our program. Although the exact percentages in each category are open to question, the underlying analysis seems valid because it recognizes that effectiveness depends in part on an appropriate matching of services and needs.

Successful participation in a Family Focus program (or indeed most other family-oriented social programs) requires a moderate level of competence, organization, available resources, and continuing motivation. One of the early analyses of Head Start concluded: "Those who have the most gain the most."

The same may apply to neighborhoods. Can family support programs operate from a neighborhood base if the neighborhood is socially and physically devastated? How much congruence is required among neighborhood-based institutions? Is it enough to have a school? A church? Is an active business community necessary? Can you operate neighborhood-based programs in a ghost town?

This leads us always to look closely at a family support program to see whether it is reaching beyond the "easy" families and the "easy" neighborhoods. There is always the danger that the program will simply open its doors and the best families will walk in—the upper third to which Weissbourd refers. The lowest third are rarely able and willing to participate in such programs. This is a particularly serious concern if we seek to employ family support to prevent child maltreatment because families involved in child maltreatment are by and large drawn from the group with the lowest levels of competence and motivation.

Consultation versus Training

To what degree is it necessary and feasible for "natural helpers"/neighbors to be "trained" to function as family support systems? This is one of the "hot" issues in the field of family support. One camp emphasizes the need for professionals to serve as "consultants" to natural neighbors or central figures. Collins and Pancoast (1976) have adopted this approach. In their day care information project, they identified women who were already the focal point of natural helping networks in the informal day care referral system. They saw as their goal facilitating these natural helpers without interfering with their operations. They emphasized the existing knowledge and skills of the natural helper and the danger of disturbing her work through overt intervention. Thus, consultation rather than training was the focus of their efforts.

In contrast, Danish and D'Augelli (1980) established a training program for preparing indigenous citizens to function on behalf of mental health promotion in their community. They emphasized the limitations of these natural helpers and the need to augment their skills and concepts. Thus, training rather than merely consultation was the focus of their efforts.

However, the use of paraprofessionals has limitations. Halpern and Larner (1987) found that paraprofessionals encountered problems in assisting clients in areas of health care, child care, and mental health services. Other problems may arise from overidentification with the client, excessive dependency on the client, projecting one's own situation onto the client, or low expectations (Austin, 1978). Parents are also at times reluctant to reveal personal matters to indigenous workers from the community because they fear a loss of privacy (Olds & Henderson, 1990).

Still other professionals (e.g., Musick & Stott, 1990) perceive that traditional staff education and training programs for paraprofessionals from the community are not adequate for promoting change in parents and optimal development in children, particularly when such psychically loaded issues as sexual abuse are involved. For example, in addition to formal training at the Ounce of Prevention Fund programs, new strategies were designed to change the service provider by transforming the way she viewed and understood parents, children, and the parent–child relationship (Musick, Bernstein, Percansky, & Stott, 1987). In the Heart-to-Heart program at the Ounce of Prevention Fund, aimed at enabling teen parents to protect their children and themselves against sexual abuse, it was discovered that many of the paraprofessionals who worked with the teen parents were also the victims of childhood sexual abuse. Therefore, the paraprofessionals received intensive training that provided opportunities for confronting their own feelings and conflicts with the issues of parenting and sexual abuse. Such opportunities for processing their experiences and feelings enabled the paraprofessionals not to confuse their own issues with the issues of the individuals with whom they were working.

The training protocol was restructured in terms of forming a relationship—to model the kinds of reciprocal, interactive roles that the professional staff expected the paraprofessional staff to fulfill vis-à-vis teen parents. Such a "chain of enablement" fosters positive growth in paraprofessional staff so that they in turn can foster such growth in teen parents. This method of training paraprofessionals is designed to result ultimately in more enabling and nurturing parenting through a structured, well-planned trickle-down effect.

"Domains of Silence"

Are there topics and issues with which neighbors and/or indigenous paraprofessionals cannot deal because they are too personally threatening or culturally taboo? This issue extends the consultation versus training issue still further and is of special relevance to any consideration of the role of social support in preventing child maltreatment.

Two of the family issues most likely to invoke personal or cultural domains of silence are sexuality and aggression. Thus, any effort that aims to prevent child maltreatment through social support systems relying on natural helpers must contend with the fact that matters of sex and violence are least likely to be addressed (or addressed successfully). The natural helpers' own experiences of victimization, teenage sexual activity, and use of corporal punishment create powerful impediments in dealing with these issues openly, as a program's formal curriculum typically dictates (Halpern, 1990a; Musick & Stott, 1990). This is not to say that these obstacles are insurmountable. Indeed, both can be addressed.

The Ounce of Prevention Fund programs dealing with sexuality and teen mothers have found it possible to deal with issues of sexuality with indigenous helpers, but only after an extensive program of education and "processing." By the same token, the North Lawndale Family Support Initiative of the National Committee for Prevention of Child Abuse in Chicago was able to open a dialogue with community members about the issue of corporal punishment, a dialogue that started from the sometimes fierce unwillingness of many parents (and natural helpers from the neighborhood) to acknowledge that a problem existed in the community with respect to corporal punishment.

Selection Effects or Genuine Impact

To what extent are neighborhood effects primarily self-selection effects and the result of exclusionary policies versus the result of the milieu represented in the neighborhood? All community and neighborhood analyses go forward potentially compromised on the basis of self-selection. Why are some people living in neighborhood A while others live in neighborhood B? Rarely is random selection the answer. The systematic grouping and exclusion of families on the basis of race, ethnicity, or income mitigates against efforts to *understand* family functioning (including child maltreatment) on the basis of neighborhood characteristics.

A study of 23 communities experiencing rapid population growth found that all but 2 communities had a disproportionate increase in crime (Freudenburg & Jones, 1991). The study suggested that changes in a community's social structure that accompany rapid growth result in a breakdown of social control. As the "density of acquaintanceship" (i.e., the proportion of a community's residents who know each other) decreases, criminal activity increases.

Another issue concerns outmigration from neighborhoods beginning to "turn bad." Such an outmigration may have debilitating effects on social networks (Fitchen, 1981) and may create still more confounding self-selection effects. Beyond even these obvious selection factors, neighborhoods differ on the basis of "ethos." Some areas are more vital and coherent, even among middle-class families (Warren, 1978).

Other neighborhoods reflect common problems. A survey in South Carolina (Melton, 1992) revealed that on a scale of 1 to 7—with 7 indicating high involvement—the average score for neighborhood residents was slightly over 2 in response to the question "How involved are you in other people's children?," and the same survey revealed that most people could not name one agency that had been particularly helpful on behalf of children.

However, if we recognize these analytic limitations, it may still be possible to go forward with prevention programs aimed at and through neighborhoods. We do know that context is important (as is self-selection and the content of treatment). For example, one recent study reported that youth whose families were relocated to subsidized housing in the suburbs were more than twice as likely to attend college (54% vs. 21%) and to find employment (75% vs. 41%) as youth who were relocated to subsidized housing in inner-city areas (Rosenbaum & Kaufman, 1991). Assuming that there were no systematic differences in who was relocated where, this result suggests a powerful social support effect on important life-course events (e.g., attending college and finding employment).

NEIGHBORHOOD-BASED RESEARCH
ON CHILD MALTREATMENT IN A SOCIAL CONTEXT

Child maltreatment takes place in a social as well as a psychological and cultural context. Prevention, treatment, and research should incorporate this social contextual orientation (Garbarino et al., 1980). Often, this means examining high-risk neighborhoods as well as high-risk families in the context of child maltreatment (Garbarino & Gilliam, 1980).

But this research focuses primarily on physical child abuse and neglect. Although psychological maltreatment is implicitly (and sometimes explicitly) included in most of this research, sexual abuse is generally not included in efforts to deal with child maltreatment through neighborhood-based family support programs and policies. We assume that neighborhood-based programs do have some relevance to sexual maltreatment (but less than their relevance to other forms of child maltreatment). Existing research on sexual abuse does indicate that it has a "social" dimension (in the sense that it is correlated with conventional socioeconomic and demographic risk factors) but that the salience of this social dimension is less than is evident with respect to other forms of child maltreatment.

Thus, aside from efforts to protect children from sexual abuse by neighborhood intruders ("strangers"), the principal neighborhood-based approach to sexual abuse is in mobilizing for reporting the early stages of sexual aggression against children by local teenagers and adults. This is largely unexplored territory from the perspective of evaluation research. However, we assume that weak neighborhoods do not engage in this mobilization while strong neighborhoods do.

Research has sought to explore and validate the concept of social impoverishment as a characteristic of high-risk family environments and as a factor in evaluating support and prevention programs aimed at child maltreatment. The starting point was identifying the environmental correlates of child maltreatment (Garbarino 1976; Garbarino & Crouter 1978), thus providing an empirical basis for "screening" neighborhoods to identify high- and low-risk areas.

The foundation for this approach is the link between low income and child maltreatment (Garbarino, 1987; National Center on Child Abuse and Neglect, 1981; Pelton, 1978, 1981, 1992). Poverty is associated with a significantly elevated risk of child maltreatment. From this flows a twofold conception of "risk" as it applies to neighborhoods and families (Garbarino & Crouter, 1978). The first refers to areas with a high absolute rate of child maltreatment (based on cases per unit of population). In this sense, concentrations of socioeconomically distressed families are most likely to be at high risk for child maltreatment. For example, in one city (Omaha, Nebraska), socioeconomic status accounted for about 40% of the variation across neighborhoods in reported rates of child maltreatment.

The magnitude of this correlation may reflect a social policy effect. It seems reasonable to hypothesize that in a society in which low income is *not* correlated with access to basic human services (e.g., maternal infant health care), this correlation would be smaller. In a society totally devoid of policies to ameliorate the impact of family-level differences in social class it might be even larger.

This hypothesis merits empirical exploration but is consistent with the observation that socioeconomic status is a more potent predictor of child development in the United States than in some European societies (Bronfenbrenner, 1979). This is evident in low infant mortality rates in some poor European countries (e.g., Ireland and Spain), rates that are lower than in the United States as a whole, and much lower than among poor communities in this country (Miller, 1987). This point emphasizes the important fact that social support is a concept operating at the macrosocial level, not just at the neighborhood level (cf. Thompson, Chapter 3, this volume).

It is a second meaning of high risk that is of greatest relevance here, however. High risk can also mean that an area has a higher rate of child maltreatment *than would be predicted knowing its socioeconomic charac-ter*. Thus, two areas with similar socioeconomic profiles may have very dif-ferent rates of child maltreatment. In this sense, one is high risk while the other is low risk, although both may have higher rates of child maltreatment than other, more affluent areas. Figure 7.1 illustrates this.

In Figure 7.1, areas A and B have high actual observed rates of child maltreatment (36 per 1,000 and 34 per 1,000, respectively). Areas C and D have lower actual rates (16 per 1,000 and 14 per 1,000). However, areas A and C have higher actual observed rates *than would be predicted* (10 per 1,000 predicted for A; 7 per 1,000 for C), while areas B and D have lower actual observed *than predicted rates* (55 per 1,000 for B; and 54 per 1,000 for D). In this sense, A and C are both high risk while B and D are both low risk. Areas E and F evidence a close approximation between predicted and actual rates. This classification system can provide the basis for identifying contrasting social environments. Unfortunately, this sort of community risk analysis is lacking in virtually all programmatic efforts aimed at preventing child maltreatment (indeed in all areas in which social support programs might be aimed at improved family functioning).

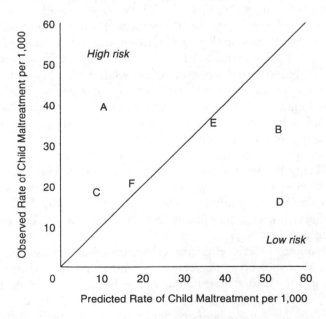

FIGURE 7.1. Two meanings of risk in assessing community areas.

The Human Significance of "Community Risk"

What do low- and high-risk social environments look like? Answering this question is important if we are to understand the essential elements and likely outcome of social support programs seeking to prevent child maltreatment. Addressing this question involves examining pairs of real neighborhoods with the same predicted but different observed rates of child maltreatment (i.e., one high risk and the other low risk for child maltreatment). This examination permits a test of the hypothesis that two such neighborhoods present contrasting environments for childrearing and thus may impose contrasting imperatives on prevention and intervention efforts.

A study of contrasting neighborhoods in Omaha, Nebraska, selected to illustrate this phenomenon provided support for this hypothesis: Relative to the low-risk area, and even though it was socioeconomically equivalent, the high-risk neighborhood was found to represent a socially impoverished human ecology (Garbarino & Sherman, 1980). It was less well socially integrated, had less positive neighboring, and represented more stressful day-to-day interactions for families.

Thus, a comprehensive strategy for obtaining information about the neighborhood-level characteristics associated with maltreatment is necessary before a neighborhood initiative can be mounted. According to Zuravin and Taylor (1987), this involves three techniques. First, a comparative mapping provides a quick visual test of how well the distribution of a particular problem correlates with the distribution of maltreatment. Second, a multiple regression analysis determines how well neighborhood characteristics predicted on the basis of theory or comparative mapping account for variation in child maltreatment rates in different neighborhoods, provides an equation for predicting the at-risk status of a neighborhood based on the characteristics identified by theory or mapping, and identifies neighborhoods whose actual degree of risk for maltreatment differs sharply from the degree of risk predicted by the regression equation. Third, random surveys of neighborhood residents provide neighborhood-specific information about correlates and possible determinants of the three types of child maltreatment (Zuravin & Taylor, 1987).

Other studies have reaffirmed the general outline of this analysis while refining the meaning of social impoverishment—away from a simple concept of social support and toward a more complex phenomenon of social integration (particularly as reflected in employment and neighboring patterns) (cf. Deccio, Horner, & Wilson, 1991; Bouchard, 1987; Sattin & Miller, 1971; Garbarino & Kostelny, 1992).

Deccio et al. (1991) replicated Garbarino and Sherman's (1980) research of Omaha neighborhoods that were economically similar but had different rates of child maltreatment. In their study of two economically similar neighborhoods in Spokane, it was found that the high-risk neighborhood had reported rates of child maltreatment more than two times the low-risk neighborhood. Although differences in perceived social support were not found, differences in social integration were. For instance, the unemployment rate in the high-risk neighborhood was three times greater than that of the low-risk neighborhood. While the average family income was a few hundred dollars higher in the high-risk neighborhood, the percentage of families living below the poverty level was larger in the high-risk neighborhood (26% vs. 17%).

Differences were also found in stability of residence, possession of a telephone, and vacancy rates. A greater percentage of families in the low-risk neighborhood had lived in their current home for more than 5 years (52% vs. 35% in the high-risk neighborhood). Moreover, there were three times as many families in the high-risk neighborhood that lacked telephones compared to those in the low-risk neighborhood. (Absence of a telephone is both a cause and effect of social isolation in the sense we are using here.) Finally, the high-risk neighborhood had more than twice as many vacant housing units as did the low-risk neighborhood (16% vs. 7%).

Thus, social integration, which connoted membership, participation, and belonging, was found to be an important factor in explaining differences in reported rates of maltreatment. More of the low-risk neighborhood's residents were employed, had incomes above the poverty level, had a history of stable residence, and were connected to friends, neighbors, and relatives by a telephone.

Perhaps the most comprehensive analysis to date concerns Chicago neighborhoods (Garbarino & Kostelny, 1992) and illustrates the challenges that must be faced in order to mount a plausible social support-oriented prevention program in the current context of extremely high levels of socioeconomic deprivation, community violence, and negative social momentum characterizing many inner-city neighborhoods where child maltreatment is a disproportionately severe problem. In this study of 77 Chicago communities, much of the variation among community rates of child maltreatment (using a composite measure that includes all forms but is largely composed of physical abuse and neglect) is linked to variations in nine socioeconomic and demographic characteristics (with the multiple correlation being .89, thus accounting for 79% of the variation). Figure 7.2 presents the results of four community areas studied in depth by plotting actual and predicted rates of child maltreatment (two predominantly poor and African-American areas, "North" and "South," and two predominantly poor and Hispanic areas, "West" and "East").

We also conducted this analysis for the 113 census tracts contained *within* our four target community areas. Figure 7.3 presents these results (multiple correlation being $r = .52$, and the proportion of variance accounted for being 27%).

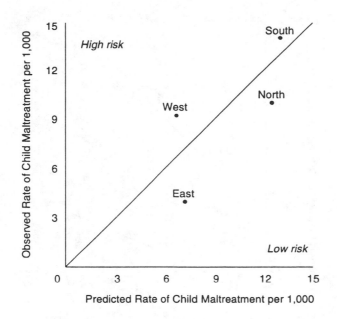

FIGURE 7.2. Actual and predicted rates of maltreatment for four community areas.

The discrepancy between the magnitude of the correlation for community areas and census tracts derives from several factors related to the statistical procedures employed and to some systematic differences among the four community areas in the direction and magnitude of some correlations. For example, the correlation between child maltreatment rates and the percentage of households headed by females is negative in the two African-American areas ($r = -.33$ and $r = -.07$) and positive in the two Hispanic areas ($r = .38$ and $r = .36$)—a difference that is statistically significant. Similarly, the correlation between maltreatment and overcrowded housing is .448 in one Hispanic area and .244 in the other (this difference is also statistically significant).

The higher proportion of variance accounted for in the results of the analysis of community areas reflects the larger units of analysis used in community areas and the apparently idiosyncratic nature of the four target areas as social environments. Because community areas encompass a greater number of individuals than does the census tract analysis, the estimates of the predictors (e.g., poverty, unemployment, and female-headed households) *and* measures of the rate of child maltreatment are more numerically stable (and thus reliable in a statistical sense) and thus more likely to produce a higher correlation. This statistical artifact is present in other studies as well (Garbarino & Crouter, 1978).

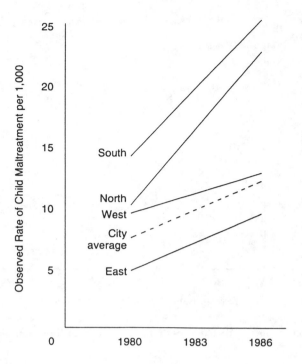

FIGURE 7.3. Child maltreatment rates in four community areas.

In addition, the variation or range of socioeconomic, demographic, and child maltreatment measures is much greater when contrasting all 77 community areas than when comparing the 113 census tracts within the four target areas—all of which have major difficulties. For example, within the two predominantly African-American areas, the census tract with the *lowest* poverty rate still has 27% living in poverty—in contrast to the full range of 77 community areas, in which 33 have poverty rates of less than 10% and 7 have more than 40%.

Child maltreatment rates for the four community areas for the years 1980, 1983, and 1986 reveal trends over time. As Figure 7.3 indicates, there is wide variation in these four areas.

In East and West, child maltreatment rates have remained stable during these 3 years. East has been consistently below the city average while West has been close to the city average. In contrast, in North and South, rates of child maltreatment have been increasing and consistently higher than the city average.

Of particular interest are the different trends observed for North in contrast to West. In 1980 these two areas had similar actual maltreatment rates. However, North's actual rate of 9.1 was below its predicted rate of

11.1, making it a low-risk area. West's actual rate of 8.4 was slightly above its predicted rate of 7.8, making it a somewhat high-risk area. However, by 1986, the two areas had changed dramatically in relation to each other: North's actual maltreatment rate had soared to 21.8 (with a predicted rate of 14.7 for 1986) while West's actual rate had increased only slightly to 10.9, but fell below its predicted rate of 12.4 for 1986.

In terms of the ratio of actual to predicted rates, North had become a very high-risk area, while West had become a low-risk area. To explore why North was deteriorating as an environment for children and families while West was not, we undertook a small set of interviews to illuminate the variable of "community climate." This case study involved interviewing seven community leaders based in human service agencies in North, a community with higher than predicted abuse, and seven in West, a community with lower than predicted abuse. An 11-item questionnaire based on prior research (Garbarino & Sherman, 1980) was used. This questionnaire included questions about perception of the area as a social environment, characteristics of neighboring, and morale.

"The View from the Trenches"

Interviews with community leaders shed some light on "community climate" in North as a "higher than predicted abuse rate" community and in West as a "lower than predicted abuse rate" community. These interviews were used to obtain answers to a series of questions.

In the high-abuse community do social service agencies mirror the high social deterioration characteristic of the families and the community? Conversely, do we observe a strong, informal support network among the social service agencies in the low-abuse community? The answer from these interviews appears to be "yes," as evident in a question-by-question analysis of the interviews (Table 7.1).

The results of this small study suggest that there is a clear difference in the climate of these two communities. The strength of this difference is perhaps best illustrated as follows: Jobs were mentioned as being of primary importance in both communities. However, they were discussed differently. In North, three respondents reported that it was important to remember that North had only an 18% employment rate; in contrast, five of the West respondents described West as a community of the working poor.

The consequences of these differences in employment are profound. Indeed, recall that Deccio et al. (1991) reported that it was precisely such a measure of employment that differentiated the low- from the high-risk neighborhoods in their study. Employment, even at low wages, is a social indicator of prosocial orientation and functionality—apart from the income implications of being employed.

The general tone of the "North" visits was depressed; people had a hard

TABLE 7.1. Interviews with Community Leaders

1. How do people in and around the community see the area?

	Very negative	Neutral	Very positive
North	6	1	0
West	2	3	2

2. What is the physical appearance of the area?

	Very negative	Neutral	Very positive
North	7	0	0
West	3	3	1

3. What are the people like who live in the area?

	Very negative	Neutral	Very positive
North	3	4	0
West	0	4	3

4. Would you say that the area is stable or changing?

	Stable	Changing
North	1	6
West	5	2

5. How would you describe the quality of life in the area?

	Very negative	Neutral	Very positive
North	7	0	0
West	3	2	2

6. How much of a problem is child abuse and neglect?

	Very serious	Neutral	Not serious
North	4	2	0
West	0	4	3

7. How active are the people in the area in community activities?

	Not active	Neutral	Very active
North	5	2	0
West	2	3	2

8. Do they participate in activities?

	No	Yes
North	6	1
West	5	2

9. How much neighboring goes on in the area?

	Not very much	Neutral	A great deal
North	4	2	1
West	0	4	3

10. What other agencies are in the area?

North	Average number listed	4.5
West	Average number listed	11.5

11. Who are the people who work at these other agencies?

	Able to name people	Not able to name people
North	2	5
West	7	0

time thinking of anything good to say about the situation. The physical spaces of the programs themselves seemed dark and depressed, and to a casual visitor, criminal activity was easily spotted. In "West," people were eager to talk about their community. While they listed serious problems, most of them felt that their communities were poor but decent places to live. One respondent described the situation as "poor but not hopeless." Although West subjects also reported drug and crime problems, these problems were not apparent to the casual visitor.

In North, the subjects knew less about the other community services and agencies that were available and demonstrated little evidence of a network or support system, either formal or informal. The one exception to this was the Family Focus program. All those interviewed in the study knew about Family Focus, and the staff at Family Focus knew people in other programs by name. In West, there were more services available, the staff at agencies knew more about what was accessible, and there were strong formal and informal social support networks. The subjects in West also reported strong political leadership from the local state senator. The North subjects did not report positive feelings about their political leaders.

In North, the leaders interviewed described a situation in which their agencies mirrored the isolation and depression of their community. In West, the agencies mirrored the strong informal support network that exists between families in their community. They seemed hopeful because many of their families were hopeful. At least in terms of this study, it seems fair to say that the social service agencies in a community mirror the problems facing the community.

The interviews with professionals complement our statistical analyses and provide further indication of the serious difficulties facing North as a social system. The extremity of the negative features of the environment— poverty, violence, poor housing—seems to be matched by negative community climate—lack of community identity and fragmented formal support system networks.

The final piece of evidence in our analysis concerns child deaths due to maltreatment. Such child deaths are a particularly telling indicator of the bottom line in a community. There were 19 child maltreatment deaths reported for the four community areas studied during 1984–1987. Eight of these deaths occurred in North, a rate of 1 death for each 2,541 children. For West, the rate was 1 death for each 5,571 children. The fact that deaths due to child maltreatment were twice as likely in "North" seems consistent with the overall findings of our statistical analyses and interviews. This is an environment in which there is truly an ecological conspiracy against children (Garbarino, 1992). Such an environment directs our attention to the need to approach the concept of social support to prevent child maltreatment with our eyes open.

Such an open-eyed approach involves refusing to accept superficial, quick, and conventional efforts. Anyone with an appreciation for the depth and pervasiveness of the social impoverishment in neighborhoods such as North understands that social support must be part of a sweeping reform of the neighborhood and its relations with the larger community.

Escalation of Social Impoverishment

Moreover, such social impoverishment has rapidly escalated in many inner-city neighborhoods. For example, up until the 1960s the social organization of many inner-city African-American neighborhoods was enhanced by the presence of working- and middle-class families. These neighborhoods featured a vertical integration of different income groups as lower-, working-, and middle-class professional African-American families lived in the same neighborhoods (Wilson, 1987). However, by the 1980s, most of the middle- and working-class population had moved from these neighborhoods, leaving behind an underclass with few mainstream role models to help maintain the traditional values of education, work, and family stability.

Likewise, there was a breakdown in social control by members of these neighborhoods. For example, DuBow and Podolefsky (1981) suggest that for informal social control to be effective, a neighborhood must have a consensus on values or norms, be able to monitor behavior, and be willing to intervene if necessary when that behavior is not acceptable. In such neighborhoods, such a consensus on values, as well as an ability to monitor behavior, is often lacking.

Thus, part and parcel of this effort must include an approach to the psychosocial factors in the community that influence the ability and willingness of both professionals and residents to make a public commitment to social support programs. Of particular concern in thinking about social support programs in socially impoverished neighborhoods is the impact of community violence on community resource people.

Community Violence and Domestic Violence

Both the general impact of poverty on the conditions of life for children and the fact that community climate variables exist that are not isomorphic with low income create both constraints and opportunities. The existence of these forces is a fact of life for those who would pursue child abuse prevention and deliver child protective services (Garbarino, Dubrow, Kostelny, & Pardo, 1992; Garbarino, Kostelny, & Dubrow, 1991a).

However, although the role of poverty is often considered in protective service decision making and child abuse and neglect program design, and the impact of community violence and social deterioration are often noted as social problems, rarely are these factors considered in relation to the stresses they place on those providing services, especially in the context of pervasive violence.

Human service workers increasingly find themselves serving children and families who live in community environments that are chronically violent. These communities include some large public housing developments and socially deteriorated low-income neighborhoods in cities across the nation.

For example, more than 100,000 children live in public housing projects in Chicago, where the rate of "serious assault" has increased 400% since the mid-1970s. An analysis of Chicago's police data (Reardon, 1988) revealed that the *officially* reported rate of violent crime victimization for residents in the housing projects was 50% higher than for the city as a whole (34 per 1,000 vs. 23 per 1,000). This means that children in public housing projects are twice as likely to be exposed to violence than are other children (because the overall 23-per-1,000 victimization rate includes the housing projects, which inflates the overall figure substantially). No one who is familiar with these data doubts that the reported rate of violent crime victimization in the housing projects is a substantial underestimate (due to the intimidation of witnesses, demoralization of individuals in these neighborhoods, and a general estrangement between residents and police).

In addition to exposure to crime, a child living in these areas is more likely to be a victim of child abuse and neglect. We have found that for census tracts having high crime rates, child maltreatment rates were up to four times higher than the city average. These incidents of domestic violence interact dynamically with the incidents of community violence. Some of the incidents outside the home are in fact related to domestic conflicts; children are exposed to violence in other families indirectly, as part of their life experience as neighbors and friends.

Implications for Social Services to Families

The fact that high-risk families live in high-risk neighborhoods is not the whole or the only story with which we must be concerned when making a commitment to prevent child maltreatment through the use of social support mechanisms. It is more than the conspiracy on the "demand" side of the equation. We must also confront the fact that the people who provide services to families in high-risk communities are also at risk for crime victimization in the course of their day-to-day work.

Thus, there is an effect on the "supply" side of the human service equation as well. For example, one of the regional directors of the Department of Children and Family Services in Chicago reported that at any given time at least 2 of his 40 caseworkers are unable to work because of injuries sustained while going to and coming from the homes of the families they serve. Many more have experienced significant trauma and live constantly with fear when investigating cases in the urban war zone.

Trauma and fear are not limited to protective service workers, of course.

We conducted a survey of 60 Head Start staff who worked in high-crime areas and asked them to describe the things that happened around the children's centers that made them fearful or upset. More than 60% of the staff had experienced shootings and gang-related activities and listed them as the things that caused them the most fear. We believe such experiences with violence undermine the foundation for neighborhood-based programs to support families.

Current research is now focusing on the routine occurrence and effects of exposure to community violence for children. In one study of children living in a public housing project in Chicago, every child in the sample had first-hand encounters with shooting by age 5 (Dubrow & Garbarino, 1989). In addition, a survey by Bell (1991) found that nearly 40% of 1,000 Chicago high school and elementary school students had witnessed a shooting, more than 33% had seen a stabbing, and 25% had seen a murder. In Alabama, 43% of a sample of inner-city children (between the ages of 7 and 19) had witnessed a homicide (*Newsweek*, 1992). Being a child in a highly stressful environment can lead to long-term mental health concerns even when the child has access to parental protection in the short term.

Living in dangerous environments affects not only the people living there but also the service providers who come into these communities to work. However, there has been little research conducted on the immediate and long-term consequences to service providers of exposure to community violence. Clarifying the stresses these workers face and illuminating the support they need will be an important addition to efforts to improve and inform services.

Our work points to additional challenges that service providers face as a result of community violence:

• In many areas, parents are afraid to attend night meetings at school. How can a neighborhood-based program succeed if families are intimidated?

• Although gunplay is an activity in which most children engage, teachers report that they can distinguish between fantasy play and reenactment of violent events in the community. If an actual shooting occurs in the community, they observe that children's play takes on a more realistic quality, reenacting the events they witnessed. But teachers do not know how to respond. How does this affect the classroom dynamics of teaching about child abuse? How does it affect the role of the school vis-à-vis the neighborhood?

• One of the social service staff who conducts home visits with parents whose children attend Head Start described how she had to take cover in the playground to avoid being hit by random bullets from two rival gang factions. She stated, "I was caught in the cross fire." She witnessed the shooting of one young man before the gunfire stopped. When it ended, she ran back to the children's center and reported the event to a coworker, who listened sympathetically. The coworker responded, "then it was over." The next day, the worker had to resume her responsibilities. There was no intervention. What are the effects of such an experience on someone faced with the prospect of reporting a case of child abuse to the protective services agency, but who knows that any such act is viewed as collaborating with the law enforcement agencies and may bring violent reprisals? How can a neighborhood function as a support system when key "players" are traumatized?

• When a teacher heard gunshots outside her classroom window, she and all 20 of the children got down on the floor. Although this teacher knew how to protect children in a crisis situation, she was unable to deal with the long-term consequences of the event (e.g., the fears of both teacher and students that this event could reoccur at any moment). How does she assess the likely impact of child abuse and neglect on children who may appear outwardly "desensitized" to violence yet who may be hypervulnerable to emotional neglect?

• At an after-school program, as some of the children were entering the building, shooting by gang members started nearby. One girl had to crawl on her hands and knees to avoid the bullets and get into the center. However, once the children were in the building, staff members were confused about whether to talk about the event or ignore it and go about planned activities. Such discussion often leads to reports of domestic violence. How can the staff respond to the community violence when they have not come to terms with the domestic violence?

Professionals who deal with these children of violence are often at a loss as how to respond to them. For example, in six training sessions involving Head Start staff from four major Chicago public housing complexes, the majority of the 60 staff participating expressed their feelings of inadequacy related to being unable to help their students deal with the violence they encounter in their daily lives. How does this relate to prevention and protective services? Many of these staff are "indigenous" to the communities they serve.

Successful child abuse prevention and child protective services must address the issues of powerlessness, traumatization, and immobilizing fear that impede effective family life and social development for a significant and growing number of children. Part of achieving success is understanding the needs of professionals who work in these environments. These professionals themselves often feel powerless, traumatized, and afraid. How do they make sense of prevention and protection missions in neighborhoods so violent they fear for their personal safety? How are they to bring messages of family safety? Does everyone concerned accept lower standards for child protection in such environments? Do they fall silent when confronted with harsh, even violent childrearing?

As noted earlier, Halpern (1990a) has identified such domains of silence as a serious impediment to the delivery of effective family services, most especially among paraprofessionals recruited from high-risk populations. One case study further amplifies this point.

After a site visit to a nationally recognized family support prevention program located in a major urban public housing project, we concluded that the interaction between program and social environment resembled what we observed in Cambodian refugee camps in eastern Thailand (cf. Garbarino, Kostelny, & Dubrow, 1991a, 1991b). In particular, we were struck by the fact that the professionals in the family support programs faced a difficult psychological and political challenge that derived from the realities of power in both settings. In both the public housing project and the refugee camp, all "outsiders" leave at the end of the business day, and after dark, the setting is controlled by the gangs (in the Cambodian situation, they are more clearly *political* gangs, but gangs nonetheless). In the public housing project, the gangs have been known to set curfews for residents as a demonstration of their power. Thus, any decisions made or action taken during the day must be reconciled with the realities of who is in charge at night. People are afraid to come out of their apartments or to contest the power of the gangs. This is hardly a desirable environment in which to promote social support programs.

NEIGHBORHOOD-BASED SOCIAL SUPPORT PROGRAMS

Setting aside for a moment the issues of context raised earlier, we can consider the issues facing neighborhood-focused social support programs regardless of their setting. This permits us to include in our analysis neighborhoods beyond the high-risk "war zone" settings identified in our research, and thus to include the broad range of settings in which U.S. children grow up, including suburban neighborhoods, and in which we seek to employ social support approaches to prevent child maltreatment (Halpern, 1990b).

The first of these issues speaks to the different orientations we refer to as "categorical" approaches (e.g., programs aimed at drug use, parent education, or some other specific problem) and "generic" approaches (i.e., programs aimed at general improvement in family functioning, child development, or community well-being). One way to address this issue is to focus on the generic role of social support in childhood resilience. If we understand this role, we can see more clearly what we need to guarantee in the neighborhood to prevent child maltreatment (and, failing that, to prevent the most deleterious consequences of child maltreatment).

Resiliency and Coping

Convergent findings from several studies of life-course responses to stressful early experience suggest a series of ameliorating factors that lead to prosocial and healthy adaptability (Lösel & Bliesener, 1990):

- Actively trying to cope with stress (rather than just reacting)
- Cognitive competence (at least an average level of intelligence)
- Experiences of self-efficacy and a corresponding self-confidence and positive self-esteem
- Temperamental characteristics that favor active coping attempts and positive relationships with others (e.g., activity, goal orientation, and sociability) rather than passive withdrawal
- A stable emotional relationship with at least one parent or other reference person
- An open, supportive educational climate and parental model of behavior that encourages constructive coping with problems
- Social support from persons outside the family

These factors have been identified as important when the stresses involved are in the "normal" range found in the mainstream of modern industrial societies (e.g., poverty, family conflict, childhood physical disability, and parental involvement in substance abuse). They provide a starting point for understanding the impact of programmatic efforts to enhance family coping and thus reduce child maltreatment.

Of the seven factors identified in the research on resiliency and coping, several are particularly relevant to our concerns (and some of the others are indirectly relevant). We are particularly interested in social support from persons outside the family; an open, supportive educational climate and parental model of behavior that encourages constructive coping with problems; and a stable emotional relationship with at last one parent or other reference person. In these three factors is the *beginning* of an agenda for neighborhood support programs to prevent child maltreatment, and, indeed, for more macrointerventions as well (cf. Thompson, Chapter 3, this volume).

The first factor is, of course, at the heart of our concern: social support from persons outside the family. We see this as a generic affirmation of the validity of a social support approach. It tells us that the importance of social support increases inversely with the inner resources of the family: The poorer *need* more help. Of course, here, as elsewhere, we expect to find a kind of "Catch-22" in operation: The more troubled and impoverished a family system *inside* its boundaries, the less effective it will be in identifying, soliciting, and making effective use of resources *outside* its boundaries.

This is the message of research on neglecting families conducted by Gaudin and Polansky (1985). Neglecting mothers are less ready, willing, and able to see and make use of social support in their neighborhoods *and* more in need of such support than are other mothers. This vicious cycle is evident repeatedly in studies of child maltreatment (Garbarino, 1977).

The second resilience factor explicitly targets the community's institutions. It is schools, religious institutions, civic organizations, and other social entities that operationalize the concept of an open, supportive educational climate. Programs and role models that teach and reward the reflective "processing" of experiences are an essential feature of social support at the neighborhood and community level.

The third resilience factor is a stable emotional relationship with at least one parent or other reference person. How does this translate into our model of generic social support? It does so through repeated findings that depth—as opposed to simply breadth—is an important feature of social support (and one often neglected in programmatic approaches). In addition to having effective social support available through friends, neighbors, coworkers, and professionals, parents (and children) need social support in its most intensive form: "someone who is absolutely crazy about them." This is clear from research on parenting (children *must* have someone in this role), but it is also important in the functioning and development of youth and adults, including those in parenting roles.

The implications are quite significant. For example, in his efforts to prevent child maltreatment among malfunctioning parent–child dyads, Wahler (1980) found that the effects of his programmatic intervention were attenuated to the point of being negligible for mothers who had no close allies who supported revisions in parenting style and practices. For poor mothers, this person is likely to be neighborhood based. Only by identifying such a maternal ally and incorporating her into the preventive intervention was Wahler able to ensure that the preventive strategies he was teaching to the mother would endure. This finding parallels other studies that emphasize social support for the goals of professional intervention (e.g., the congruence of residential treatment goals for youth in the postrelease social environment) (cf. Whittaker, Garbarino, & Associates, 1983).

It is important to remember that social support has at least two distinct dimensions. The first is its role in simply making the individual feel connected—which is important in its own right. The second is its role in promoting prosocial behavior (e.g., avoiding child maltreatment even under stressful conditions).

This explains the finding that under conditions of social stress, families whose only social network is kin are more likely to abuse children than families whose network includes nonkin (Gelles & Straus, 1988). Kin-only networks are more likely than more diverse networks to offer consensus support for an interpretation of child behavior and a corresponding rationale for parent behavior. Considering the structure of social support without regard to its value and cultural content is insufficient. We can see further evidence of this by explicitly focusing on socially maladaptive methods of coping.

Maladaptive Coping

Families forced to cope with highly stressful situations (such as the chronic danger and social impoverishment of many low-income neighborhoods or the unstable and alienated neighborhoods that reflect community disruption even in the absence of poverty) may adapt in ways that are dysfunctional.

The psychopathological dimensions of such adaptation are now widely recognized—most notably posttraumatic stress disorder in the case of traumatic environments. The social dimensions are equally worthy of attention, however.

Families may cope with highly stressful conditions by adopting a world view or persona that may be dysfunctional in any "normal" situations in which they are expected to participate (e.g., in school and in other settings of the larger community). For example, aggressive behavior may in the short run appear to be adaptive behavior in the abnormal situation of chronic crisis in which they live. However, such aggressive behavior may be maladaptive to school success, as it stimulates rejection at school.

Moreover, some reactions to chronic threat and social impoverishment (such as emotional withdrawal) may be socially adaptive in the short run but may become a danger to the next generation when the individual becomes a parent. This phenomenon has been observed in studies of families of Holocaust survivors (Danieli, 1988). The family's ability to be a good neighbor and to make use of social support (let alone to serve as a source of social support to others) may be one of the casualties of this developmental process.

Even in the absence of this intergenerational process, however, the links between threat and stress on the one hand and social support on the other may operate directly on families. Their adaptations to socially impoverished and threatening environments may produce childrearing strategies that impede normal development. For example, the parent who prohibits the child from playing outside for fear of shooting incidents may be denying the child a chance to engage in social and athletic play, an undesirable side effect of protecting the child from assault.

Similarly, the fear felt by parents of children in high-crime environments may manifest itself as a restrictive and punitive style of discipline (including physical assault) in an effort to protect the child from falling under the influence of negative forces in the neighborhood (e.g., gangs). This "adaptive" strategy (which may be socially supported in the neighborhood) can be a significant impediment to efforts aimed at preventing child maltreatment (which seek to foster a more open, less punitive childrearing style).

Moreover, punitive childrearing is likely to result in heightening aggression on the child's part, with one consequence being difficulty in succeeding in social contexts that provide alternatives to the "culture" of the highly stressed and socially impoverished neighborhood environment. In addition, punitive childrearing can lead to endorsing and accepting violence as the modus operandi for social control (which in turn rationalizes the "culture of aggression" that further impedes efforts to prevent child maltreatment).

Holding the child back from negative forces through punitive restrictiveness is generally much less successful a strategy than promoting positive alternatives to the negative subculture feared by the parent (Scheinfeld, 1983). This finding parallels more generic conceptions of social influence that emphasize the need to communicate empowerment as a resource in coping (as is evident in the list of resources in resilience noted earlier).

All this highlights an important dilemma. Over time, negative neighborhoods stimulate and reinforce negative individual behavior (on the part of newcomers—new residents or children growing up). Thus, eventually we see negative *individual* behavior and attitudes as the cause and effect of negative neighborhoods. Accordingly, attempting to change neighborhoods without changing individuals may be foolhardy. Therefore, we must design and implement efforts that restructure the social and physical environment of the neighborhood in ways that induce and reinforce changed individual behavior. Such efforts are necessary to create a climate in which more conventional educational and therapeutic innovations can take root. A strategy that incorporates economic initiatives with social and psychological interventions seems most suitable to meeting these objectives.

Participation, and the ethos that supports it, is a major component of social support interventions. What do we know about the factors that enhance and sustain participation in neighborhoods and their social institutions?

Origins of Participation

Wandersman and his colleagues (Wandersman, Jakubs, & Giamartino, 1981; Wandersman, Florin, Friedmann, & Meier, 1987) conducted research to identify the factors that enhance participation in neighborhood organizations, particularly "block organizations." This research is highly relevant to our concern because any effort to stimulate social support through neighborhood organization must accommodate to these factors.

A community development project conducted by Chavis and Wandersman (1990) found that participation in block organizations is related to being "rooted" in place demographically: older, married, homeowner, female, long-term resident. This confirms Collins and Pancoast's (1976) observations concerning natural helping networks. It is primarily older women (whose children are grown) who have a long history in the neighborhood who serve as central figures and natural helpers.

Beyond these demographic factors, Wandersman and his colleagues have identified some "psychological variables" that predict participation. These include a sense of civic duty and political efficacy, a perception that problems are within the realm of local control, a strong sense of community, and a high level of self-esteem. Once again, there is a congruence between these findings and what Collins and Pancoast observed: Demographic position alone is insufficient; an individual must have attributes that translate opportunity into actual participation.

These findings are important as we consider the role of neighborhood social support in preventing child maltreatment. Such programs must seek out self-confident, public-spirited older married women who are long-term residents of the neighborhood. In the high-risk neighborhoods, these women are often already carrying a heavy load of family responsibility—often caring for their grandchildren (and sometimes providing a home and financial support for their adult children). In some areas these women may be overwhelmed with their responsibilities—rather than "free from drain" as are the usual candidates for leadership roles in social support networks identified by Collins and Pancoast (1976).

As ever, we face a Catch-22 situation. The neighborhoods most in need of preventive intervention are those in which the attributes cited by Wandersman are in shortest supply. They are by no means absent, but any effort must begin with the recognition that special efforts and investment will be required to identify existing resources for participation and to enhance these resources. We must keep this in mind as we examine specific programs.

Program Reviews

Elmira, New York, Home Health Visiting Program

Olds et al. (1986) conducted a family support program that combined significant intervention with a sophisticated research design. Home health visitors (registered nurses) were assigned to a family during the mother's pregnancy and continuing for the first 2 years of the child's life.

These nurse practitioners provided parent education regarding fetal and infant development, involved family members and friends in child care and support of the mother, and linked family members with other health and human services to 400 first-time mothers in a small county of 100,000 residents in the Appalachian region of New York State. The mothers were teenagers, unmarried, or of low socioeconomic status. Initially, visits were weekly and then tapered off to monthly. Three smaller forms of intervention incorporated a prenatal health visitor, free transportation to health clinics, and screening/diagnostic testing. There was a significant reduction of child maltreatment for poor, unmarried mothers 19 years of age or younger (4% for the longer home health visitor treatment vs. 19% for the other intervention conditions). Olds et al. (1986) speculated that the long-term home health visitors developed a relationship with their young clients characterized by both nurturance and feedback. The young mothers also punished their children less frequently and brought them to the emergency room less often, and their children were seen by physicians less frequently for accidents and poisonings.

The Minnesota Early Learning Demonstration

The Minnesota Early Learning Demonstration (MELD) is one of the most widely disseminated group-based models of parent education and support. MELD's mission is to eliminate the potential for maltreatment by never letting abusive or neglectful patterns begin. MELD uses an individualized and empowerment model in which parents are given solid parenting information and alternative methods to address different childrearing issues. An evaluation by the Child Welfare League of America found that 80% of the participants had finished or were completing high school (compared to 20% for the general adolescent parent population), and that the repeat pregnancy rate was 10–15% (compared to 25% of all teenage mothers). Finally, the percentage of parents who used corporal punishment on their children went from 56% at the beginning of the program to 12% at the end (Ellwood, 1988).

North Lawndale Family Support Initiative

The Chicago-based North Lawndale Family Support Initiative (NLFSI), sponsored by the National Committee for Prevention of Child Abuse (Lauderdale & Savage, 1991), highlights the strengths and limitations of neighborhood-oriented programming aimed at preventing child maltreatment. In 1989, out of 77 Chicago communities, the community of North Lawndale had the second highest rate of child fatalities over a 7-year period. The total number of reported cases of child abuse also rose 65% in an 18-month period from June 1986 to December 1987. Although North Lawndale's population is only 0.5% of the state's population, it experienced 13% of all Illinois substantiated child abuse fatalities during that same period.

The NLFSI, started in 1989, is a 5-year demonstration project to establish a community-based prevention strategy. The NLFSI first identified neighborhood leaders and secured their cooperation to support child abuse prevention efforts. These community leaders then identified those individuals and groups (e.g., civic groups, elected officials, religious officials, professionals, schools, and organized labor) that also could be enlisted in their efforts to prevent child abuse. The leaders provided valuable perspectives on the causes of child abuse and neglect in the community, opened doors to needed human resources in the community, and sanctioned the actual planning and implementation of prevention programs and activities.

After the completion of a neighborhood needs assessment, strategies were developed to address prevention education needs of school-age children, education and support needs of parents, treatment programs for victims of abuse, substance abuse treatment, and perinatal support. Outcome data are not yet available—impeding efforts to assess the impact of child maltreatment prevention programs.

Avance

The Avance Educational Programs for Parents and Teens is a community-based parent education program for low-income Mexican-American families in San Antonio, Texas. The 9-month program provides bilingual discussions and child development, toy-making classes, day care practica, and referral services. Evaluation by Rodriguez and Corez (1988) found that participants were more hopeful about their future, more willing to assume the role of educator with their children, less likely to hold severe conceptions of punishment, and more willing to utilize social supports to gain help.

Parents Too Soon

The Ounce of Prevention Fund's Parents Too Soon is a neighborhood-based program that has as its overall goal the reduction of child maltreatment. Parents Too Soon addresses adolescent parenting through 32 programs—21 focused on pregnant teens and 11 on nonpregnant teens. The mean age is 15; the average stay is 8–12 months. Some 90% of the staff are paraprofessionals. Parents Too Soon is a "strength" model, built on the assumption that most people want to be good parents. Parents Too Soon provides parent education and support as well as day care services and primary prevention services. In addition to preventing child abuse and neglect, other goals include improving developmental outcomes of children, improving parenting skills, promoting basic physical health in mother and child, promoting self sufficiency, supporting vocational issues, and preventing subsequent pregnancy during adolescence. However, the difficulty in achieving these goals is apparent: 50–60% of teen mothers become pregnant again within 2 years of their first child.

Heart to Heart

Heart to Heart, a program started by the Ounce of Prevention Fund in 1985, is an effort both to provide effective interventions for teen parents and to prevent child sexual abuse. It was created as a public–private agency for the purpose of preventing family problems that result in child abuse and neglect, infant mortality, delayed development in children, and repeated cycles of teenage pregnancy and parenthood. The program also strives to involve members of the community in the shared responsibility of child sexual abuse prevention.

Heart to Heart was begun in response to dissatisfaction with traditional parenting and sexual abuse prevention programs that had limited outcomes (Halpern, 1991), as well as the recognition of the extent to which young mothers in parent support groups had experienced sexual abuse. For example, in one survey of 445 Ounce of Prevention participants, 61% had an unwanted sexual experience. Many others reported that they were child victims of sexual abuse. The children of teen parents are at greater risk for sexual abuse both because of their parents' history of abuse and because teen parents may not know how to provide safe and appropriate child care.

Group meetings are held weekly to inform and discuss such topics as personal history of abuse, inappropriate child care arrangements, and current abuse relationships. Participants also are given journals in which they write about their thoughts and feelings.

Heart to Heart is offered in conjunction with a 2-year MELD's Young Moms (MYM) parent support group. MYM groups are guided peer self-help groups specifically developed for pregnant teens and teen parents, and focusing on preventive health, family planning, nutritional guidelines, and child guidance. Group leaders are often former teen mothers. In addition to the peer leader, there is a clinical group leader who can make appropriate referrals and be responsive to clinical issues that may arise.

The participants who experienced sexual abuse are provided with three options for processing their experiences: group discussion, journal writing, and one-to-one interviews. Heart to Heart also helps the teen parent draw on community resources. A local advisory council is created to support a community effort to prevent child sexual abuse.

Group leaders receive extensive training on sexual abuse and related topics. Such training allows the group leaders to examine their own feelings and conflicts around sexuality, sexual abuse, and parenting and gives them permission to be reflective about their personal values and experiences.

Neighborhood Parenting Support Project

The Neighborhood Parenting Support Project was developed in 1988 in two neighborhoods in Winnipeg that had three to four times the city average of child maltreatment cases. The premise of the program was that if social support for parenting was strengthened at the neighborhood level, the risk for child maltreatment would be reduced.

After identifying and mapping neighborhood and parent social networks, project staff initiated a social network intervention. Through a neighborhood parenting support worker, parents were helped to change their personal social networks—reinforcing positive connections and weakening destructive connections. For example, in order to help parents reduce high family stress, the parent would be helped to weaken stressful ties with family members and to reinforce ties with neighbors who might be less critical of the parent and better able to help the parent by providing child care support in emergencies or emotional support in a crisis.

The neighborhood parenting support worker provided social support in problem identification and solving, networking skills, parenting skills, support and help-seeking skills, communication skills, and support-giving skills. The neighborhood parenting support worker would join with and support neighborhood central figures, natural helpers, and network "connectors" in an effort to develop a referral network and neighborhood parenting support network structures. She "connected" with people in settings frequented by parents and children, such as family centers, day care centers, and playgrounds, as well as such places as coffee shops, laundromats, and churches.

The Child Development Specialist Program

The Child Development Specialist Program provides parent education to families living in rural communities in Oklahoma. The program emphasizes teaching effective childrearing practices, reducing stress in parent–child relationships, and enhancing the home environment. In addition to providing services to individual families through groups and workshops, services are offered in other community settings—such as schools, libraries, churches, Head Start, and community centers.

Family Support Services of West Hawaii

The Family Support Services of West Hawaii was founded in 1979 by members of the community concerned with the prevention of child abuse and neglect. Its goal is to promote healthy families by providing support services to strengthen families and foster the optimal development of children (Marrack, 1992). Prevention programs are Family Support Services' main focus. These include Healthy Start, a nationally acclaimed community-based maternal and child health program, and the Oihana Ohana Respite Nursery Program, providing planned and emergency respite care services and parent support groups. Family Support Services offers parent education classes and adapts to community needs. A community liaison committee made up of parents, service providers, and community leaders develops policy and programs.

William Penn Prevention Initiative

The William Penn Prevention Initiative was designed to achieve a reduction in the risk for child abuse and neglect among families residing in some of the most at-risk communities in the Greater Philadelphia area. Fourteen demonstration projects composed of different service types (e.g., home health visitors, parent education, and parent support) were evaluated across services by the National Committee for Prevention of Child Abuse (1992).

Issues evaluated were the extent that the initiative changed specific parenting practices, personal functioning, and parent–child interactions.

As a group, the 14 demonstration projects significantly reduced their clients' levels of risk for maltreatment as measured by the Child Abuse Potential Inventory and staff assessments. Overall, participants showed a decrease in their potential for child abuse. Moreover, staff rated nearly 70% of all participants as having benefited from services. In terms of specific at-risk behaviors, clients were significantly less likely to use corporal punishment, to inadequately supervise their children, or to ignore their child's emotional needs.

In addition, these gains were retained and enhanced over time. Participants reported continued changes in their methods of discipline and an increase in positive interactions with their children. Furthermore, a significant decrease in the likelihood for maltreatment was observed.

The most powerful predictor of client outcomes was the intensity with which services were provided. The greater the number of weekly contacts a client had with a program, the less likely parents were to engage in child maltreatment. Moreover, the high-risk clients who received multiple types of interventions were more likely than similar clients who received a single intervention to have a reduced risk for maltreatment.

Moving beyond the small range of neighborhood-based programs specifically designed to prevent child maltreatment, an examination of other early intervention programs at the neighborhood level can be of value.

Head Start

Head Start addresses social, political, and psychological concerns of individuals at the neighborhood level. Coming out of the civil rights movement, it emphasizes community organizing and allows for the transfer of power and control to community residents through self-help and collective action. Through Head Start, parents become agents of broader change in their community. Moreover, the small size and nonbureaucratic atmosphere in the programs, as well as the fact that the centers primarily serve children from the local neighborhood, help ensure Head Start success at the neighborhood level (Valentine & Stark, 1979; Beller, 1979).

Head Start programs function as multipurpose community centers, providing a range of educational, medical, and social services. In addition to providing employment opportunities for community members, Head Start centers also offer respite to parents, especially young mothers who feel isolated in their apartments. Many centers have "parents' rooms" where mothers can socialize once their children have been left with their teachers. There are also special outings and activities exclusively for parents. The opportunity to get out and meet other parents is an important feature of Head Start that has helped it put down roots in neighborhoods across the nation (Skerry, 1983).

Reaching the Hard-to-Reach

These programs served isolated and depressed mothers with infants in the community. The target population was multirisk, low-income mothers in the Cambridge, Massachusetts, community who had difficulty relating to and caring for their infants (Lyons-Ruth, Botein, & Grunebaum, 1984). Mothers and their infants were randomly assigned to one of two treatment conditions. A matched control group of mothers and infants from the community with no psychiatric histories participated in the research assessments. The first program, the Neighborhood Support Systems for Infants project, was a home-visiting program staffed by working-class mothers from the community. The professional staff included a nurse practitioner, an occupational therapist, and an early childhood educator. The second program, the family support service, was both a home-visiting and support group program staffed by psychologists, most of whom were mothers. Each psychologist acted as both a home visitor and a group facilitator for mothers on her case load.

Although no major differences were found between the two programs, Lyons concluded that the data showed clearly that a home-visiting intervention would reach greater numbers of depressed, isolated, high-risk mothers and their infants than would a center-based group treatment.

The Community Infant Project

The Community Infant Project (CIP), in Boulder, Colorado, is an interdisciplinary, early-intervention program that has as its goal the prevention of parenting dysfunction in high-risk families from the prenatal period through the child's first 3 years of life. The main aim of the CIP is to prevent parenting dysfunction and resulting child abuse and neglect, failure to thrive, developmental delay, and failure in bonding. The staff consists of public health nurses, mental health professionals, a psychiatrist, and a number of paraprofessional volunteers. The program is home based and geared to the needs of the family.

Nurse–clinician teams provide case management, psychotherapy, and education in maternal and infant health, child development, nutrition, safety, infant stimulation techniques, and mother–infant bonding. Psychiatric treatment, including psychiatric evaluation, medication, and hospitalization, is provided when needed, and referrals are made for other forms of medical care as well. CIP staff coordinate the activity of multiple agencies and, working intensively in the family home, focus on parents' emotional problems, family conflict, confidence, and self-esteem. Staff provide training in the care of the infant, including helping the parent develop appropriate expectations of the infant's behavior.

In a research study designed to measure outcomes, 20 families treated by the CIP were matched with a control group of 20 families referred to the

CIP but not treated because the program was full. Outcome measures were obtained on parental attitudes (Adult/Adolescent Parenting Inventory), the home environment (HOME Scale), family use of health care and other services, and child maltreatment reports.

Results indicate that the program was successful in producing better outcomes in treated cases than in the control group—mothers in the group that received intervention displayed significantly more emotional and verbal responsiveness and involvement with their children and provided their children with more appropriate play materials than the control group. The mothers who received intervention also used less physical punishment on their children and less services through other community agencies, including hospital emergency rooms. In addition, there were fewer verified episodes of reported child abuse (one vs. four). The results of this investigation support the possibility that integrated, intensive, home-based services aimed at preventing parenting dysfunction can change parental attitudes and practices, reduce the use of other community health and social services, and decrease child abuse.

Community Partnerships for Substance Abuse Prevention

The Community Partnerships for Substance Abuse Prevention has been initiated in approximately 250 communities throughout the United States (Wandersman & Goodman, 1991). This reflects the fact that in many communities, residents identify drugs as the number one concern. A study in South Carolina (Melton, 1992) highlighted the nature of this problem, finding that this number one ranking was evident even in neighborhoods with no drug arrests or residents in long-term drug rehabilitation programs.

The Office for Substance Abuse Prevention has provided 5 years of funding to each community to form a partnership of influential leaders and community members to develop a comprehensive plan for reducing alcohol and drug abuse. At initiation, the lead agency in each community convenes an ad hoc committee of community leaders representing different sectors of the community and nominates influential citizens to sit on committees representing schools, businesses, religious institutions, the media, health, academic, government, criminal justice, and grass-roots organizations. Each committee conducts a needs assessment and recommends strategies for community action. Then the chairpersons of each committee integrate all the strategies into one comprehensive plan which is then implemented through the coalition of organizations that were involved in developing the community plan.

Important issues that will be addressed are whether the coalition's efforts increase communitywide knowledge of drugs and the perceived risk of drugs and whether they produce a reduction in overall drug use, decrease in DUI (driving under the influence) arrests, decrease in school disciplinary actions for drug or alcohol offenses, and reduction in rate of new students starting drug use. Outcome data are not yet available.

Community Violence Prevention

Boston's Violence Prevention Project (Prothrow-Stith, 1991) is a community-based primary prevention program that seeks to change individual behavior and community attitudes about violence through outreach and education in an effort to reduce the incidence of violent behavior and associated social and medical hazards for adolescents. The project is presently concentrating its efforts in Boston's two poorest neighborhoods. One neighborhood, Roxbury, is predominantly African-American and has the highest adolescent homicide rate in Boston. The other neighborhood, South Boston, is predominantly white and has the most rapidly rising adolescent homicide rate.

A supportive network of secondary therapeutic services and a hospital-based secondary prevention service project, directed toward patients with intentional injuries, supplements the primary prevention activities to provide a comprehensive program. A violence prevention curriculum used in high schools is at the core of the intervention. The project is geared to individual behavior modification using descriptive information on the risks of violence and homicide. It also provides conflict resolution techniques and implements a nonviolent classroom ethos.

The school curriculum is also presented in less traditional educational settings (e.g., alternative schools, recreational programs, public housing developments, Sunday schools, boys and girls clubs, YMCAs, and neighborhood health centers) in the community. Clergy and police have been recruited to spread violence prevention education through their contact with adolescents, their families, and other significant adults in the community. By using many and varied community settings to communicate the message of violence prevention, the community becomes "saturated."

Because some youth need more than primary prevention efforts and a medical setting is often the only place that troubled youth go for help, the project has begun working with adolescents admitted to the Boston City Hospital with intentional injuries. Because adolescents do not return for follow-up services and are difficult to contact, a new strategy that uses pediatric nurses trained by the project to work with seriously injured adolescents, their friends, and family over the course of hospitalization and afterwards has been developed. Support groups are also conducted for young people as well as for their parents. In addition, the clinical setting was made more responsive to the needs of youth engaging in violent behavior by developing a protocol for health care providers on how to deal with adolescents who engage in such violence.

The limitations of this project centered around the notion among the general public that violence is inevitable and not preventable. To counteract this attitude, it was necessary to educate everyone in the community, not just the targeted adolescents. Media-based efforts and peer education strategies were essential in this process.

The Coalition for Alternatives to Violence and Abuse

In 1982, more than 20 community agencies in Contra Costa County, California, concerned with violence prevention, formed a communitywide violence prevention coalition, Alternatives to Violence and Abuse Coalition (AVAC). AVAC implemented a violence prevention curriculum in several district high schools (Cohen, 1991). Included in this curriculum were education about interpersonal violence and a peer counseling program. Another program was directed at parents and established violence prevention programs in workplaces, providing education and resources on a variety of violence-related issues (e.g., drug and alcohol abuse and teen suicide). Currently, the program is utilizing these building blocks in broadening the community's response to violence.

As in the case of the Boston project, the most difficult obstacle to overcome was the pervasive idea in the community that violence is normal and not preventable. Moreover, among people who believed violence is potentially preventable, there was little agreement on the skills and approaches that would work. Success came slowly and was mixed with substantial failures and disappointments.

GENERAL PRINCIPLES DERIVED FROM EXISTING
PROGRAMS AND RESEARCH

Children in conditions of developmental risk (e.g., risk associated with the conditions that produce child maltreatment) need relationships with adults—"teaching" relationships to help them process their experiences in a way that prevents developmental harm. Vygotsky (1986) referred to this developmental space between what the child can do alone and what the child can do with the help of a teacher as the "zone of proximal development."

Developmentalists have come to recognize that it is this zone of proximal development between the child and a guiding teacher that leads the child to forward movement. Children who experience child maltreatment are generally denied that processing within the family. Indeed, they receive just the opposite of what they need, particularly in conditions of social risk derived from the social environment outside the home. This is one reason why the problem of child maltreatment in the context of high-stress/low-support social environments deserves the highest priority as a matter of social policy; these are the children who can least tolerate maltreatment.

The critical function of mediation and processing seems particularly important in the case of moral development—which is inextricably linked to the problem of child maltreatment both as an interpersonal issue within families and as a social issue in communities. The key is a process of "optimal discrepancy" in which the child's moral teachers (be they adults or peers) lead the child toward higher-order thinking by presenting positions that are one stage above the child's characteristic mode of responding to social events as moral issues.

When this process occurs in the context of a nurturant affective system—a warm family, for example—the result is ever-advancing moral development, the development of a principled ethic of caring (Gilligan, 1982). Moreover, even if the parents create a rigid, noninteractive "authoritarian" family context (and thus block moral development), the larger community may compensate: "The child of authoritarian parents may function in a larger more democratic society whose varied patterns provide the requisite experiences for conceptualizing an egalitarian model of distributive justice" (Fields, 1987, p. 5).

If schoolteachers, neighbors, and other adult representatives of the community are unable or disinclined to model higher-order moral reasoning, the process of moral truncation that is "natural" to situations of family and community violence will proceed unimpeded.

This may well be happening in many urban school systems in which teachers are demoralized, parents incapacitated, and students apathetic. The result is to permit the natural socialization of the depleted community to proceed, with its consequences in intergenerational aggression, neighborhood deterioration, and family malfunction (e.g., child maltreatment).

Families can provide the emotional context for the necessary "processing" to make positive moral sense of social experience outside the home. But to do so they must be functioning well to start with. This is hardly the case when child maltreatment is present. Thus, in cases of child maltreatment within families, neighbors and professionals in communities usually must carry things to the next step (i.e., stimulating higher-order moral development and compensatory socialization).

They do this by presenting a supportive and democratic milieu (e.g., in schools, churches, neighborhood associations, and local political parties). Without these efforts, the result is likely to be impaired social and moral development, particularly among boys, who are more vulnerable to this consequence of living "at risk," as they are to most other risks (Werner, 1990). This analysis leads to an appreciation for the relevance of four principles.

1. *Social class differences in the relevance of neighborhood.* There appears to be an inverse relationship between social class and the relevance of

neighborhood (Lewis, 1978). Poor families and individuals are more dependent on local resources than are affluent families. This dependence has at
least two important implications.

The first implication is that middle-class professionals and policymakers
are likely to underestimate the importance of neighborhood factors because
they themselves depend less on such factors in their personal life. A survey
in South Carolina (Melton, 1992) reported that middle-class families were
particularly likely to indicate that when facing a problem with their child,
they would go directly to professional specialists rather than rely on the social
network. This implies the need for special training and sensitization for professionals (including on-site "walkarounds") to emphasize the salience of
neighborhood geography in family life.

The second implication is that advocacy efforts will be needed to preserve and enhance not just neighborhoods in general but neighborhoods for
poor families in particular. One facet of this intervention is financial. Part of
the process of neighborhood decline with which we are concerned derives
from the draining of banks and other financially stabilizing influences (e.g.,
the net outflow of insurance premiums starves investment).

2. *Community differences in the positive and negative "social momentum" occurring within neighborhoods.* Some neighborhoods engender negative social momentum, which attracts antisocial and deteriorating individuals and families while discouraging and displacing prosocial and functional
families (Rutter, Cox, Tupling, Berger, & Yule, 1975). Reversing such a
downward spiral may require outside intervention—"neighborhood revital-
ization"—to create a process of positive social momentum that attracts functional families and improves the social environment for children.

The mechanics and logistics of such efforts require the coordination of
economic investment, social services, political mobilization, and law enforcement: Jobs, housing, and safety are basics of community well-being. Efforts
to promote community cooperation to produce community self-reliance are
essential (Stokes, 1981). Programs such as Adopt a School and I Have a
Dream can serve as vehicles to involve private philanthropy in this effort.
Although largely unevaluated, in this context "neighborhood watch" and
"block parents" seem likely to contribute to this process.

3. *Social class homogeneity in promoting neighborhood interaction and
integration.* Social class homogeneity is an observed correlate of higher levels
of neighborhood interaction (Unger & Wandersman, 1982). Similarity increases integration (in the sense of being a cohesive group rather than in the
sense of combining different groups). This finding presents an obstacle to
many initiatives that seek to promote neighborhood *heterogeneity* as a way
to increase the availability of diverse role models and resource patterns within
neighborhoods.

Of course, in some "pathogenic" neighborhoods the facilitating effects
of homogeneity may be exceeded in importance by the negative momentum

present. That is, in very poor, high-stress, low-support neighborhoods, homogeneity may facilitate more intensive neighboring that leads to *greater* rather than lesser social pathology (Garbarino, 1992). "Support" can enhance negative rather than positive child outcomes; the key is prosocial support. All this has an important bearing on the role of schools in promoting neighborhood-based family support.

The local school (most notably the elementary school) can serve as a focal point for family support systems—particularly if it defines its social mission broadly. However, policies that dilute the neighborhood character of schools (e.g., busing to achieve racial balance or to serve other social goals) dilute this role. Local school councils (such as those instituted in Chicago) may serve to energize the school as a center for family support systems and neighborhood mobilization. However, simple bureaucratic reform is insufficient. The communities most in need often lack the organizational resources and motivation to seize this opportunity effectively.

4. *Mediators of motivation to participate.* Research on neighborhood organization illuminates the individual decision-making process that governs participation and involvement in formal groups. The identified mediators include perceived connection to the issue, problem-focused coping style, and family consensus (Unger, Wandersman, & Hallman, 1991).

These factors are relevant to assessing the potential of neighborhood social support as a force in dealing with the problem of child maltreatment. The strong themes of family autonomy and privacy evident in American culture mitigate against neighbors recognizing a connection between themselves and the dynamics of child maltreatment. This suggests the need to promote a definition of child maltreatment as a collective problem of the neighborhood, not simply as a problem of individual parents or families. Demonstration projects are needed to field test alternative approaches to accomplishing this goal.

By the same token, it is necessary to understand how individual coping styles affect the likelihood of participation in neighborhood-based family support programs aimed at child maltreatment. In general, the more "empowered" neighbors are—in their lives as workers, citizens, parents, and so forth—the more likely they will bring an assumption of effectiveness and potency to neighborhood activities. Once again, we seem to face a dilemma: The neighborhoods most in need of social support programs aimed at child maltreatment are generally composed of individuals least likely to define themselves in ways that facilitate participation in such efforts. In general, then, programming of this sort will work best in areas least in need of it and will require the greatest potency to succeed in the areas most in need.

The role of family consensus in facilitating neighborhood participation tells a parallel story. Families involved in child maltreatment are not good candidates for family consensus on issues related to social support in the neighborhood (at least not in terms of facilitating such support, given the likelihood that they have an orientation that has been described as "isolated and distancing"). On the other hand, the most well-functioning families in the neighborhood are good candidates for neighborhood activity for this same reason. They are likely to have family consensus concerning the "normal" needs and processes of families.

All in all, this review of factors that affect neighboring highlights the need for special investments in high-stress, low-resource neighborhoods. Such investments are necessary in order to reverse negative social momentum as a *precondition* for relying on neighborhood-based social support efforts to deal with the problem of child maltreatment. In well-functioning (i.e., high-resource, low-stress) environments, however, it should prove easier to turn the neighborhood's focus to dealing with child maltreatment if organizers can deal successfully with the issues of family autonomy and privacy. Of course, such neighborhoods account for relatively little of the total child maltreatment problem, so the net effect on the overall problem of abuse and neglect will be small.

RESEARCH AND DEMONSTRATION NEEDS

The situation of neighborhoods at risk for child maltreatment due to a deterioration of economic and social supports bears a relationship to situations of "acute disaster," in which there is a *dramatic* destruction of the infrastructure of daily life. However, neighborhoods at risk for child maltreatment usually have experienced a chronic deterioration rather than an abrupt calamity.

Erikson's (1976) study of an Appalachian community devastated by flood speaks to one of the fundamental similarities. Young children are confronted with vivid and concrete evidence of their vulnerability. In the case of the flood, their homes were destroyed and their parents demoralized and socially powerless: "The major problem, for adults and children alike, is that the fears haunting them are prompted not only by the memory of past terrors but by a wholly realistic assessment of present dangers" (p. 238).

The plight of families in some high-risk areas might well be termed a social catastrophe, and maltreatment is a special risk factor for children in such situations. These children have access to neither the buffering of parents through the context of their positive attachments nor the ameliorating and compensating influences of the community beyond the family. The quality of life for young children—and their reservoirs of resilience—thus becomes a "social indicator" of the balance of social supports for parents and parental capacity to buffer social stress in the lives of children (Garbarino & Associates, 1992).

After reviewing a large body of research dealing with violence and aggression, Goldstein concluded that "aggressive behavior used to achieve a personal goal, such as wealth and power, and that may be perceived by the actor as justified (or even as non-aggressive) is a primary cause of the aggressive and criminal behavior of others" (Goldstein, 1986, p. ix). The social deterioration of many neighborhoods raises troubling questions about the existence of sufficient *social* identity to provide a meaningful context for any assertion of power and authority. Without such a framework of collective meaning, *all* actions and goals become personal (in the sense used by Goldstein).

This analysis places child abuse squarely in the center as a threat to socialization that has clear community and neighborhood dimensions. As a "personal" use of violence, child abuse is a prime stimulator of aggression, aggression that resonates and conspires with the extrafamilial experiences of the child living in a dangerous environment. At present, we know little about how this conspiracy works against the child's development and child protection and child abuse prevention efforts. That it should become the focus of research and policy initiatives is clear.

The U.S. Advisory Board on Child Abuse and Neglect (1991) concluded that our nation faces a child maltreatment "emergency." Rates of child maltreatment continue to increase in many areas, and public agencies are pushed beyond their capacity to respond. The link between poverty and child maltreatment continues as a powerful feature of the problem. In the current socioeconomic climate, poverty for families has been increasing, and in urban areas becoming ever more geographically concentrated in segregated neighborhoods (Garbarino & Associates, 1992). That being the case, it is little wonder that the problem of child maltreatment is worsening in urban areas of concentrated poverty.

Our analysis of neighborhood-based social support programs and policies calls attention to an important reality about neighborhood life: Social momentum is a powerful force. When things are going badly, the tendency is for all the social systems to be pulled down. It takes extraordinary energy and effort to resist such negative social momentum (e.g., a political leader of special talent, commitment, and resources or a powerful social program that creates its own positive momentum in the neighborhood).

Child maltreatment is a symptom not just of individual or family trouble but of neighborhood and community trouble as well. *And*, it may well conspire with those negative community forces to jeopardize still further the development of children. We know that many children can absorb and overcome an experience with one or two risk factors. But when the risk factors add up, they may well precipitate developmental impairment (Sameroff & Fiese, 1990). This, we believe, is the situation faced by abused and neglected children living in the most devastated neighborhoods.

The challenge is to deal with the conspiracy of negative social indicators. But, as social indicators, they can be responsive to social change (e.g., the energizing effect of community mobilization). As we plan and implement child abuse prevention initiatives, we must recognize that the task is not easy. Indeed, if we hope to have a significant effect when addressing neighborhoods of concentrated poverty and social disorganization, we must introduce powerful efforts to reverse negative social momentum. And we must do so with an appreciation of the compounding of problems engendered by community violence in the lives of victimized children.

This is the difficult course to follow. Translating this broad conclusion into specific policy and programming is a challenge. One appealing approach for research/demonstration projects is to identify prevention zones, which can become the target for comprehensive, sustained intervention by a wide range of public and private agencies. Only in this way, it would seem, can we hope to reverse the destructive pressure of negative social momentum observed in some poor neighborhoods and replace it with the positive momentum observed in others.

In so doing, policy and programming must contend with several major unresolved issues and design research/demonstration projects accordingly:

• Neighborhood-based programs remain an underutilized resource in dealing with child maltreatment. The Catch-22 of efforts to review the research on neighborhood-based support to prevent child maltreatment is that there is so little directly relevant information to review. This low utilization level of neighborhood models makes it difficult to evaluate the overall validity, limitations, and "best practice" (Unger & Powell, 1991).

• Funders who support neighborhood-based programming to prevent child maltreatment have not made adequate investments in the evaluation of these programs. One element of this unmet need concerns the use of quantitative and qualitative evaluation models. A second concerns the value of a general focus on the concept of empowerment as a unifying theme in understanding the supportive functions of neighborhood life for families (Whitmore, 1991).

• We have yet to document fully the potential and probable magnitude of neighborhood effects on family functioning related to child maltreatment. We do not have clear guidance as to reasonable expectations for the role of neighborhood-based programming in contrast to other manipulable factors such as income maintenance, housing policy, law enforcement, centralized professional human service delivery systems, and national media campaigns.

As families in the group most at risk for child maltreatment deteriorate (e.g., become characterized by deeply rooted, often multigenerational problems of drug or alcohol abuse, poverty, illiteracy, and psychological trauma) the relevance of easy neighborhood-based approaches to social support may diminish while the need for a powerful neighborhood-based approach increases (Halpern, 1991). Thus, we should be both encouraged to consider further efforts at exploring the implementation of neighborhood-based family support and warned to recognize that superficial investments and commitments are unlikely to resolve the issues faced by high-risk families in multiproblem neighborhoods.

REFERENCES

Alinsky, S. (1970). Citizen participation and community organization in planning and urban renewal. In F. Cox, J. Erlich, J. Rothman, & J. Tropman (Eds.), *Strategies of community organization* (pp. 216–226). Itasca, IL: Peacock.

Austin, M. (1978). *Professionals and paraprofessionals.* New York: Human Science Press.

Barry, F. (1991). *Neighborhood-based approach—What is it?* Background Paper for the U.S. Advisory Board on Child Abuse and Neglect. Cornell University, Family Life Development Center, Ithaca, NY.

Bell, C. (1991). Traumatic stress and children in danger. *Journal of Health Care for the Poor and Underserved, 2*(1), 175–188.

Belle, D. (Ed.). (1989). *Children's social networks and social supports.* New York: Wiley.

Beller, K. (1979). Early intervention programs. In J. Osofsky (Ed.), *Handbook of infant development* (pp. 852–894). New York: Wiley.

Bouchard, C. (1987). *Child maltreatment in Montreal.* Unpublished manuscript, University of Quebec, Montreal.

Bronfenbrenner, U. (1979). *The ecology of human development: Experiments by nature and design.* Cambridge, MA: Harvard University Press.

Bryant, B. (1985). The neighborhood walk: Sources of support in middle childhood. *Monographs of the Society for Research in Child Development, 50*(3), 1–115.

Caplan, G., & Killilea, M. (Eds.). (1976). *Support systems and mutual help: Multidisciplinary explorations.* New York: Grune & Stratton.

Chavis, D., & Wandersman, A. (1990). Sense of community in the urban environment: A catalyst for participation and community development. *American Journal of Community Psychology, 18,* 55–81.

Cohen, L. (1991, December 10–12). The coalition for alternatives to violence and abuse. [Summary]. *Forum on Youth Violence in Minority Communities: Setting the Agenda for Prevention.* Atlanta, GA.

Collins, A., & Pancoast, D. (1976). *Natural helping networks.* Washington, DC: National Association of Social Workers.

Danieli, Y. (1988). The treatment and prevention of long-term effects and intergenerational transmission of victimization: A lesson from Holocaust survivors and their children. In C. Figley (Ed.), *Trauma and its wake* (pp. 295–313). New York: Brunner/Mazel.

Danish, S., & D'Augelli. (1980). *Helping skills: A basic training program*. New York: Human Sciences Press.

Deccio, G., Horner, B., & Wilson, D. (1991). *High-risk neighborhoods and high-risk families: Replication research related to the human ecology of child maltreatment*. Unpublished manuscript, Eastern Washington University, Cheney.

DuBow, F., & Podolefsky, A. (1981). Citizen participation in community crime prevention. *Human Organization, 41*, 307–314.

Dubrow, N., & Garbarino, J. (1989). Living in the war zone: Mothers and young children in a public housing development. *Child Welfare, 68*(1), 3–20.

Ellwood, A. (1988). Prove to me that MELD makes a difference. In H. Weiss & F. Jacobs (Eds.), *Evaluating family programs* (pp. 303–314). Hawthorne, NY: Aldine de Gruyter.

Erikson, K. (1976). *Everything in its path: Destruction of community in the Buffalo Creek flood*. New York: Simon & Schuster.

Fields, R. (1987). *Terrorized into terrorist: Sequelae of PTSD in young victims*. Paper presented at the meeting of the Society for Traumatic Stress Studies, New York.

Fitchen, J. (1981). *Poverty in rural America: A case study*. Boulder, CO: Westview.

Freudenburg, W., & Jones, R. (1991). Criminal behavior and rapid community growth: Examining the evidence. *Rural Sociology, 56*, 619–645.

Froland, C., Pancoast, D., Chapman, N., & Kimboko, P. (1981). *Helping networks and human services*. Beverly Hills, CA: Sage.

Garbarino, J. (1976). A preliminary study of some ecological correlates of child abuse: The impact of socioeconomic stress on mothers. *Child Development, 47*, 178–185.

Garbarino, J. (1977). The human ecology of child maltreatment: A conceptual model for research. *Journal of Marriage and the Family, 39*, 721–736.

Garbarino, J. (1987). Family support and the prevention of child maltreatment. In S. Kagan, R. Powell, B. Weissbourd, & E. Zigler (Eds.), *America's family support programs*. New Haven: Yale University Press.

Garbarino, J. (1992). *Towards a sustainable society: An economic, social and environmental agenda for our children's future*. Chicago: Noble Press.

Garbarino, J., & Associates. (1992). *Children and families in the social environment* (2nd ed.). Hawthorne, NY: Aldine de Gruyter.

Garbarino, J., Dubrow, N., Kostelny, K., & Pardo, C. (1992). *Children in danger: Coping with the consequences of community violence*. San Francisco: Jossey-Bass.

Garbarino, J., & Crouter, A. (1978). Defining the community context of parent–child relations. *Child Development, 49*, 604–616.

Garbarino, J., & Gilliam, G. (1980). Understanding abusive families. Lexington, MA: Lexington Books.

Garbarino, J., & Kostelny, K. (1992). Child maltreatment as a community problem. *International Journal of Child Abuse and Neglect, 16*, 455–464.

Garbarino, J., Kostelny, K., & Dubrow, N. (1991a). *No place to be a child: Growing up in a war zone*. Lexington, MA: Lexington Books.

Garbarino, J., Kostelny, K., & Dubrow, N. (1991b). What children can tell us about living in danger. *American Psychologist, 46*(4), 376–383.

Garbarino, J., & Sherman, D. (1980). High-risk neighborhoods and high-risk families: The human ecology of child maltreatment. *Child Development*, 51, 188–198.

Garbarino, J., Stocking, H., & Associates. (1980). *Protecting children from abuse and neglect: Developing and maintaining effective support systems for families*. San Francisco: Jossey-Bass.

Gaudin, J., & Polansky, N. (1985). Social distancing of the neglectful family: Sex, race, and social class influences. *Social Service Review*, 58, 245–253.

Gelles, R., & Straus, M. (1988). *Intimate violence: The definitive study of the causes and consequences of abuse in the American family*. New York: Simon and Schuster.

Gilligan, C. (1982). *In a different voice*. Cambridge, MA: Harvard University Press.

Goldstein, J. (1986). *Aggression and crimes of violence*. New York: Oxford University Press.

Halpern, R. (1990a). Community-based early intervention. In S. Meisels & J. Shonkoff (Eds.), *Handbook of early childhood intervention* (pp. 469–498). New York: Cambridge University Press.

Halpern, R. (1990b). Parent support and education programs. *Children and Youth Services Review*, 12, 285–308.

Halpern, R. (1991). *Neighborhood-based initiative to address poverty: Lessons from experience*. Chicago: Erikson Institute.

Halpern, R., & Larner, M. (1987). Lay family support during pregnancy and infancy: The child survival/fair start initiative. *Infant Mental Health Journal*, 8(2), 130–143.

Hawley, A. (1950). *Human ecology: A theory of community structure*. New York: Ronald Press.

Kagan, S., Powell, D., Weissbourd, B., & Zigler, E. (Eds.). (1987). *America's family support programs: Perspectives and prospects*. New Haven: Yale University Press.

Lauderdale, M., & Savage, C. (1991, June 6–7). *Prevention strategies in the neighborhood environment*. Paper presented at the NCCAN Prevention Conference, Washington, DC.

Lewis, M. (1978). Nearest neighbor analysis of epidemiological and community variables. *Psychological Bulletin*, 85(6), 1302–1308.

Losel, F., & Bliesner, T. (1990). Resilience in adolescence: A study on the generalizability of protective factors. In K. Hurrelmann & F. Losel (Eds.), *Health hazards in adolescence* (pp. 299–320). Berlin: Walter de Gruyter.

Lyons-Ruth, K., Botein, S., & Grunebaum, J. (1984). Reaching the hard-to-reach: Serving isolated and depressed mothers with infants in the community. In B. Cohler & J. Musick (Eds.), *Intervention with psychiatrically disabled parents and their young children* (pp. 95–122). San Francisco: Jossey Bass.

Marrack, J. (1992). The West Hawaii Family Center: Centralizing services to combat isolation. *Family Resource Coalition Report*, 11(1), 14.

Melton, G. (1992). It's time for neighborhood research and action. *Child Abuse and Neglect*, 16(4), 909–913.

Miller, A. (1987). *Maternal health and infant survival: An analysis of medical and social services to pregnant women, newborns, and their families in ten*

European countries. Washington, DC: National Center for Clinical Infant Programs.

Mitchell, M. (1991, December 10–12). The Kansas City Project [Summary]. *Forum on Youth Violence in Minority Communities: Setting the Agenda for Prevention*. Atlanta, GA.

Musick, J., Bernstein, V., Percansky, C., & Stott, F. (1987, December). A chain of enablement: Using community-based programs to strengthen relationships between teen parents and their infants. *Zero to Three, 8*(2), 1–7.

Musick, J., & Stott, F. (1990). Paraprofessionals, parenting and child development: Understanding the problems and seeking solutions. In S. Meisels & J. Shonkoff (Eds.), *Handbook of early intervention* (pp. 651–667). New York: Cambridge University Press.

Myers-Walls, J. (1992). Natural helping networks: Using local human resources to support families. *Family Resource Coalition Report, 11*(1), 10–11.

National Committee for Prevention of Child Abuse. (1992). *Evaluation of the William Penn Foundation Child Abuse Prevention Initiative*. Chicago: Author.

Newsweek. (1992, March 9). p. 29.

Olds, D., & Henderson, C. (1990). The prevention of maltreatment. In D. Cicchetti, & V. Carlson (Eds.), *Child maltreatment* (pp. 722–763). New York: Cambridge University Press.

Olds, D., Henderson, C., Tatelbaum, R., & Chamberlain, R. (1986). Preventing child abuse and neglect: A randomized trial of nurse home visitation. *Pediatrics, 78*, 65–78.

Pelton, L. (1978). Child abuse and neglect: The myth of classlessness. *American Journal of Orthopsychiatry, 48*, 608–617.

Pelton, L. (1992). *The role of material factors in child abuse and neglect*. Washington, DC: U.S. Advisory Board on Child Abuse and Neglect.

Pelton, L. (1981). *The social context of child abuse and neglect*. New York: Human Sciences Press.

Pfannesntiel, J., & Seltzer, D. (1989). New parents as teachers: Evaluation of an early parent education program. *Early Childhood Research Quarterly, 4*(1), 1–18.

Prothrow-Stith, D. (1991, December 10–12). Boston's Violence Prevention Project [Summary]. *Forum on Youth Violence in Minority Communities: Setting the Agenda for Prevention*. Atlanta, GA.

Reardon, P. (1988, June 22). CHA violent crimes up 9% for year. *Chicago Tribune*, p. 1.

Rodriguez, G., & Corez, C. (1988). Evaluation experience of Avance Parent Child Education Program. In H. Weiss & S. Jacobs (Eds.), *Evaluating family programs* (pp. 287–301). Hawthorne, NY: Aldine de Gruyter.

Rosenbaum, J., & Kaufman, J. (1991). *Educational and occuaptional achievements of low income black youth in white suburbs*. Paper presented at the Annual meeting of the American Sociological Association, Cincinnati.

Rutter, M., Cox, A., Tupling, C., Berger, M., & Yule, W. (1975). Attainment and adjustment in two geographical areas. *British Journal of Psychiatry, 126*, 493–509.

Sameroff, A., & Fiese, B. (1990). Transactional regulation and early intervention.

In S. J. Meisels & J. P. Shonkoff (Eds.), *Handbook of early childhood intervention* (pp. 119–149). Cambridge, England: Cambridge University Press.

Sattin, D., & Miller, J. (1971). The ecology of child abuse within a military community. *American Journal of Orthopsychiatry, 41*(4), 675–678.

Scheinfeld, D. (1983). Family relationships and school achievement among boys of lower-income urban black families. *American Journal of Orthopsychiatry, 53*(1), 127–143.

Skerry, P. (1983). The charmed life of Head Start. *Public Interest, 73*, 18–39.

Stokes, B. (1981). *Helping ourselves: Local solutions to global problems*. New York: Norton.

Unger, D., & Powell, D. (1991). *Families as nurturing systems: Support across the life span*. New York: Haworth Press.

Unger, D., & Wandersman, A. (1982). Neighboring in an urban environment. *American Journal of Community Psychology, 10*, 493–509.

Unger, D., & Wandersman, A. (1985). The importance of neighbors: The social, cognitive, and affective components of neighboring. *American Journal of Community Psychology, 13*(2), 139–169.

Unger, D., Wandersman, A., & Hallman, W. (1991). Coping with living near a hazardous waste facility: Individual and family distress. *American Journal of Orthopsychiatry, 62*, 55–70.

U.S. Advisory Board on Child Abuse and Neglect. (1991). *Creating caring communities: Blueprint for an effective federal policy on child abuse and neglect*. Washington, DC: U.S. Government Printing Office.

Valentine, J., & Stark, E. (1979). The social context of parent involvement in Head Start. In E. Zigler & J. Valentine (Eds.), *Head Start: Legacy of the War on Poverty* (pp. 291–313). New York: Free Press.

Vgotsky, L. (1986). *Thought and language*. Cambridge, MA: MIT Press.

Wahler, R. (1980). The insular mother: Her problems in parent–child treatment. *Journal of Applied Behavior Analysis, 13*, 207–219.

Wandersman, A., Florin, P., Friedmann, R., & Meier, R. (1987). Who participates, who does not, and why? An analysis of voluntary neighborhood organizations in the United States and Israel. *Sociological Forum, 2*, 534–555.

Wandersman, A., & Goodman, R. (1991, September). *Community partnerships for substance abuse prevention*. Family Resource Coalition Special Issue on Substance Abuse Prevention.

Wandersman, A., Jakubs, J., & Glamartino, G. (1981). Participation in block organizations. *Journal of Community Action, 1*, 40–47.

Wandersman, A., & Moos, R. (1981). Assessing and evaluating residential environments. *Environment and Behavior, 13*(4), 481–508.

Warren, R. (1978). *The community in America*. Boston: Houghton Mifflin.

Weiss, H., & Halpern, R. (1991). *Community-based family support and education programs: Something old or something new?* New York: Columbia University.

Weissbourd, B., & Kagan, S. (Eds.). (1994). *Putting families first: America's family support movement and the challenge of change*. San Francisco: Jossey-Bass.

Wellman, B. (1979). The community question: The intimate networks of East Yonkers. *American Journal of Sociology, 84*, 1201–1231.

Werner, E. (1990). Protective factors and individual resilience. In S. J. Meisels &

J. P. Shonkoff (Eds.), *Handbook of early childhood intervention* (pp. 97–116). Cambridge, England: Cambridge University Press.

Whitmore, E. (1991, September). Evaluation and empowerment: It's the process that counts. *Networking Bulletin: Empowerment and Family Support*, 2(2), 1–7.

Whittaker, J. Garbarino, J., & Associates. (1983). *Social support networks on informal helping in the human services*. Hawthorne, NY: Aldine de Gruyter.

Wilson, W. J. (1987). *The truly disadvantaged*. Chicago : University of Chicago Press.

Zuravin, S., & Taylor, R. (1987). The ecology of child maltreatment: Identifying and characterizing high-risk neighborhoods. *Child Welfare*, 66(6), 497–506.

Chapter 8

Child Protection and Out-of-Home Care: System Reforms and Regulating Placements

Paul Lerman

Children and youth who have experienced abuse or neglect can be found in substantial numbers in out-of-home placements associated with the fields of mental health, child welfare, and juvenile corrections (Silver, 1990; Dembo et al.,1989; Young, Pappenfort, & Marlow, 1983). While residing in residential treatment centers, group homes, or detention centers, they are at risk once again of abuse or neglect by staff or other peer residents. Evidence exists, on a national scale, that children and youth, with and without prior experiences of abuse or neglect have an equal or greater chance of being a victim of an incident of abuse or neglect in out-of-home placements than do children residing in families (Rindfleisch & Rabb, 1984a; Rindfleisch & Nunno, 1992). Therefore, the diminution of institutional abuse by reducing out-of-home placements and regulating facilities associated with the major systems dealing with children and youth (i.e., mental health, child welfare, and juvenile corrections) is the logical target of any prevention strategy. This chapter assesses the research and service literature for broad strategies that can reduce placements and improve the regulation of out-of-home-settings. More specifically, the strategies are pursued by the following:

1. Describing and examining leading examples of comprehensive service system reforms that possess the potential—by design and implementation—to yield services that can provide care, protection, and treatment while reducing placements or providing alternatives to restrictive out-of-home settings.
2. Describing and examining leading examples of regulatory reforms that possess the potential—by design and implementation—to symbolize and enforce the goals of child protection for children at risk of placement or in a placement of any duration.

ANALYTIC ASSUMPTIONS

The descriptions and assessments of exemplars of comprehensive service system and regulatory reforms are guided by a set of specific analytic assumptions. These assumptions pertain to the definitions of child protection, choice of target groups, choice of exemplars, ranking of residential options and location of services, and research design preferences. These assumptions are important to highlight and briefly discuss so that the values underlying the choice of exemplars and the accompanying assessments can be openly and directly addressed.

1. *Definition of child protection.* The definitions and declarations in the National Child Protection Policy set forth by the U.S. Advisory Board on Child Abuse and Neglect (1991) provide the initial starting point of this chapter's analytic stance. Child protection refers to the multiple systems that "facilitate comprehensive community efforts to ensure the safe and healthy development of children and youth" (p. 37). A comprehensive child protection policy would attempt to integrate the varied contributions of public, civic, religious, and professional services and organizations. Ideally, the services would be "child-centered" as a first priority, oriented toward "strengthening families" wherever possible, and "focused at the level of urban and suburban neighborhoods and rural communities" (pp. 41–42).

2. *Choice of prevention targets.* A major focus of a comprehensive child protection policy would be to reduce the likelihood of maltreatment. As noted earlier, it has been well established that children in out-of-home placements are at a high risk of experiencing incidents of abuse and/or neglect. Regardless of the system associated with, authorizing, or finding the placement, all children living away from their families face a high risk of maltreatment (Harrell & Orem, 1980; Rindfleisch & Rabb, 1984b; Weithorn, 1988; Rindfleisch & Nunno, 1992). A high priority of a child protection strategy would include the reduction in the frequency and duration of out-of-home placements. Therefore, the target groups are *all* children at risk of being placed away from their families for 24 hours or more, including children and youth who have not previously experienced child abuse or neglect but might if they were placed and children who have been victimized within their own families and face the risk of additional maltreatment in an out-of-home placement.

3. *Choice of exemplars.* Since the 1960s, communities throughout the country have experimented with a variety of community-based program demonstrations or "institutional alternatives" (see, e.g., Lerman, 1975, 1982). This chapter analyzes those efforts that are closest in philosophy and practice with a child care protection policy. I particularly sought efforts that targeted preventing and limiting out-of-home care, treatment, and custody while also providing a wide range of nonresidential services within a community.

Service system efforts that created explicit mechanisms for coordinating and integrating services with other public and private organizations, monitored or evaluated services and outcomes, and were designed to operate beyond a short-term period received special attention. Attempts at reforming a community's entire service system for children and youth—especially across the major fields—received greater scrutiny than did specific types of program innovations.

Programs that are components of service systems have historically attracted the greatest amount of evaluation resources and attention. However, service system reforms that attempt to incorporate program innovations within a broader, more closely coordinated network of services may offer a unique contribution to a national child protection strategy. The nuts and bolts of more comprehensive service system reforms within the three major fields, therefore, receive a greater amount of analytic attention than do the component programs. However, many of the component programs are discussed by Wolfe (Chapter 6, this volume).

4. *Ranking of residential options.* The primary exemplars of system reforms seem to opt for placement policies—when utilized—that are guided by beliefs that rank-order out-of-home placements from least to most restrictive. Detention centers, training schools, and psychiatric wards and hospitals are generally perceived to be more restrictive than are residential treatment centers, and the treatment centers tend to be ranked as more restrictive than group homes, crisis and shelter residences, and foster homes. National empirical data offer support for an ordering of preferred placement types. In a national survey of *all* residential facilities, conducted in 1981 by researchers at the University of Chicago, the administrators of over 3,900 facilities were asked questions of how "open" the facilities were relative to a normal home and ecological environment. Going outside the facility to attend school and visiting friends in their homes were used as two indicators of relative access and openness to the community (Young et al., 1983; Lerman, 1990). Youth in correctional and psychiatric facilities were least likely to go to local schools (12% and 8%, respectively) or visit friends at local homes (4% and 18%, respectively). Residents of group homes, by contrast had much greater access to schools and visiting friends (78% and 48%, respectively). Nonhospital facilities for the emotionally disturbed permitted much less access to local schools (35%) or visiting local homes (27%). Using these empirical results, it seems reasonable to define juvenile correctional and psychiatric facilities as the most restrictive, least "normal" placements, followed by residential treatment centers and then group homes and foster care facilities. Assessments of success in reducing the risks associated with out-of-home placement can use this rank-ordering of residential types as an evaluative template.

5. *Research design preferences.* Most social scientists engaged in evaluation research would agree that the most trustworthy assessments of service

system and program innovations include the emulation of a clinical trial research design. In this type of ideal evaluation design, recipients of innovations are randomly assigned to an experimental "treatment" group or a nontreatment control group. In this way, if comparable outcome measures are utilized to assess each equivalent sample of service recipients, at a similar time after treatment (or nontreatment), there is greater confidence that any "success" can be attributed to the innovation and not to differences associated with the recipients. A recent program component innovation, "family preservation" services provided to parents and children in their own homes, for example, was subjected to experimental-type designs in three states: New Jersey (Feldman, 1991), California (McDonald & Associates, 1990), and Minnesota (Au Claire & Schwartz, 1986). The results provided sobering findings that yield a more realistic image of the potential of time-limited, intensive, home-based services. Without the clinical trials, less sophisticated findings might have remained part of the service literatures (see Wells & Biegel, 1992; Wolfe, Chapter 6, this volume, for the most recent assessment).

It may be unfair that recent innovative services are being held to a high standard of evaluation whereas the older, most heavily reimbursed, and restrictive settings—such as psychiatric hospitals and residential treatment centers—are associated with the least amount of research (Burns & Friedman, 1990). Psychiatric hospitalization, the fastest growing residential type, can boast of only one clinical trial in the literature on mental health services for children, but this was conducted over a decade ago and failed to support hospitalization after a diagnostic evaluation stay (Burns & Friedman, 1990). Residential treatment centers, actively endorsed in official reports and the professional literature until recently, are still unable to provide research reports that include a clinical trial that demonstrates their superiority to less costly and restrictive alternatives (Lerman, 1968; Joint Commission on Mental Health of Children, 1969; President's Commission on Mental Health, 1978; Maluccio & Marlow, 1972; Whittaker & Maluccio, 1989; Burns & Friedman, 1990).

The absence of an empirically sound basis for relying on psychiatric hospitalization and residential treatment centers, two of the most widely used models of restrictive care for children and youth, does not justify relaxing evaluative standards for component programs. However, it does legitimate a greater amount of latitude in assessing the recent attempts to redesign entire systems of service that are based on avoiding or reducing the more restrictive and less normalized forms of residential care, treatment, and custody. At present, there is no reasonable basis for believing that the most restrictive and costly models of residential treatment are any more effective than the nonresidential or less intrusive alternatives in changing youth behaviors. Instead of relying solely on the standard of effectiveness, we can rely on the values of least harm and greater efficiency of resources as the initial bases for assessing service system reforms. These initial findings concerning reduced harms and efficiency can be part of a strategy of "incremental search" (Lerman, 1975). An incremental search strategy is willing to rely on research studies that start with baseline and expected outcome comparisons, proceed to research designs with explicit comparison groups, and then attempt to replicate outcomes with new samples in new communities. Finally, we can expect an array of experimental studies that accumulate in the literature over time, with the expectation that the older the innovation, the higher the standards of cumulative evidence based on tighter research designs (Wells & Biegel, 1992; Burns & Friedman, 1990).

In a broad sense, the assessments of system reforms can be guided by this general research hypothesis: The new programs of care and services, if provided in sufficient range and number with competent staff to youth at risk of placement, and coordinated for maximum impact, offer the best likelihood of implementing a service system design for youth that is client centered, less restrictive, more normal, and least likely to produce incidents of abuse and neglect at home or in out-of-home placements. Exemplars of reform are assessed here in order to determine whether counterfactual evidence exists that would not support this general hypothesis. These initial assessments could change over time, as cumulative studies continue to appear in the research and service literature.

ESTIMATES OF YOUTH AT HIGH RISK

It is useful to set forth a conceptual and numerical standard for assessing the population of high-risk youth so that the magnitude of a national strategy can be guided by facts rather than conjecture. The most conservative empirical estimate can be based on an enumeration of the number of youth who actually reside in an out-of-home placement during a calendar year. Presumably, all youth actually placed were, in fact, at high risk of leaving their families during the year. If we are interested in reducing the frequency and duration of placements, we must identify the major fields associated with residential episodes. For the purposes of the analysis that follows, out-of-home, residential episodes of care include residence in a facility type on the last day of a census year *plus* admission during the subsequent year. In this manner, facilities that have a high turnover of beds (e.g., shelters, psychiatric wards, and detention facilities) will be counted much more accurately than if we relied only on one-day counts. The National Institute of Mental Health (NIMH) has used the episode method for all ages for many years (see, e.g., NIMH, 1967–1980). I adapted the episode method for use with national surveys of facilities in child welfare, juvenile corrections,and mental health, but I use the phrase "episodes of care, treatment, and custody" to refer to the multiple functions performed (in varying degrees) by all facility types (for an initial use with 1970s data see Lerman, 1982).

The best estimates for the number of episodes of care, treatment and custody of youth under 18 for each major system, is as follows, for the mid-1980s (based on Lerman, 1990):

Mental health	361,000 episodes
Juvenile corrections	713,000
Jails and prisons	102,000
Child welfare facilities	54,000
Foster care	190,000
Total	1,400,000

The reporting systems associated with residential counts are notoriously tardy and inefficient in publishing results, so it is impossible to produce an accurate count for the 1990s at this time (Lerman, 1991). There are an unknown number of readmissions for each system, and a counting overlap probably exists to an unknown degree between the major systems. These potential duplicate counts are offset, to an appreciable—but unknown—degree by the absence of any admissions data for foster care and facilities associated exclusively with child welfare; data for these two residential types refer only to one-day resident counts. Taking all of these caveats into account, it is unlikely that the unduplicated number of youth experiencing an episode of care, treatment, and custody was less than 1 million per year during the mid-1980s; the 1.4 million episodes can serve as the upper limit of an annual estimate of youth at risk.

The more conservative figure of 1 million is *twice* as large as the number offered in 1990 by the Select Committee on Children, Youth, and Families of the U.S. House of Representatives (see, e.g., Wells & Biegel, 1992, citing the select committee's figure). This difference is due to the fact that this official body, like many professionals, refers only to one-day counts. But this approach, as noted, misses all the youth during a year who will occupy the bed vacated by those counted on a census day. For our purposes, 1 million to 1.4 million youth is much closer to the mark and refers to all youth who actually experienced the risk and lived away from families, relatives, and friends, during the year.

If we use the lower and upper estimates of unduplicated youth living in out-of-home residences in the 1980s, and settle on 1987 as a midpoint between 1985 and 1990, it is also possible to calculate a national estimate of the proportion of youth at risk. The U.S. Bureau of Census reported that about 67 million youth under age 18 lived in the country on July 1, 1987. Using this figure as a base, and the 1–1.4 million unduplicated youth as the numerator, the estimated at-risk rate is about 1.5–2.0% each year (U.S. Bureau of Census, 1988). At a minimum, a national strategy of preventing institutional abuse and neglect during a single year would need to target at least 1.5% of America's under-18 population. With better reporting data, it is conceivable that the rate could, of course, be higher and surpass the upper limit estimate of 2% (Lerman, 1991). Even in the absence of better, more recent, information, we can be confident that the usual figure of 500,000 at-risk youth is off the mark by at least 100% (as are the rates of risk).

SERVICE SYSTEM REFORMS: MENTAL HEALTH

The past decade has witnessed an upsurge of interest in reshaping the design of service delivery systems for children and adolescents. Rather than just adding new technical therapeutic procedures and service programs to existing efforts, many states and localities began to experiment with mechanisms for integrating and coordinating "old" programs with "new" human service models. Examples of systems that strive to be client centered and neighborhood based and attempt to provide a continuum of services from least restrictive and normal care arrangements to secure, more controlling residences can be found in the following fields of service and locations:

1. *Mental health.* California (Jordan & Hernandez, 1990; Attkisson, Dresser, & Rosenblatt, 1991), North Carolina (Behar, 1985, 1991), Alaska (Van Den Berg, 1989; Schlenger, Etheridge, Hansen, & Fairbank, 1990), and Vermont (Burchard & Clarke, 1990) have new system designs that are led by mental health administrators but involve collaborations with juvenile justice, child welfare, and local school systems.

2. *Child welfare.* Four Iowa counties have new system designs led by child welfare administrators but also involving collaborations with juvenile justice, mental health, and local school systems (Bruner, 1989; Kassar, 1991).

3. *Juvenile corrections.* The new system design conceived and implemented in Massachusetts in the 1970s (Ohlin, Coates, & Miller, 1977; Austin, Elms, Krisberg, & Steele, 1991) and emulated elsewhere (Butts & Streit, 1988; Barton, Streit, & Schwartz, 1991; Schwartz & Loughran, 1991) is led by state correctional officials but also involves contractual collaboration with public and private providers in mental health and child welfare.

Besides attempting to promote a more rational and effective service design via contractual promises of collaboration and other administrative and fiscal mechanisms, each new system design was initiated to reduce the fiscal and social costs associated with extensive utilization of out-of-home placements in restrictive, less normal, and distant locations. The reports on the system innovations disclose an effort to contain and/or reduce reliance on the following types of costs associated with the more restrictive out-of-home placements:

1. *Psychiatric hospitals:* as high as $106,200 per year in California (Jordan & Hernandez, 1990).
2. *Residential treatment centers:* as high as $75,000 per stay for the children of military personnel living in Ft. Bragg, North Carolina (Behar, 1991).
3. *Correctional training schools:* as high as $45,000 per year for operational costs in many states (Austin et al., 1990).

The persons planning and guiding the system design efforts tend to share a philosophy about emphasizing nonresidential services wherever possible. However, because attempts at innovation are confronted with specific local or state problems, constraints, and fiscal realities, each demonstration site created distinctive arrangements. An assessment of the similarities and differences between the various system designs by service fields can be instructive, provided it is grounded on an understanding of the philosophy of each attempt at reform and the specific goals, target populations, and fiscal circumstances influencing the local efforts. This section focuses on service system reforms in mental health; the following section discusses system change in child welfare and juvenile corrections.

Ideal Design, Values, and Principles

The general philosophy of the new look in mental health service system design is best captured by a widely cited paper disseminated by the Child and Adolescent Service System Program (CASSP) of the NIMH (Stroul & Friedman, 1986). The paper sets forth a design based on a set of "core values" and "principles" that should ideally govern the delivery of services in a community. The core values set forth by Stroul and Friedman (1986) are based on the following beliefs: (1) a system of care should be child centered, with the needs of the child and family guiding the types and mix of services provided, and (2) a system of care should be community based, with the responsibility for management and decision making residing at the local level. Based on these core values, Stroul and Friedman (1986) set forth 10 "guiding principles" for a local system:

1) Emotionally disturbed children should have access to a comprehensive array of services that address the child's physical, emotional, social, and educational needs;

2) Emotionally disturbed children should receive individualized services in accordance with the unique needs and potentials of each child and guided by an individualized service plan;

3) Emotionally disturbed children should receive services within the least restrictive, most normative environment that is clinically appropriate;

4) The families and surrogate families of emotionally disturbed children should be full participants in all aspects of the planning and delivery of services;

5) Emotionally disturbed children should receive services that are integrated, with linkages between child-caring agencies and programs and mechanisms for planning, developing, and coordinating services;

6) Emotionally disturbed children should be provided with case management or similar mechanisms to ensure that multiple services are delivered in a coordinated and therapeutic manner and that they can move through the system of services in accordance with their changing needs;

7) Early identification and intervention for children with emotional problems should be promoted by the system of care in order to enhance the likelihood of positive outcomes;

8) Emotionally disturbed children should be ensured smooth transitions to the adult service system as they reach maturity;

9) The rights of emotionally disturbed children should be protected, and effective advocacy efforts for emotionally disturbed children and youth should be promoted;

10) Emotionally disturbed children should receive services without regard to race, religion, national origin, sex, physical disability, or other characteristics, and services should be sensitive and responsive to cultural differences and special needs. (as summarized in Stroul & Goldman, 1990, p. 63)

Stroul and Friedman (1986) present a specific set of mental health "program components" that a fully adequate mental health service delivery system should be able to provide, consisting of nonresidential and residential service types as follows:

Nonresidential programs	Residential programs
1. Assessment	1. Therapeutic foster care
2. Early identification/intervention	2. Therapeutic group care
3. Prevention	3. Therapeutic camps
4. Outpatient treatment	4. Independent living services
5. Home-based services	5. Crisis residential services
6. Day treatment	6. Residential treatment
	7. Psychiatric inpatient services

An implicit assumption of this ideal system design is that the new system arrangements and their component programs would be more effective in dealing with youth problems and less costly than the more restrictive alternatives (Burns & Friedman, 1990). In an unpublished manuscript, Friedman (1987) attempted to specify the actual amounts of distinct treatment resources that a system would need in order to have a continuum of services with a "proper balance." According to Friedman, a well-designed mental health service system would have ratio of 12 nonresidential service slots and 4 case management places available to every single out-of-home residential slot. For planning purposes, the 12 nonresidential services would provide slots in the following ratios: 8:1 for outpatient, 2:1 for day treatment, and 2:1 for home-based services. These estimates are based on the experiences of North Carolina mental health planners in devising a new service system for about 1,100 youth declared eligible for mental health services by a federal class action suit (Behar, 1985). The estimate includes the assumption that a public mental health sector would provide mental health services for 1–2% of children and adolescents in a local youth population; further, only $1/10$ of 1% (0.1%) would require residential services because of serious emotional problems. There are probably few communities ready to muster the fiscal resources necessary to fully implement Friedman's ideal configuration of services. However, a unique demonstration is currently occurring in a military community in North Carolina that can furnish empirical data about the reality of creating an ideal mental health system for an entire community of children and adolescents. The implementation of the Ft. Bragg/CHAMPUS 4-year demonstration project, funded by a generous allocation from the military budget, can have profound implications for civilian, as well as military, families. There are about 41,600 children under the age of 18 residing in the Ft. Bragg, North Carolina, community, and they experience family and developmental problems comparable to those faced in communities across America.

The Ft. Bragg/CHAMPUS Demonstration Project

The goals of the Ft. Bragg/CHAMPUS project, as reported by Behar (1991), are as follows: (1) to provide a "full continuum" of mental health services for all children of military personnel stationed at Ft. Bragg displaying mental health problems diagnosed by a clinician; (2) to deliver the most appropriate and cost-effective services, with particular emphasis on providing "alternatives to inpatient and residential treatment to those in need"; and (3) to serve as a "major effort at cost containment of CHAMPUS costs" (Behar, 1991, p. 3). The demonstration project is fully funded by the U.S. Army, as part of the Civilian Hospital and Medical Program of the Unified Services (CHAMPUS). The military funders were particularly alarmed at the "dramatic increase of 154% in CHAMPUS hospital and residential treatment costs for children and adolescents during the FY 86 to FY 89 period" (Behar, 1991, p. 2).

The Ft. Bragg/CHAMPUS project is administered under a 5-year contract by the North Carolina Division of Mental Health and Developmental Disabilities. This state agency has had a decade of experience in directing and supervising services to aggressive youth with serious psychiatric problems (Behar, 1985, 1986). The clinical services are offered at the General Jones Rumbaugh Clinic, located at Ft. Bragg. The demonstration project began in

June 1990 and is scheduled to conclude at the end of May 1994. From June 1990 to mid-April, 1991—10.5 months—the active case load of clinic patients at the Rumbaugh Clinic grew from 282 to 1,382. This large increase in active cases provides evidence that the provision of a full continuum of clinic services was, in fact, utilized by Ft. Bragg military families. Detailed assessment of the first 10.5 months reveals that a total of 2,403 children were actually referred for services, but not all met the admissions criteria of a bona fide clinical diagnosis according to the third revised edition of the *Diagnostic and Statistical Manual of Mental Disorders* (DSM-III-R) (1987). The disposition of cases was handled as follows (data from Behar, 1991):

	Number	%
Screened out prior to admissions	360	15.0
Screened out after admissions	121	5.0
Diagnosis pending	167	7.0
Active clients	1,352	56.3
Completed treatment	403	16.7
Total	2,403	100.0

The 1st-year flow of referrals indicates that about 20% of the referrals are rejected as not meeting the clinical intake criteria of a DSM-III-R diagnosis. If the results of the first 10.5 months are projected on an annual basis, the Ft. Bragg demonstration reveals that about 6.6% of the total youth population under age 18 (41,600) were referred for services; about 5.3% met the DSM-III-R criteria and were admitted to receive mental health services. The 5.3% rate is far above the rate estimated by Friedman (1987) in creating an ideal design, but his projection of 1–2% needing services is based on "serious" cases; however, the Ft. Bragg clinic population is not screened on the basis of seriousness. The Ft. Bragg/CHAMPUS utilization rate of 5.3% is also far above the actual 1986 national rate of new admissions to outpatient mental health services of youth under 18—less than 1% (calculated from data in Sunshine, Witkin, Atay, & Manderscheid, 1991; U.S. Bureau of Census, 1988).

The 5.3% Ft. Bragg clinic rate is, however, below the estimate of 13.6% needing services, provided by the Joint Commission on the Mental Health of Children (1969) or the recent 12% estimate of the Institute of Medicine's (1989) expert "Committee for the Study of Research on Child and Adolescent Disorders" (p. 33). If the Institute of Medicine's expert committee is near the mark, the Ft. Bragg/CHAMPUS project may be attracting only about one half of the potential target group. However, if the Ft. Bragg services continue to be used at a comparable rate in subsequent years, even when a full range of services is made available at little or no cost, it is possible that the expert epidemiological estimates may have to be revised.

The Ft. Bragg evidence indicates that medical practitioners (particularly pediatricians) are a strong referral source (about 30% of all referrals), as are families (about 30%), mental health practitioners (about 20%), and schools (about 16%). The strong involvement of medical practitioners in Ft. Bragg referrals appears quite striking when compared to the best available national data—youth admissions to inpatient psychiatric services in 1980—where doctors were involved in only 8% of the cases (calculated from Milazzo-Sayre, Benson, Rosenstein, Manderscheid, 1986). Ft. Bragg receives few referrals from police or court officials (less than 3%), whereas these correctional screeners accounted for about 15% of the 1980 national inpatient psychiatric admissions (Milazzo-Sayre et al., 1986).

During the 1st-year of the project, the following continuum of services were provided (or were soon to be provided) (Behar, 1991):

1. *Outpatient services*
   a. Full intake and assessment services for about 6.6% of the child population of Ft. Bragg, referred by local schools, child welfare and social services, health care providers, police, and family members.
   b. Individualized treatment plans within a limited time period.
   c. Emergency crisis available 24 hours per day.
   d. Youth and family treatment provided in offices or at home with project staff or contract providers.
   e. In-school support.

2. *Family preservation services*
   a. In-home crisis stabilization on call around the clock for up to 6–8 weeks.
   b. Short-term crisis-emergency services.
   c. Day parenting.

3. *Day treatment*
   a. Therapeutic preschool.
   b. Moderate management with public school for half day.
   c. Moderate management for full day.
   d. High management for full day.
   e. Therapeutic vocational placement.
   f. After school or work in evening for half day equivalent.

4. *Therapeutic camping*
   a. Week-end.
   b. Summer.
   c. Year-round.

5. *Out-of-home residence*
   a. Therapeutic foster care for emergencies and lengthier stays.
   b. Therapeutic group homes for emergencies and lengthier stays.

      c. Residential treatment centers.
      d. Supervised independent living.

6. *Hospitalization*
      a. Crisis stabilization primarily.

7. *Casework management for all active cases*
      a. Out-patient care coordination—65 cases per staff.
      b. All other service modalities—20 cases per staff.

8. *Special substance abuse evaluation and services*

    The Ft. Bragg/CHAMPUS delivery system relies on newly hired clinical staff, as well as a variety of local nonresidential and residential providers, to implement the treatment plans devised by the intake and assessment staff. The project's complex system of services is founded on the belief that the provision of professional care management must be accompanied by the coordination and monitoring of the quality of services, whether delivered inside or outside the premises of the Rumbaugh Clinic. Case management is specifically divided into two categories: (1) typical outpatient-level cases, staffed by eight bachelor's-level outpatient case coordinators; and (2) more seriously disturbed cases, staffed by six master's-level clinical case managers. A careful reading of the plan and simple calculations reveal that at any particular time the project will be able to coordinate and monitor a maximum of about 520 typical outpatient cases (based on eight coordinators serving an average case load of 65 cases) and about 120 intensive-service cases (based on six clinicians case managing an average case load of 20 clients). As of April 1991 (the date when other useful information was available), with an active case load of 1,404 youth, the number of cases not covered by a case manager could have amounted to 764 cases (i.e., 1,404 minus 640 "coordinated" and "clinically case managed" cases). A reasonable inference is that these 764 cases present fewer problems and require fewer services and can be handled in a more traditional manner, without coordination or management. Because the project relied heavily on outside contract providers for the vast majority of outpatient services, the project also relies on contract renewal and direct coordination and case management as mechanisms for directly monitoring the provision and quality of services.

    The coordinators and case managers participate in the clinical treatment team meetings that review moderate and serious cases every 45 days subsequent to the initial screening and planning. Rumbaugh Clinic staff, either at intake or at team reviews, control all residential placement decisions. At the 45-day review, all members are expected to focus on whether the planned services—inside or outside the clinic and inside or outside the home—have enhanced and reinforced "adaptive competencies" within the client and family. Besides the varied internal mechanisms for assessing type and quality of service and indicators of improvement, the project is also undergoing a formal external evaluation by Dr. Leonard Brickman of Vanderbilt University. The formal evaluation is jointly funded by the Army and the NIMH and will include a comparison with two "control sites," Fort Campbell and Fort Stewart. The goals of the external evaluation are to assess the quality, costs, and impact of the services (Behar, 1991).

The 1991 progress report provides initial information that is useful in assessing headway in (1) implementing a full continuum of services, (2) reducing reliance on more restrictive residential services, and (3) promoting cost-effective services. The limited secondary analyses presented in Tables 8.1, 8.2, and 8.3 are based on an extrapolation of information contained in the April 29, 1992, report of the first 9 months. The analysis of the full continuum (reported in Table 8.1) contains information about most of the major components of the Ft. Bragg/CHAMPUS service system that were actually in place (or would soon be implemented) and compares the design in action with the ideal set forth by Friedman (1987). However, the analysis of residential services (reported in Table 8.2) refers only to the utilization of hospitals and residential treatment centers and does not include any calculations concerning changes in the use of group homes and foster care; nor does it include any information about any impact on the utilization of residential placements associated with the child welfare or juvenile correctional system. The secondary analysis of cost-effectiveness (reported in Table 8.3) refers

TABLE 8.1. Implementation of a Full Continuum of Mental Health Services: A Comparison of an Ideal Design and Ft. Bragg/CHAMPUS

	Number of slots	
	Friedman ideal design (for 40,000 youth)[a]	Ft. Bragg actual (for 41,600 youth)[b]
A. *Residential Types*		
Hospital	04	15
Residential treatment center	04	07
Therapeutic group home	16	18
Therapeutic foster care	16	12
Subtotal	40	52
B. *Nonresidential Services*		
In-home treatment	80	40
Day treatment	80	31
Outpatient servcices only	320	1,281
Subtotal	480	1,352
Ratio of nonresidential:residential	12:1	26:1
Case management services	160	640
Ratio of case management:residential	4:1	12:1

[a]Data from Friedman (1987), for 10,000 youth multipled by 4.
[b]Data from Behar (1991), actual and planned descriptions of an active case load of 1,404 youth.

TABLE 8.2. Utilization of Hospitals and RTCs over a 9-Month Period by Ft. Bragg/CHAMPUS Youth

	Date	No. active clients	Hospital	RTC	Total
A. Utilization rates (by residence type) per 100 active clients for 1 month	June 1990 February 1991	284 1,404	3.8 1.1	3.2 0.5	7.0 1.6
B. Average beds used (per day)	June 1990 February 1991	284 1,404	10.9 15.3	9.1 6.8	20.0 22.1
C. Annual beds used (estimated days per year	June 1990 February 1991	284 1,404	3,979 5,585	3,321 2,482	7,300 8,067
D. Annual beds used (estimated days per child served)	June 1990 February 1991	284 1,404	14.01 3.98	11.69 1.77	25.70 5.75

Note. Estimations are based on data from Behar, 1991, Attachment 1, table on utilization.

only to the costs associated with the utilization of hospitals and residential treatment centers and does not include estimates of any potential shifts in other residential or nonresidential costs of services.

Table 8.1 presents estimates of the actual and planned implementation of a full continuum of services. The actual Ft. Bragg/CHAMPUS project's delivery system is compared to Friedman's ideal design for a smaller target group of "seriously emotionally disturbed" youth. The total number of residential slots projected by Friedman (1987) is fairly similar to that achieved by Ft. Bragg/CHAMPUS (40 vs. 50 slots). The major difference is that Ft. Bragg/CHAMPUS places a much stronger reliance on the use of psychiatric hospital services. This may be due to the fact that a private psychiatric facility is located nearby, which makes it easier to contract for crisis stabilization services and evaluation/diagnostic services and still maintain family links (Behar, 1991, Attachment 2, p. 11). It is conceivable, too, that the inclusion of substance abuse evaluations for all youth 11 years or older, as well as treatment services, may also be linked to the higher utilization of hospital slots. Perhaps the Brickman evaluation will be able to distinguish hospital use by type of social problem, as well as clinical diagnoses, and pinpoint the characteristics of cases associated with hospitalization.

Part B of Table 8.1 discloses, as expected, that Ft. Bragg/CHAMPUS has an unusually high number of outpatient slots used and/or reserved for its broad target population compared to the more limited group addressed by Friedman (1987) (320 vs. 1,281 slots). Ft. Bragg/CHAMPUS has a lower capacity of family preservation treatment slots (of the Homebuilders type), even though the 10.5-month availability of a maximum of 16 slots is due to be augmented by an additional 24 slots during the last part of the first year

TABLE 8.3. Cost Estimates of Hospital and RTC Use, by Annual Bed Days per Child Served and Annual Bed Days Used by Placed Youth

A. *Cost estimates by annual bed days per child served in month[a]*

	Hospital costs		RTC costs		
Date	Daily cost	Cost/child served	Daily cost	Cost/child served	Total costs/ child served
June 1990	$721	$10,101	$410	$4,793	$14,894
February 1991	721	2,870	410	726	3,596
Cost change	$ 0	–$ 7,231	$ 0	–$4,067	–$11,298

B. *Cost estimates by annual bed days used by placed youth[b]*

	Hospital costs		RTC costs		
Date	Daily cost	Annual cost of bed days	Daily cost	Annual cost of bed days	Total annual bed days cost
June 1990	$721	$2,868,859	$410	$1,361,610	$4,230,469
February 1991	721	4,026,785	410	1,077,620	5,044,405
Cost change	$ 0	+$1,157,926	$ 0	–$ 343,990	+$ 813,936

[a]Estimated annual bed days per child served from Table 8.2, part D, is multiplied by daily cost of bed.
[b]Estimated annual bed days actually used by placed youth from part C, Table 8.2, is multiplied by daily cost of bed.

(80 vs. 40 slots). There is also a lower reliance on day-treatment programming than envisaged by Friedman, even when after-school slots are added to nonschool day services (80 vs. 31 slots).

Part C indicates that the ratio of nonresident to resident slots is quite high in Ft. Bragg/CHAMPUS—26:1 versus 12:1—due primarily to the high utilization of outpatient services provided by the private sector. Ft. Bragg/ CHAMPUS also relies on case management services (all types) to a much greater extent than might be expected for such a broad target group—12:1 versus 4:1 slots. In general, it is quite evident that the Ft. Bragg/CHAMPUS project has been quite successful in implementing a full continuum of services for 5.3% of the community's youth population.

Assessing progress toward reducing reliance on more restrictive residential services over the first 9 months is presented from four perspectives in Table 8.2. Part A documents that the utilization rates of hospitals and residential treatment centers (RTC) were reduced from June 1990 to February 1991—from a total rate of 7 per 100 active cases during a month to 1.6 per 100 active cases. However, part B documents that the enormous increase in the number of active cases is associated with a higher average bed use for hospitals over the 9-month period (15.3 beds used per day vs. 10.9). Part B also documents that the RTC bed use was reduced (9.1 vs. 6.8) despite the increase in active cases. The total average bed use per day in both facility types combined was slightly greater in February 1991 than in June 1990 (20.0 vs. 22.1 per day). However, if the small increase in daily average bed use is extrapolated via a secondary analysis for an entire year (as in part C), the consequences are appreciable—an increase in the annual bed days per year of 767 (i.e., 8,067 minus 7,300 estimated annual bed days). Part D makes it clear, however, that while the total number of bed days probably increased over the first year, there has been a sizable increase in the efficiency of the use in beds as measured by annual bed use per child served (from a high of 25.07 bed days in a year per child served in June 1990 to 5.75 in February 1991). In summary, the data in Table 8.2 provide evidence that the Ft. Bragg/CHAMPUS has become more efficient in the use of residential placements, but that the total number of residential days has continued to increase. There are two reasons: (1) there was an enormous increase in active cases served by the project and (2) the utilization of hospital beds did not keep pace with the decrease in the use of RTC beds.

These divergent trends—increased efficiency in the use of residential placements and the expansion in total residential days on a daily and annual basis—have implications for a preliminary assessment of cost-effectiveness. If by cost-effectiveness we mean the residential cost per child served, then part A of Table 8.3 provides strong evidence that the mental health services provided to Ft. Bragg/CHAMPUS youth have become much more cost-efficient. There are savings per child served in the total program on an annual basis for each residential type. Although the Ft. Bragg/CHAMPUS project has probably become much more cost-efficient in the use of out-of-home placements, it is quite likely that the Army will actually pay more for the use of hospitals by the end of the year (about $1,157,926). The estimated savings from the reduced reliance on RTC annual bed days is, as depicted in part B, not sufficient to offset the increase the residential bill by over $800,000.

This complex outcome should caution us against prematurely concluding that a gain in social and economic efficiency will automatically be associated with actual social and fiscal savings. Besides the cost of a new non-residential system, there are divergent trends that cannot be ignored. When the number of targeted youth receiving services increases appreciably, as has definitely occurred, the increased supply of youth to be served may offset the reduction in residential service utilization. This is particularly the case if the most expensive residential type—the psychiatric hospital—has an actual increase in the number of daily slots. It is possible of course that the total Ft. Bragg model will prove less costly than the comparison programs at Fort Campbell and Stewart. It is also possible, that by the end of the 4th year the Ft. Bragg/CHAMPUS project will be able to further reduce reliance on psychiatric hospitals and increase alternative residential and nonresidential services. If it cannot accomplish this ideal design goal effectively, an overall assessment may have to await empirical evidence that the increase in youth served and the implementation of a full-service continuum produces social benefits in the form of improved functioning by youth at home, in school, and in the community. The Brickman evaluation may help to assess these and related policy issues when a fuller analysis is conducted that includes more information about the demonstration's social impacts and fiscal costs as well as comparisons with two comparable military communities.

The Ventura County Cost-Offset Model

The designers of California's Ventura County model, in contrast to the planners of the Ft. Bragg/CHAMPUS project, are *not* interested in creating a "full continuum" of care based on an ideal service system (Feltman & Essex, 1989). They believe that an ideal model approach toward improving mental health services has the following "major shortcomings": (1) It "ignores the variations across localities and populations," which require varying mixes of types and amounts of services; (2) it sets standards that are absolute, without prescribing specific outcome measures of benefit, and, therefore, "does not provide a rationale for policy makers to fund those services"; and (3) the ideal standards of service that are proposed by professionals are so vastly different from current standards that "policy makers simply have not taken the standards seriously" (Jordan & Hernandez, 1990, pp. 27–28).

In contrast to the ideal standards model, the Ventura Planning Model was conceived as a strategic approach for capturing more state funds for mental health services at a time of "tight fiscal constraints on human service programs" (Jordan & Hernandez, 1990, p. 28) in California (and other states). The Ventura designers believe that more funds can be captured if mental health organizations can offer policy makers a "return on their investment." On the basis of their own positive experience with an earlier small demonstration project to reduce state hospital utilization, Jordan and Hernandez (1990) offer the following planning strategy: A state legislature will "respond positively to the concept of 'cost-offsets' or 'cost avoidance' which defines cost-benefits in terms of avoiding expenditures in other funding categories due to the services provided" (p. 28). The evidence offered by the Ventura cost-offset model has been accepted by the California state legislature and approved by a conservative governor to such an extent that the initial Children's Demonstration Project in Ventura County was provided with permanent funding, and additional funds were provided for projects in three other counties in California via the Children's Mental Health Service Act of 1987 (Jordan & Hernandez, 1990). In addition, Ventura County was provided with a $16 million grant to extend the Ventura County Planning Model to adults and seniors.

The evidence for conceiving the Ventura County Planning Model as a "success" was assembled, analyzed, and presented by the county's evaluation staff, using methods to calculate outcomes "negotiated in a series of meetings with the State Department of Finance" (Jordan & Hernandez, 1990, p. 42). Using criteria similar to those employed by Ventura County, the California Department of Mental Health has contracted with researchers at the University of California, San Francisco, to assess the replication of Ventura's results in three other counties: San Mateo (youth population of 142,486), Santa Cruz (youth population of 54,704), and Riverside (youth population of 333,261). Research reports describing the target populations and services added by the three new counties have begun to appear in unpublished and published papers and are referred to where appropriate (Rosenblatt & Attkisson, 1992; Attkisson et al., 1991).

The designers of the Ventura County model did not start with a formal planning guide to mental health programming. As the designers readily admit, the approach began as a specific set of programs to function as an alternative to reducing state hospitalization, evolved into "subsystems of care," and then finally as a set of planning procedures. Jordan and Hernandez (1990) believe that the procedures are now "designed to be generic" and are applicable to other localities, where specific local needs and program interests can produce "widely different systems of care" (p. 28). The Ventura model combines five major planning components, or steps, which are set forth as a framework for planning systems of care: (1) define the target population precisely, (2) define goals that are objective and measurable, (3) develop interagency coalitions and agreements, (4) develop new services and program standards, and (5) evaluate the social and cost effectiveness of the system.

Define the Target Population Precisely

It is critical to use criteria that give first priority to children removed, or at-risk of removal, from their homes. Planners should identify by individual cases the subpopulation within this at-risk population that are seriously emotionally disordered *and* at higher risk of becoming the legal responsibility or fiscal liability of the public sector. Operationally, Ventura used three combined criteria to identify individuals who have first priority: Each youth must (1) have a DSM-III-R diagnosis; (2) have a severe functional impairment in the home, community, and school; and (3) be in an out-of-home foster home placement or at risk of placement in a group, residential home, or psychiatric hospital. It is important to note that the at-risk placements are those where *state* funding is substantial. The at-risk concept is a limited one. Local detention halls, county correctional facilities, and local psychiatric units of general hospitals, disproportionately funded by local or private insurance funds, are not included in the at-risk definitions. The total annual at-risk case load consisted of about 1,200 youths, representing less than 1% (0.6% of the under-18 population). Juvenile court wards, dependents, and special education pupils each accounted for about 30% of the total case load, and about 10% were other youth at risk of placement.

Define Goals That Are Objective and Measurable

The county's "overarching goal" was to help youth remain with their families and their communities, if possible. This goal was accompanied by the aim of utilizing placements that were the least restrictive and least costly consistent with the youth's needs. County staff reached agreement with state legislative staff that goal achievement could be achieved by meeting the following outcome: either 100% offset of state costs or 50% offset of state costs plus a list of beneficial social outcomes (e.g., improvements in school attendance and performance and reduction in out-of-county placements).

Develop Interagency Coalitions and Agreements

The achievement of the goals required extensive interagency collaboration in the use of staff, funds, and program resources. New mental health dollars—about $1.5 million per year—were used as a "catalyst for the blending of services." Formal agreements specifying each agency's responsibility at points of system entry, intervention, and aftercare were specified in contracts between mental health and special education, public social services, and local correction agencies. Besides these interagency agreements, an Interagency Case Management Council was created as a placement regulatory mechanism and as a forum to "assess, plan, link monitor, and advocate for particularly difficult cases" (Jordan & Hernandez, 1990, p. 38). The county also created a private-sector "Youth Correction Board" to acquire additional resources on behalf of targeted youth; examples of private donations achieved through this novel mechanism included a dentist contributing one examination and a set of fillings and a retailer contributing one set of clothes per year.

Develop New Services and Program Standards

At the outset, new funds helped to develop extra services attached to existing programs. Over time, the new services were conceived into categories of services that were deemed useful by interagency members. Between 1985 and 1990, an array of discrete services was developed; later, the services were assigned to three categories of programs and services. The programs associated with each category constitute the Ventura version of a continuum of services for seriously disturbed youth at risk of placement in a state-funded facility. Jordan and Hernandez (1990) describe the programs as follows:*

> I. *Family Preservation Programs*—Mental health programs which serve as
>   alternatives to residential placement.
>   1. Intensive outpatient services (up to eight hours a week, community or
>   clinic based)

*Copyright 1990 by the Association of Mental Health Administrators. Reprinted by permission.

2. Enriched classes for the seriously emotionally disturbed (mental health staff work in the schools)
3. Juvenile sex offender program (Outpatient services for juvenile justice wards)
4. Genesis Crisis Program (Intensive-up to 20 hours a week-in-home services)
5. Phoenix School Day Care (School site jointly operated by Ventura County Schools and Mental Health)
6. VIP Day Care (School site jointly operated by Ventura County Schools and Mental Health)
7. Shomair Enriched Foster Care (Mental health services provided to dependents in foster care)
8. Youth Connection Resources Project (Outreach to the private sector to get needed resources for children and youth. Each private provider is asked to donate "one unit" of goods or services, e.g., one dental exam and set of fillings, one set of clothing, one medical treatment)

II. *Family Reunification Programs*—Time-limited, local residential alternatives to long-term AFDC-FC Group Home placement and state hospitalization.
   1. Colston Intensive Intervention Program (Corrections residential facility with on-site mental health day treatment for juvenile justice wards)
   2. Interface Crisis Residential Home (contract service funded by the mental health department)
   3. Santa Rosa Treatment Home (contract service funded by the mental health department)
   4. Hobbs Landing

III. *Case Management*—Monitoring and control of residential placements and state hospital utilization.
   1. Mental Health case Management Team (10 staff)
   2. Juvenile Justice Placement Screening Committee (resolves disagreements between agencies regarding specific seriously emotionally disturbed juvenile justice wards)
   3. Protective Services Placement Screening Committee (resolves disagreements between agencies regarding specific seriously emotionally disturbed dependents)
   4. Expanded special education IEP (Individualized Education Plan) teams for residential candidates
   5. Interagency Case Management Council (sets overall policy and resolves differences between agencies) (pp. 39–40)

Probably the most unique characteristic of these services are the labels provided for categories II and III. Category II might be reasonably conceived to refer to postresidence services, but in the Ventura model the components refer to four county-based and locally funded out-of-home placements, used as alternatives to out-of-county, state-funded placements. Category III might be reasonably conceived to refer to individual case management of cases, but in the Ventura model the components refer primarily to organizational mechanisms for screening the use and location of out-of-home placements for three referral sources: (1) the juvenile court, (2) the local child welfare system, and (3) the special education teams. The "screening committees" appear to be a critical ingredient for ensuring that improper placements—especially to state-funded systems—do not occur without explicit legitimation by interagency personnel.

Evaluate the Social and Cost Effectiveness of the System

The county attempted to implement a dual evaluation system. The first evaluation was designed to provide information to external funding agencies, and it focused on the social and cost effectiveness of new mental health funds. The second evaluation was designed to provide internal information for those organizations and staff collaborating in the demonstration project.

The social and fiscal evaluations, developed by the county to persuade state funding sources to permanently fund the Ventura model and to replicate the reform in other counties, are reproduced in Tables 8.4 and 8.5. Table 8.4 summarizes the treatment and outcome goals achieved over a 3-year period.

The left-hand column of Table 8.4 specifies the specific outcome goals that the county promised to the state legislature, the State Department of Finance, and the State Department of Mental Health. All the major goals were actually exceeded, except for the recidivism of juvenile offenders. Rates of incarceration were actually lower for the jointly operated, and locally based, Colston Youth Center, but the number of bed days increased. Jordan and Hernandez (1990) claim that the local judge tended to give longer sentences since the demonstration project began. Recently, a new judge was appointed and he has implemented an even tougher sentencing policy than previous judges had. Evidently, the planning model collaborators were unable to persuade these judges to become cooperative members of the Juvenile Justice Placement Screening Committee.

Despite the difficulty in assessing the juvenile corrections goal, it is evident that the county was quite successful in reducing out-of-county placements for all the other social groups listed in Table 8.4. In addition, the demonstration project was associated with improved school attendance at the school-based day-treatment program and had an impact on academic performance. All the social comparisons of Table 8.4 are based on assessments of change of the youth acting as their own control, with before measures functioning as a baseline for evaluating success.

Table 8.5 provides the fiscal data associated with the levels of success reported in Table 8.4. The second column—costs avoided—actually refers to state costs avoided. The dollar amounts related to each category are the amounts associated with the reductions in out-of-county placements. The third column calculates the percentage of the project's state funding that the cost avoided represents as a "cost-offset." Even with the juvenile incarcera-

TABLE 8.4. Treatment and Outcome Goals Required by Ventura Project

Treatment-oriented goals to be met	Project outcome	Was substantial compliance achieved?
A 20% reduction in out-of-county court-ordered placements of juvenile justice wards and social service dependents	Down 47%	Exceeded
A statistically significant reduction in rate of recidivism by juvenile offenders participating in the demonstration project	Episodes down 22%, days up 28%	Met[a]
A 25% reduction in rate of state hospitalization of minors from the 1980–1981 level	Down 68%[b]	Exceeded
A 10% reduction in rate of out-of-county nonpublic school residential placements of special education pupils	Down 21%	Exceeded
Allow at least 50% of children at risk of imminent placement served by the intensive in-home crisis treatment program to remain at home at least 6 months	85% have stayed at home more than 6 months	Exceeded
Statistically significant improvement in school attendance and academic performance, of mentally disordered special education pupils treated in the demonstration project's day treatment program	Significant gains in attendance and academic performance	Exceeded

[a]Please see text.
[b]7-year average.

tion costs omitted, the overall offset is 66.4%—a figure higher than the 50% figure agreed to by the state legislature.

From a societal perspective, we lack any information about whether the county increased any additional fiscal costs as a result of the demonstration project. We also lack information on the noncorrectional rates and duration of local out-of-home placements before and after the project, which is necessary in order to assess whether *overall* utilizations of out-of-home placement also decreased. We know that the new funds supported local residential alternatives, but we are not in a position to assess whether these placements were less restrictive and balanced out-of-county reductions. Finally, we lack information about the consequences of the county's policies on incidents of abuse or neglect in homes or institutions.

TABLE 8.5. Cost Avoidance Outcomes Required by AB 377

Costs avoided	State costs avoided	Percentage of project costs ($1,528,265)
Group home costs paid by Aid to Families with Dependent Children (AFDC)	$ 410,775	26.9
Child and adolescent state hospital programs	415,178	27.2
Nonpublic school residential placement costs	109,229	7.2
Juvenile justice incarceration costs	NA[a]	NA[a]
Other savings: special education placement	78,130	5.1
Total short- and long-term cost avoidance	$1,013,852	66.4

Note. NA = not available.
[a]Please see text.

It is possible that the evaluations of the replications in the three new counties will provide more detailed information on the actual residential and treatment experiences and costs of the target youth in their home counties and not just focus on the avoidance of out-of-county placements and costs. Early reports by Attkisson and his colleagues have not yet provided implementation and outcome data, but they have yielded information on the characteristics of the target groups chosen and the new services that emerged from the planning process. The target populations range from 0.39% of youth population in San Mateo to 0.94% in Santa Cruz to 1.5% in Riverside. The youth tend to be older, with low scores on adaptive functioning, and DSM-III-R diagnoses that indicate a high involvement in antisocial activities. Diagnoses referring to "disruptive behavior," "adjustment disorders," and "substance abuse" refer to about 58% of the youth, and "mood disorders" for about 22% (Rosenblatt & Attkisson, 1992).

Attkisson and his colleagues report that the three counties have developed services similar to Ventura County's even though they were free to develop individual programs. All three provide case management to link and coordinate services. All make placement decisions though interagency screening committees, as was done in Ventura County. And all three counties provide mental health services within other local systems. For example, they have therapeutic day-treatment programs in schools, in-home services to foster parents, mental health programs in detention halls, and mental health programs within the county correctional residential facilities operated by probation departments. The "specific characteristics" of these service offerings may vary (like a Wilderness program in mountainous Santa Cruz), but on the whole there appears to be a consensus on providing case management services for Ventura-type services within other systems and mechanisms for controlling out-of-county placements. It is quite likely that if the three replicating counties are successful in reducing out-of-county placements—particularly in group homes—there will be a disproportionate impact on abused and neglected youth. A companion study of a control county, San Francisco, revealed that approximately two thirds of a sample of "multiple placement youth" had definitely or possibly experienced some type of abuse and neglect (Cornsweet, Rosenblatt, Harris, & Attkisson, 1991). If these findings occur in the replication counties, and if the analyses focus special attention on these youth, the final evaluation by Attkisson and his colleagues will have impact beyond the field of mental health.

The Alaska Youth Initiative

The discussion and assessments of the Ft. Bragg/CHAMPUS and Ventura system reforms highlighted the differences between changes based on an ideal versus a cost-offset design of mental health services for children and youth. While the differences between the ideal and cost-offset designs are quite apparent regarding the target group served and evaluational criteria, they both rely on a varied number of specific program components as the necessary building blocks of a comprehensive and responsive service system. In contrast, the Alaska Youth Initiative (AYI) is based on creating unique service packages to "wrap around" each individual that may not include existing program components. The leaders of this distinct system reform describe their "new services model" as follows:

> In the traditional "categorical" model of services, children are brought into preexisting programs and intervention models. When their needs are not met, they are referred elsewhere. In an "individualized" model of services, an interdisciplinary team of persons (including the parents) sit down and ask the question "What does this youth need so that they can get better?" The team looks at not only the medical areas, but family, friends, vocational, educational, psychological, safety, economic, and other areas of need. The team agrees that they will offer the youth unconditional care. This means that if his or her needs are not met, their individualized program will be changed, and that the youth cannot be "kicked out." Individualized services programs such as AYI are not totally state run nor totally privately run, but are partnerships of state and private agencies. (Van Den Berg, Sewall, & Kubley, 1991, pp. 2–3)

Examples of individualized care include the following cases:

1. A 15-year-old boy with schizophrenia was at risk for out-of-state placement. AYI made a commitment to keep the youth in his home community in Alaska. The boy had lost all his friends because of his bizarre and frightening behaviors. The local treatment team decided to hire a teenager to spend time with the boy. The "hired friend" was trained by a psychiatrist in understanding the illness, including the identification of the behaviors that might signal the need for special help. After several months, the two boys

became friends and other teenagers become less fearful of interacting with the mentally ill boy. Gradually, the financial arrangements with the hired friend and the training sessions with the psychiatrist were phased out (Moran, 1991, p. 9).

2. A 16-year-old girl had been in several group and foster homes before being considered for out-of-state placement. She first came to the attention of school authorities because she had arrived at school unbathed and disheveled and had minimal social skills. AYI found a concerned grandmother, went to court to help her gain custody, and then trained the grandmother in how to deal with the girl's "negativistic, hostile, and defiant" behaviors. AYI furnished tutoring and crisis services and the team was made available on a daily basis. The girl began attending classes regularly and had good prospects for completing high school and perhaps attending college (Moran, 1991, p. 9).

3. A 16-year-old Eskimo boy uninterested in school and at risk of out-of-state placement for deviant behaviors was found to have an interest in fishing. The team contracted with a 25-year-old Eskimo male to house the youth and teach him how to become a commercial fisherman. The youth accepted the arrangement and now has a career goal (Van Den Berg, 1989, p. 17).

These cases illustrate the meaning of individualized care in action. As might be expected, the cost of tailor-made efforts, designed to last as long as necessary to maintain youths in normal settings, can be quite costly. The 1st-year cost for designing individual service packages amounted to $40,000 per year per child. The cost per capita has reportedly been reduced since 1986, but 1990 data still disclose a cost of over $40,000 per year for each of the 65 active cases (Burchard & Clarke, 1990; and analysis of data reported in Van Den Berg et al., 1991). While the cost is a high one, especially in the 1st year of care, it is not as high as the $72,000 per year that Alaska paid for sending youth out of state when the project began in 1986. If the individualized care model had not been implemented to keep youth in Alaska, the 1990 cost might have been well over $100,000 per year for out-of-state care (Van Den Berg et al., 1991).

The state of Alaska believes it is saving money by funding AYI on a permanent basis as a unique service system. In addition, the legislature authorized more than $600,000 to develop individualized care services for developmentally disabled adults and children. Adult programs for mentally ill adults with special problems are also being modified to include individualized care services. The NIMH is sufficiently interested in AYI and similar individualized service systems that it is funding a 5-year longitudinal study to track and evaluate 240 youth in six states (including Alaska). The study will be led by the University of Southern Florida's Mental Health Institutes (Van Den Berg, 1989).

In order to fully understand the ingredients and potential worth of the AYI model, a brief account of its origins and development will be useful.

Otherwise, the model could appear as unusually idealistic and devoid of political, fiscal, and interorganizational realities. Prior to the 1970s, Alaska had close to 200 youth in out-of-state care at any one time. By the late 1970s this figure was reduced to 90 youth, primarily because Alaska had developed in-state residential facilities for seriously disturbed youth. During the early 1980s, the number of youth that the new in-state residential system could not handle—and was referring for out-of-state treatment, care, and custody—fluctuated between 40 and 90. According to Van Den Berg, coordinator of both AYI and Child and Mental Health Services for the state, the fluctuations were primarily due to the relative availability of residential placement funds from three state-level departments: (1) the Division of Family and Youth Services (DFYS), serving youth associated with the child welfare and juvenile justice system; (2) the Department of Education (DOE), serving youth unable to function in local school programs; and (3) the Division of Mental Health and Developmental Disabilities (DMHDD). During restrictive budget cycles, youth were actually retrieved from out-of-state placements and "put back into their communities without additional services" (Van Den Berg, 1989, p. 11). If youth turned 18 while in out-of-state placement, they were voluntarily or involuntarily returned to Alaska.

By 1985, there was sufficient pressure from schools, child welfare officials, and juvenile justice agencies to place greater numbers of youth out of state that a state-level interdepartmental team (IDT) was formed, composed of senior staff from DFYS, DOE, and DMHDD. The IDT members decided to conduct a national search for programs that appeared successful in returning out-of-state youth to their own communities. They found a promising service system model in Illinois, named Kaleidoscope, to capture its multifaceted approach to serving over 2,000 youth living in out-of-state facilities. Kaleidoscope served as the initial model for the IDT staff. The Illinois service model provided the following component services: home-based supportive services, therapeutic foster care, vocational services, group homes, and case management. In addition, Kaleidoscope had a program philosophy that emphasized three basic tenets: (1) "unconditional care," defined as "never giving up on a youth"; (2) "normalization," defined as living in a family or family-like environment; and (3) individual programming, regardless of problem severity or disability (Van Den Berg, 1989).

The IDT believed that Kaleidoscope was effective in serving disturbed youth even though the program had no published or unpublished outcome data. Kaleidoscope staff came to Alaska, under contract, to demonstrate the applicability of the Illinois model to Alaska's out-of-state youth population. The first efforts to emulate Kaleidoscope's types of alternative residential facilities and services for returning youth were soon proven unsuccessful. The IDT staff then began pragmatically to construct a "totally individually configured intervention" for each youth. These new efforts were guided by the belief of the IDT staff that the philosophy of Kaleidoscope was still valid— unconditional care, normalization, and individual programming—but the preconceived program models were a failure if applied in a stereotypical fashion. The new model for out-of-state youth was given the specific title "Alaska Youth Initiative" in 1986. The title of "coordinator" was given to Van Den Berg, who had been hired (with federal seed money) to become the state's first head of children and adolescent mental health services in DMHDD.

An external federal review team, reporting in 1990, contended that the choice of Van Den Berg was important to Alaska's success in creating an improved mental health system for youth. According to the review team, Van Den Berg's role in creating AYI was part of a broad "articulated strategy for system development" that included the following "principles":

> 1) *Start Small*—Establish new programs on a small scale at specific sites in order to demonstrate that innovations can be developed and that they are useful to participants;
> 2) *Flexible Funds*—Create pools of funds that can be used to buy services for specific cases, rather than spending funds to create and maintain categorical service programs;
> 3) *Collaborate Around Specific Cases*—Improve interagency collaboration and coordination by focusing on providing services for specific cases, relying on the assumption that agencies will collaborate more frequently when they learn that it is in their interest. (Schlenger et al., 1990, p. 5)

Under Van Den Berg's leadership, the IDT established goals and operational guidelines and functioned as a statewide referral screening board and monitoring team for AYI. As of 1986, AYI had three paramount goals, which were still on the agenda in the 1990 annual report:

> Limit further inappropriate institutional and out-of-state placements; . . .
> Transition back our youth who have been placed out-of- state; . . .
> Provide special individualized case planning, monitoring, program development, and funding for youth and their families. (Van Den Berg et al., 1991, p. 2)

The first operational decision, in 1986, involved an agreement by the three major state agencies that youth would be brought back to the state with funds that were currently subsidizing out-of-state placements. The "dollars would follow the children" and could be used flexibly for any type of service that would meet the needs of youth; the only formal exception was that funds could not be used to pay a parent to care for their own children. A second operational decision was that DMHDD would fund the administrative costs for managing AYI. While the funds were flexibly assigned on a case-by-case basis by each state agency, there was no single AYI fund budgeted and managed as a distinct entity at the beginning of 1991 (Van Den Berg et al., 1991, p. 20).

The third major decision involved the assumption of a high risk to AYI.

Instead of screening for the easiest cases, the IDT staff decided to bring back youth from out-of-state in the relative order of the severity of their disability. By starting with the most disabled first, the IDT staff reasoned that if AYI was effective with these youth, critics could not contend that it worked for "easy" cases but it could never work for more "severe kids" (Van Den Berg, 1989, p. 14).

A fourth area of early decision making focused on reducing the financial incentives to child-serving agencies to promote out-of-community placement. Local school districts, prior to 1986, were encouraged to promote placements because their responsibility for education was ended if youth were placed out of district. Using the power of administrative regulations, the leaders of DOE promulgated new rules that stated that school districts would continue to be responsible for educating local youth, regardless of whether the youth was placed out of district. According to Van Den Berg, fiscal contingencies also operated within the child welfare and juvenile justice system, and these incentives encouraged referrals for out-of-state care. The AYI staff were unable to change the fiscal incentives, but they were successful in persuading state officials in DFYS to administratively order the regional office not to recommend out-of-state placements (Van Den Berg, 1989, p. 15).

As the number of cases scheduled to return increased, AYI's administrative structure decentralized to include three regional coordinators, located in Anchorage, Fairbanks, and Juneau. The regional coordinators became responsible for assembling the local "treatment and education team" for each youth. These teams can include "influentials in the child's life" such as relatives, parents, attorneys, social workers, teachers, or any one else deemed appropriate. The teams are encouraged to seek solutions "uninhibited by cost or practicality of the suggestions" (Van Den Berg, 1989, p. 17).

By the beginning of the 2nd year, pressures began to build from local communities to serve youth who could qualify to be placed out of state but were prevented by DFYS and DOE regulations. They argued that with the funds saved from bringing youth back home, additional youth could be served. The IDT staff agreed but had to confront the issue of choosing criteria other than qualifying as an out-of-state youth. According to recent reports, deciding on eligibility for AYI services continues to be "a complex problem to solve" (Van Den Berg, 1989, p. 20). The IDT staff—at a state level—still make all acceptance decisions but do not use DSM-III-R or other specific diagnostic criteria or instruments. The staff contend that local political pressures to get rid of local troublemakers and fiscal contingencies can still operate, so each case must be assessed on a case-by-case basis. In the first 2 years, IDT staff relied on consensus, but as cases increased they began to rely on majority vote. In 1989, about 60% of AYI referrals were rejected (Van Den Berg, 1989, p. 21).

According to a participant in eligibility determinations, the IDT staff relied mainly on this central question for deciding AYI eligibility: Is there clear and convincing evidence that the key decision makers for a given youth have exhausted the entire array of relevant "component" services within that youth's community-of-tie such that the youth now already is, or stands at imminent risk for being placed, in unduly restrictive out-of-region placement? If the answer is yes to this question, the youth is found AYI eligible (Sewall, 1990). It appears that the IDT screening decisions are operationally guided by the availability and prior utilization of all local services as well as the "imminent risk" of out-of-region placements. In effect, AYI is conceding that its service model relies on the existence of an entire array of relevant component services. Burchard and Clarke (1990), developers of a Vermont version of "wraparound" services, concur in this viewpoint, by arguing that "individualized care should be used to supplement the component care system and to target those children who are falling through the cracks" (p. 58). The pragmatic availability of funding resources, as well as program philosophy, guides eligibility decisions.

By the end of 1990, the referral rate to AYI had grown much faster than had the available resources. AYI now accepts more youth for individualized services than it can fund. If deemed eligible by IDT staff but not served, the accepted referrals are placed on a list of "unfunded youth." A team is formed and prepares a tentative plan and budget for each unfunded youth. AYI attempts to use this mechanism to notify the appropriate division directors providing funds (i.e., DOE, DFYS, and DMHDD) of the "status of the fiscal need [for services] for Alaska's most disturbed youth" (Van Den Berg et al., 1991, pp. 11–12).

As of January 1991, AYI served about 65 youth and had an unfunded list of 15 youth (Van Den Berg et al., 1991, p. 1). Alaska natives and other minorities comprise over 50% of the active AYI case load. The average age of acceptance has been reduced from 15.2 in 1987 to 14.2 in 1991. Youth with "conduct disorders" constitute a large proportion of the most difficult cases (Van Den Berg, 1991, p. 13, 18).

As AYI began to develop from an initiative into an ongoing service model, the leadership attempted to articulate the principal features that had emerged in the development of a philosophy of individualized, or wraparound, services. Ten features have now been identified:

1. Building and maintaining normative lifestyles.
2. Insuring that services are client-centered.
3. Providing unconditional care.
4. Planning for the long term.
5. Working toward less restrictive alternatives.
6. Achieving provider competencies.
7. Establishing consensus among key decision makers.
8. Funding services with flexible budgets.
9. Installing a "gatekeeper" function
10. Developing measurable accountability. (Van Den Berg et al., 1991, p. 5)

By the beginning of 1991, AYI claimed that implementation of these principal features had achieved the following positive program outcomes:

1. Only 2 out of 117 AYI youth have been placed out-of-state, and both of these occurred in the first two years;
2. No youth returned to Alaska through AYI has had to go back;
3. AYI has established itself as a "viable alternative" to institutionalization, and is now recognized as a national leader in developing the individualized care model. (Van Den Berg et al., 1991, p. 2)

Besides establishing a viable alternative to out-of-state placements, Van Den Berg and his colleagues in mental health could also point to the development of less intrusive component services for youth who need not be candidates for AYI. In 1985, the year planning for AYI began, the total number of youth in Alaska receiving an outpatient assessment or treatment was about 1,000; by 1989, this figure increased to about 1,900. While nearly doubling the capability of the mental health system to function as a first step in the delivery of services to youth, the following services were added: (1) day treatment (from 0 to 85 slots), (2) home-based services (from 0 to 90 slots), (3) therapeutic foster care (from 2 to 40 slots), (4) therapeutic camping (from 0 to 35 slots), (5) independent living service (from 0 to 40 slots), and flexible-funded services within mental health centers (from 0 to 80 slots). This sizable extension of the component care system was accompanied by a drop in the use of hospitals and residential treatment centers—from a total of 81 admissions for 1,000 youth to 77 admissions for 1,900 youth (or from 8.1% to 4.1% of the potential case load) (Schlenger et al., 1990, p. A-4).

Although AYI leaders are aware of their success in expanding the component care system and in virtually eliminating out-of-state care with a much less restrictive, more normalized mode of service, they are also aware of AYI implementation problems. Some of the deficiencies were noted by parents, advocates, and providers, whereas others were disclosed as part of a major external review by Burchard (the Vermont developer of an individualized care model). The following problems were noted in the 1991 annual report (Van Den Berg et al., 1991):

1. AYI has had less success with youth who entered the program at age 17 or older and youth who have an extensive involvement with the juvenile justice system.
2. The philosophy of the model is not always followed in practice by providers, indicating that they need "better and more frequent" training about "how to" deliver individualized services and that providers need to be monitored on a more frequent schedule.
3. AYI local staff also require more frequent and systematic training.

4. Fiscal management and budgeting procedures for each case are sometime careless and need to be systematized in a procedures manual.
5. Policies and procedures for providing liability protection for staff and providers need improvement and should be part of the AYI procedures manual.
6. Records and documents are not handled in an orderly manner and require systematic filing procedures.
7. Methods for tracking and measuring services outcome need to be improved.
8. Methods for recruiting, training, and maintaining "specialized foster parents" need to be more adequately implemented and improved.
9. Explicit policies for how and when youth are discharged have to be identified, so that new service slots can be opened for unfunded youth.
10. Better methods for recruiting agencies to be providers have to be developed.

Comparable problems of dealing with program integrity, training, monitoring, and administration can be ascribed to many service delivery systems. However, the leadership of AYI have begun to accept and work on these problems (Van Den Berg et al., 1991; Burchard & Clarke, 1990). Maintaining an open, self-critical, and nondefensive stance toward service delivery issues is an important organizational ingredient possessed by AYI under Van Den Berg's leadership. Whether a spirit of organizational openness will continue under a new generation of leaders remains to be seen.

Summary and Conclusions

Each mental health system reform discussed in this chapter has a distinct philosophy, target population, and referral sources. Yet each reform model is also guided by the objective of reducing reliance on restrictive types of institutions and providing a comprehensive array of services at a local level. Besides providing alternative services as one aspect of reducing out-of-home placements, each system relies on internal control mechanisms to screen placement decisions, in order to make certain that placements are in fact reduced. The Ft. Bragg/CHAMPUS project uses the treatment assessment team, Ventura uses a screening committee for each major residential system, and AYI uses a state-level IDT to make certain that youth are not placed out of state. The screening mechanisms of each system appear as critical to the "success" of reducing out-of-home placements as the provision of alternative services. The screeners may need to believe that alternative services exist and can replace a residential-type placement, and the service personnel may need a screening mechanism in place in order to ensure that results are actually achieved. Without devising organizational controls for regulating discretionary decisions to place, systems run the risk of merely adding on services and costs without showing results that justify them.

Besides incorporating screening mechanisms to deter placements by judges, clinicians, and social workers, each system has devised mechanisms for obtaining high degrees of flexibility in spending funds. Ft. Bragg/ CHAMPUS administrators have access to funds that can be used for any mix of service approved by the treatment team, as long as utilization of hospitals and RTCs is monitored and controlled. Ventura's mental health money is blended with other funds and allocated according to the decision of the case management council members. The AYI deliberately obtains funds from multiple state-level, categorical funding sources and then blends them into a single pool of funds to be used by regional treatment teams. The flexibility of funding makes it easier not only to deliver a less stereotypical package of services, but also to provide incentives for interagency cooperation and coordination. Appealing to ideals of client-centered services and cooperation is undoubtedly made easier when incentives are forthcoming.

States and communities interested in reforming their mental health services to achieve a reduction of out-of-home placements can be attracted to each model for solving local problems. If there is interest and available resources to create an "ideal system" of services, the CHAMPUS model for delivering services and regulating placement could prove quite useful. If there is interest in achieving more specific types of institutional reduction outside the mental health system within a limited time period, the Ventura cost-offset model could prove attractive. And if there are youth who cannot be served adequately by either an ideal or cost-offset component-type system, the AYI individualized care approach could be useful. It is quite conceivable that a reconceptualized ideal system could use elements of each approach in designing models that can achieve multiple objectives for multiple targets of youth in trouble.

It is prudent to remember, however, that the evidence on behalf of each model is provisional and requires further evaluation and replication. Particularly necessary are research assessments that can determine whether the mix of new services—either component or individually tailored—has an impact on the precipitating behavioral, social, cognitive, emotional, and relational problems that trigger referrals to a mental health system. Current evaluations tend to emphasize out-of-home placement reductions and fiscal savings per capita served, but there is still insufficient empirical evidence that youth are really "better off" for having been clients of the referred systems. Ventura County has made the biggest strides in terms of assessing school behaviors, but much more is needed to yield convincing evidence that families function more smoothly, youth are less deviant, and presenting psychiatric symptoms have been reduced.

While we await better empirical evidence concerning the efficacy of each model, it is important to remember that the alternatives—psychiatric hospitals, RTCs, and training schools—have yet to prove effective in changing behaviors. Given the risks of institutional abuse, higher fiscal costs, and an unproven record of empirical accomplishments, continued experimentation with the three system reforms is warranted and promising.

SERVICE SYSTEM REFORM: CHILD WELFARE AND JUVENILE CORRECTIONS

About 20 years ago, Massachusetts reformed its juvenile corrections system by taking an unprecedented action: All long-term, custodial training schools were closed. This drastic step was taken after a new commissioner of youth services, Jerome Miller, concluded that the old system—which included staff beatings, uniform dress codes, short haircuts, and other dehumanizing acts—was incapable of being reformed into a "therapeutic" community. Almost overnight, Massachusetts created a number of state-funded, administratively decentralized, community-based residential units that were small, mainly privately operated, and more humane in spirit and practice. Since 1972, the community-based system has endured even though there have been four commissioners and a change in political climate subsequent to the Miller era. The Massachusetts model of juvenile corrections continues to function as the national exemplar of humane treatment of juvenile offenders. The most recent version, and its replication in Utah, is certainly worth consideration as a component of a comprehensive child care protection policy (Coates, Miller, & Ohlin, 1978; Austin et al., 1991; Schwartz & Loughran, 1991).

While not as dramatic as the overnight closing of a state training school, Iowa's decategorization of state-funded child welfare service may soon become another exemplar for delivering services in a less centralized fashion. By deregulating 30 child welfare funding categories into one pool of flexible funds, the state of Iowa is offering counties an opportunity to tailor local child and family services to the preferences of community policymakers and providers—rather than to the criteria associated with state-promulgated regulations (Bruner, 1989). The origins and implementation of the Iowa model will be discussed first, followed by a discussion of the Massachusetts corrections model of system reform.

Decategorization of Child Welfare Services in Iowa

Between 1982 and 1987 the rate of foster care placements of Iowa youth increased by about 40%. During the same period, the state's youth population declined by 8%. During this time many placements occurred out of state because Iowa lacked the foster parents and residential facilities to match the out-of-home demand. Policymakers in the state legislature were concerned about the transfer of $750,000 out of state and the loss of jobs, as well as the attenuation of family and community ties by the displaced youth. The state's policymakers were also concerned that by 1987, fully 90% of the child welfare budget was absorbed by out-of-home placement costs, while only 10% could be used for family-based services. In response to these considerations, the state was quite receptive to funding the initiation of family preservation services—of the Home builders type—as a new component program within the county-based child welfare systems (Bruner, 1989).

The Homebuilder projects were evaluated by the counties as being quite successful in helping families remain intact a year after receiving services (Kassar, 1991). Perceiving a success rate of 66%, planners sought increased funds for family preservation services. However, they discovered that "the traditional funding system placed severe constraints on investing in placement-prevention services and, in fact, often rewarded placement responses to families in crises" (Kassar, 1991, p. 6). For example, maximum federal funds were contributed only when children entered foster care and not for placement-prevention services.

In order to locate funds for more home-centered services, without having to vote for additional revenues from the state treasury, creative policymakers sought to capture existing funds for new services. They identified 30 specific funding categories that had 30 sets of rules and regulations concerning eligibility criteria. These included child welfare funds associated with (1) the state portion of subsidized foster care; (2) in-home services; (3) direct Department of Human Service (DHS) services; (4) day care; (5) adoption; and (6) institutional care for delinquents, mentally ill, and disabled youth. A decision was made to decategorize the 30 funding streams at the state level, merge them into a single pool of funds, and allocate the newly defined money to local counties. (Kassar, 1991, p. 3). No new funds were to be added to the decategorized pool of money. The policy was designed from the outset to be fiscally neutral.

The designers of the decategorization concept were well aware of the Ventura County approach to flexible use of state funds but decided to incorporate a unique set of planning reforms in the 1987 legislation. These reforms can be identified as follows:

1. *A bottom-up implementation strategy.* The state desired funds to be used to expand child-centered and family-centered services, but it did not want to engage in "top-down" directives regarding specific goals or the means for achieving those goals. Instead, the legislative drafters (led by Bruner) reasoned that local counties that designed and implemented a service delivery system, based on local needs and interests, would assume "own-

ership" of their reforms. The drafters appeared aware that the policy implementation literature offered strong empirical support for the success of a "bottom-up" implementation strategy (Elmore, 1978, 1979).

2. *Fiscal incentive strategy.* By giving counties one pool of funds—rather than 30 categories—each county would be free to utilize the funds in any way it sought, as there were to be few state regulations attached to the expenditure allocations. If the counties believed in home preservation and other less restrictive services, they could spend less on foster care and residential placements and use the "savings" for the preferred services. It was to the advantage of the counties to be cost-effective in allocating funds to fit their own priorities and to cooperate in order to function efficiently.

3. *Use a pilot strategy.* While the decategorization reform appeared promising, there were a host of implementation problems to be addressed at the state and local level. By dealing with only two counties, on a pilot basis (for 3 years), problems could be identified and dealt with without reforming the state at one fell swoop.

4. *Specify the planning governance structure at each level.* The 1987 legislation chose the responsible child welfare agency at the state level, the DHS, to serve as the lead agency. The DHS would plan the decategorization of funds and regulations in 1987–1988, before receiving county applications. A statewide advisory committee, composed of other state agencies and statewide child welfare interest groups, was designated to offer the state DHS advice. The local level was designated to function quite differently. Any plans to be submitted to the state had to be *cosigned* by three county officials: the county DHS director, the chief juvenile court judge, and the county board of supervisors. By requiring these signatories to the plan, the state would involve critical interests that would have a stake in the way funds were allocated at a county level. The three planning leaders would jointly select a project coordinator. They were expected to expand their executive committee to include others and would also involve a variety of local public and private providers and interests to participate in the work of planning task forces. The final plan might have technical components, but it was expected that it would also be a political and financial document expressing the "needs" and interests of the county.

5. *Choose strategic counties.* The first two counties chosen were Polk and Scott. The former contains the state capital of Des Moines and the latter, the city of Davenport. The counties represented 15% of the state's population and possessed the local personnel and motivation to engage in the reform process (Bruner, 1989; Kassar, 1991).

Planning in the initial two counties began in Fall 1988 and were completed by July 1989. In 1990, two more counties were added. The four counties were allocated $26 million in fiscal year 1991. Each of the first two counties spent hundreds of hours of intensive discussions to arrive at its operational plans for using the decategorized funds. According to Bruner (a former state legislator), these discussions culminated in the following types of decisions:

1. *Common goals.* Both counties agreed that the services should be client centered and should involve interagency coordination.

2. *Ongoing governance structure for spending funds.* Each county decided that all allocation decisions would be by the agreement of all three key decision makers.

3. *Redesign of existing services.* Both counties wanted to add more prevention and early intervention services but discovered that they could obtain these services only if they reallocated funds from high-cost family services. Each county discovered the concept of cost-effectiveness.

4. *Improve information and accountability.* Before decategorization, clients were tracked by their eligibility status. Instead, each county decided to employ a client tracking system, based on a family unit, that captured information on the basis of services provided and types of outcomes.

5. *Improve functioning of line workers.* By increasing responsibility for delivering local services, workers would need more on-the-job training and greater backup support. Multiproblem and multiagency families would require fewer assigned workers and greater case coordination efforts. Workers also needed to have "flexible" funds for special service needs.

6. *Identify service gaps for costly clients.* In order to reduce costs, it was necessary to specify target client populations that could benefit from more "intensive," but less restrictive and costly, services. New services with specific outcome expectations were to be developed.

7. *Continue planning and problem solving.* Both counties planned to upgrade their client tracking systems in order to evaluate services and identify new high-problem families requiring special efforts.

According to the state official responsible for monitoring the project, the two early pilot counties reported specific types of goal achievements. However, they appeared to differ in the extent of their achievement by the end of the first year of implementation. The reported accomplishments can be compared as follows (from Kassar, 1991, p. 9):

Scott achievements	Polk achievements
"Increased Funding for family-based services by 23%"	"Enhanced funding for family-centered services and *accelerated* implementation of family preservation"
"Reduced the average number of children in foster care by 11%"	
"Reduced state institutional placements of delinquent males by 22%"	"Reduced projected foster care spending by 10%"

The 1st-year comparison of self-reported outcomes discloses that Polk is unable to identify a reduction of clients experiencing institutional care or to report a reduction in foster care numbers. Instead, the report focuses on expansion of services or reduction of foster care funding. It appears that Scott County is more outcome oriented whereas Polk County is associated with services and dollars. The Polk emphasis may shift in subsequent reports, but meanwhile early results indicate one of the potential consequences of a bottom-up design approach that does not require the setting of specific targets. If the top does not require the bottom to set minimal goals—or set them as a state condition—it is possible that funds and services can be reshuffled or even expanded without minimal indicators of outcome.

In addition, specification of outcomes without evidence that the alternative services are indeed more client centered and less restrictive can yield an inconclusive image of what has been accomplished. For example, the report about Scott's goal achievements also reports that Scott County has added an array of new services that includes a "secure local residential unit" (besides adolescent day treatment, expanded day care, and family assistance dollars for "concrete" services). Without more information that the number of youth residing inside the local service unit on a census day, or during the year, is less than the reported reduction of state institutional placements, readers are unable to determine whether the county's youth have a higher, lower, or equal chance of being confined after decategorization than before.

The state leaders do not appear to have these types of concerns (or report them in writing). Instead, when identifying "obstacles" encountered in implementing the program, the following local difficulties were identified (Kassar, 1991):

1. Lack of initial seed money to start up the project, pay for technical assistance, and train staff;
2. Project coordination;
3. Inadequate data information;
4. Limited capacity for outcome-oriented evaluation;
5. Difficulty in obtaining agreements on methods of budgeting and tracking expenditures;
6. Lack of funds for an external project evaluation.

The lack of seed money was partially overcome with the assistance of funds from the Edna McConnell Clark Foundation. The Clark Foundation paid for the county project coordinator positions in the two pilot counties and subsidized technical assistance from the Center for the Study of Social Policy and the National Conference of State Legislatures (Bruner, 1989, p. 16).

As of the spring of 1992, the problems associated with initiating a new mode of administering and budgeting pooled funds at both state and local levels have been addressed and coped with, if not completely solved. A tele-phone conversation with a responsible state official revealed that the state of Iowa believed that decategorization had proven its practicality in the four counties (plus another one added after 1990) and could even be adapted for smaller, rural counties if they banded together on a regional basis. While the counties had differed regarding the achievement of explicit goals in out-of-home placements, as a 1st-year analysis indicated, state officials and legisla-tors were accepting of the variable outcome.

From a state perspective, a stabilization of funding for out-of-home placements was achieved, with a devolution of responsibility to the county level. In a sense, decategorization assisted the state in "capping" child wel-fare funding. In-depth evaluations would be necessary to determine whether the type, frequency, and duration of out-of-home placements were reduced to a significant degree in one or more of the participating counties. As of the spring of 1992, the funds for such an evaluation were not yet budgeted by the state legislature or forthcoming from private foundations.

System Reform in Juvenile Corrections: An Ideal Blueprint

When Massachusetts closed its training schools in 1971–1972, the leaders were guided by the desire to divert youth from inhumane organizations and practices. The plans for creating an alternative, community-based set of ar-rangements were sketchy indeed, and it took several years for a functioning system to be created and stabilized (Coates et al., 1978; Rutherford, 1974). Since the 1970s, there have been efforts to conceptualize a model of juvenile corrections that would capture the humanistic values of Miller and his col-leagues, and combine them with a set of guidelines for specific reform out-comes that other states could emulate. The most thoughtful model, built on the basis of prior efforts and empirical assessments, is the *Blueprint for Cor-rections* (Barton et al., 1991). This section summarizes the blueprint; the next section describes and assesses the system components of the Massachusetts model as it functioned in 1974 and 1990.

Barton et al. (1991) believe that the overuse of state training schools—the most restrictive long-term facility—is a result of the following factors: (1) a lack of *clear goals* for the system as a whole, (2) a lack of clarity about the *principles* or values that can balance the competing goals, (3) a lack of specificity about the *system characteristics* necessary to effectively achieve the goals, and (4) *inadequate decision making* in creating disposition options. The logic of their approach will become clear as each factor is discussed:

Goal Clarity

A "balanced approach" to juvenile corrections must pay attention to achiev-ing three major goals:

1. Offender accountability for past illegal behaviors, by an "equitable use of sanctions";
2. Public safety protection from future illegal behaviors, by identifying "which youths require what degree of restrictive control and providing that control efficiently"; and
3. Development of competencies among youth, so they can be provided with "the skills and resources needed to function positively in mainstream society" (Barton et al., 1991, p. 4).

Principles of Good Public Practice

Given that the youth corrections system accepts the goals of attaining accountability for past harms, safety for future risks, and competency development for reintegration into society, there must be a set of values that guides goal attainment. These values are:

1. *Equity:* decisions to punish must be "fair, consistent, and subject to appeal";
2. *Cost efficiency:* employ the "least costly means necessary to achieve the most effective outcome"; and
3. *Performance accountability:* engage in "monitoring and evaluation at all levels of responsibility and to all constituents and client groups" (Barton et al., 1991, p. 5).

Barton et al. (1991) argue that being concerned about each principle can help balance an emphasis on one goal over another. For example, an "overemphasis on offender accountability could result in the inefficient incarceration of large numbers of youths who could be handled adequately in less costly settings" (p. 5). Further, an exaggerated emphasis on competency development could result in an undervaluing of concerns for public safety, and thereby provide inadequate performance accountability to the public.

System Characteristics

Barton et al. (1991) believe that "at the heart of the blueprint is a series of characteristics" (p. 5) that must also be developed to effectively pursue the three major goals in a balanced fashion:

1. *Coordination.* This must be sought at the individual case level, as well as at a program, and interagency level.
2. *Rational decision making.* Dispositions should be guided by "objective assessments" using information relevant to achieving the three major goals, so that the "right youths" are assigned to appropriate levels of restrictiveness.

3. *Array of services.* To meet the varied identifiable needs of youth, the following options should be available: basic supervision and supports; special treatment for substance abuse, mental health problems, and sexual deviance; a variety of living arrangements; job training and placement services; other competency development services that include education, social skills building, recreation, and special programming; and family intervention services.

4. *Flexible funds.* Reduce or merge "categorical funding schemes" so that funds can be allocated according to a good assessment of individual youth needs.

5. *Advocacy.* In order to ensure fairness in dispositions and meeting individual competency needs, youth require legal and case management advocates, preferably persons not responsible for policing behavioral compliance with program rules and regulations.

6. *Evaluation.* Implementation of policies and practices requires a decent information system and evaluative feedback.

Classification and Assessment in Dispositions

Before deciding on a treatment plan, it is necessary to make a decision about restrictiveness. Classification and assessment decisions could be guided by the following considerations, in the following order:

1. *Offender accountability.* Punishment decisions refer to the type, degree, and duration of restrictiveness—or deprivation of liberty, rights, and privileges. Punishments should be guided by the value of "just deserts"—so that serious, violent, chronic offenders would be dealt with more seriously than youth committing minor offenses. Besides using "proportionality" to assess sanctions for past behaviors, an efficient use of resources would *limit severe placements* primarily to seriously violent and chronic felony offenders. Less serious offenders would not be placed in secure facilities.

2. *Public safety protection/risk control.* Empirical research has identified factors that predict better than chance the likelihood of *reoffending* in the future. Assessing the risk profile of offenders and designing ways to control that future risk can guide how youths are supervised within the level of restrictive living that has already been decided on the basis of past deeds. Assessments about *future* behaviors cannot justify the abandonment of just deserts decisions about *past* behaviors.

3. *Competency development/services.* Rather than pretend that all youth can be served with one or two approaches (as often occurs in traditional corrections), a service plan should be based on comprehensive assessment of needs.

This approach to classification and assessment could provide three specific sets of guidelines: (1) restrictiveness, (2) level of risk, and (3) areas of need. *Restrictiveness guidelines* refer to five levels: (1) maximum security for the most serious and/or chronic offenders, (2) medium security for chronic serious property offenders, (3) intensive community supervision for less serious offenders, (4) regular community supervision for relatively minor offenders, and (5) minimal supervision for youth with very few offenses. Offender accountability could also be reinforced by community service work, curfews, and restitution.

Risk control strategies can vary by setting—residential and nonresidential. These strategies include architecture, staff ratios, size of living units, and tracking mechanisms and procedures.

Needs-based guidelines would include a "generic" list that would be optimally considered for every youth. Needs areas that require appropriate resources or services include basic food and shelter; medical/dental; mental health; substance abuse; family environment; peer environment; leisure time; learning disabilities; school adjustment; vocational; developmental disabilities; sexual adjustment; and independent living skills.

Barton et al. (1991) believe that following their blueprint is a way for the youth corrections system to get "smart" by providing a cost-effective means for dealing with juvenile delinquency. By clearly setting forth the primary goals and by explicitly linking assessment and intervention procedures to these goals, it is possible to create a youth corrections system that is equitable, efficient, and accountable. A summary of the Massachusetts model as it functioned in 1990 can provide insights into how the ideal might look in practice.

System Reform in Massachusetts: The Blueprint in Action

Prior to the initiation of a community-based juvenile corrections system by the state of Massachusetts, the Department of Youth Services (DYS) operated a traditional system of four training schools (separated by age and sex), a secure psychiatric unit for the most "dangerous acting out youth," and a forestry camp. In addition, DYS operated all the state's pretrial detention facilities (four units). During the last half of the 1960s, the inhumane conditions occurring in the system became widely publicized and stimulated a series of outside investigations. The investigations "generally deplored the abusive conditions, the lack of programming, and the lack of training and administrative support for the staff" (Coates et al., 1978, p. 23). Physical abuse of a youth by a staff member at the psychiatric unit precipitated the appointment of a new commissioner, who gave instructions to reform the system (Ohlin et al., 1977).

Dr. Jerome Miller, the new commissioner was trained in England (while in the Army) by Maxwell Jones, the originator of "milieu therapy." Miller brought his belief in the efficacy of milieu therapy to Massachusetts and attempted to retrain a traditional staff into therapeutic enablers of change. In addition, he closed the psychiatric wing and issued administrative orders forbidding the threat or use of force, disciplinary haircuts, and military-type regimentation of cottage life (Rutherford, 1974; Ohlin et al., 1977). Many custodial staff and supervisors resisted complying with the central administration directives and substituting coercive controls with interpersonal measures associated with milieu therapy. After struggling with a recalcitrant staff for over a year, Miller initiated a radical action in 1972—he depopulated the training schools and placed the youths in a variety of hastily prepared community settings (Rutherford, 1974; Ohlin et al., 1977). He was aided in his efforts by political support from the governor and private interest groups, as well as federal funds for the initiation of 20 group homes throughout the state (Coates et al., 1978, pp. 24–26).

In 1973, Miller resigned in order to accept an offer to reform the Illinois system of juvenile corrections. The new commissioner remained in the job for about 2 years. His administration of the decentralized system of DYS programs was continually criticized for poor fiscal controls, inappropriate programs, deficient tracking procedures, and an inattention to the problems presented by "dangerous" youth. Conservative legislators and interests fought to reinstitute the creation of large, secure facilities. At about the time the counterattack occurred, the DYS effort created the following distribution of program responses for youth entrusted to its care, treatment, and custody (as of July 1974): 132 youths in secure care, 399 in nonsecure group homes, 171 in foster care, 724 in nonresidential programs, and 941 on minimal supervision parole. Of a total of 2,367 youths, there were 1,426 in active programs. Of those in active programs, fewer than 10% (132) were in secure facilities. In contrast, in 1968, the 833 youth in active programs were in "secure" training schools or the psychiatric wing of a state hospital (Coates el al., 1978, pp. 22, 30). Critics argued there were too few in secure programs.

Critics of the DYS policy of drastic deinstitutionalization could also highlight the fact that the percentage of youths over 16 years of age increased from 33% to 58%—a sizable increase. In addition, the relative mix of offender types and sex ratios began to change markedly. The removal of status offenders (in Massachusetts, children in need of supervision—or CHINS) from DYS began in 1973 and resulted in fewer girls and noncriminal offenders. From 1968 to 1974, the proportion of youths committed to DYS for a crime against persons had risen from 2% to 10% (Coates et al., 1978).

The third reform commissioner responded to his critics by strengthening fiscal accountability, tracking youths more systematically, and supervising the regional managers more closely. Unfortunately, what he could not provide were empirical data that demonstrated that the community-based system was more effective in reducing renewed delinquency. Harvard researchers published an empirical evaluation of a 1974 cohort of youth and compared their rates of reappearance in court and reconvictions with a 1968

cohort of training school youth. The overall comparison favored the training school cohort, but this difference could be accounted for by the demographic and offense characteristics that had shifted between 1968 and 1974
(Coates et al., 1978, pp. 147–175). The Harvard team concluded that while
the outcome rates of the new system were probably comparable to the training school system, there were social benefits that were associated with the
reforms: (1) youth received more humane care, (2) a few of the new programs demonstrated that they were high in creating a "normalized" living
environment, and (3) the overall juvenile crime rate of the state was unaffected by DYS policies and programs. In addition, the fiscal cost of the added
social benefits (and comparable postsystem outcomes) was quite similar to
the costs of operating a 1968–type training school system. They concluded
that the reforms toward normalization of programs and linkages to schools,
jobs, and local community resources had "not gone far enough." If reform
efforts went further, even better results might occur in the future (Coates
et al., 1978, pp. 175–198).

In 1991, the National Council on Crime and Delinquency (NCCD)
(funded by the Edna McConnell Clark Foundation) published an empirical
update on the Massachusetts reform, using data from a cohort of 819 youth
formally admitted to DYS and released between 1984 and 1985 (Austin et al.,
1991). The NCCD study found that the 1980s cohort appeared to reflect
more favorably on the DYS system than did the 1970s cohort. Using court
arraignment as an indicator of reoffending while at risk in the community,
the 1984–1985 cohort was followed for all the time the youth were not in
secure custody for a period of 12 months; this procedure was comparable to
the method used by the Harvard researchers.

The NCCD study also used rates of conviction and reincarceration as
indicators of effectiveness. However, these indicators are less trustworthy
than court arraignments because official policies and practices regarding sus-
pensions and revocations by the correctional organizational per se can influence the extent to which cases are handled internally rather than by a court.
Court arraignments also present difficulties (as discussed later), but this
measure is closest to the least biased indicator of reoffending—the arrest by
a law enforcement officer who is unaware of the commitment or parole status of a youth. Unfortunately, the NCCD study team did not obtain arrest
data, so arraignments will be used in this analysis as the best measure of
assessing outcomes (see Lerman, 1975, pp. 58–67, for an earlier analysis of
the difficulties in using "recidivism indicators" that are potentially influenced
by correctional decision-making and practices).

The 1984–1985 cohort had a 51% rate of rearraignments, compared
to the 1974 cohort rate of 74% for early community-based efforts and 66%
for a 1968 training school cohort (Austin et al., 1991, p. 15). Austin et al.
(1991) concluded that the results were not attributable to the 1984–1985
DYS cohort containing fewer serious offenders or to changes in local law

enforcement practices. They concluded that the more mature DYS system came "closer to its stated goals of reform—a rich diversity of community-based services permitting youth normal experiences in school, work, and family settings" (p. 15). The researchers also provided evidence that the DYS had done so without increasing the state's overall risk of juvenile delinquency.

Although the outcomes of the mid-1980s may prove to be superior to the results of the early 1970s, it would be premature to allocate the positive difference as due entirely to the "rich diversity" of services. Compared to the 1970s, the DYS had also changed its use of social controls in response to antireform critics. Instead of fewer than 10% of active cases being assigned to secure facilities, the proportion increased to over 20% (see Figure 8.1). In addition, the DYS system became accustomed to using "intermittent and relatively short periods of secure confinement" as part of its community-based corrections programming (Austin et al., 1991, p. 5). The widespread use of intermittent detention may add a confounding factor to the use of court arraignments as an indicator of success. The DYS system that has actually evolved is much more complex and requires a careful analysis in order to understand what the blueprint looks like in practice, as well as to understand the fiscal and social effectiveness of the correctional reform.

To begin to appreciate the combined control-treatment program as it probably functioned in the mid-1980s, I have prepared two charts based on recent information contained in the NCCD report and a monograph coauthored by Edward Loughran, the 1991 Commissioner of DYS (Schwartz & Loughran, 1991). The first, Figure 8.1, presents a flow diagram of decision making for 830 youth actually committed to DYS in 1990. Using this figure, the initial classification and assessment guidelines are discussed. The second, Table 8.6, presents the distribution of residential beds in order to assess the allocation of resources for secure facilities by residential type.

According to Schwartz and Loughran (1991), there were 2,993 admissions to the DYS-run detention facilities located in five regions of the state. There were 7 secure (i.e., physically locked) and 6 nonsecure, 24–hour staff, shelter units operated throughout the state. Unlike other states, there are no detention facilities operated by local communities or counties. The 13 detention sites contained 250 beds; for 2,993 admissions there are approximately 11.97 admissions per bed during the year with an estimated average stay of 30 days (i.e., 365 days divided by 11.97). Of these 2,993 admissions, about 28% (i.e., 830 youth) were committed to DYS in 1990; the remaining 72% of the admissions (2,163 cases) were given non-DYS local correctional dispositions (or perhaps dismissed).

After being formally committed to DYS, all youth receive a case manager. The case manager refers about 30% of the new commitments to a classification panel for possible assignment to a secure treatment facility. There are two categories of mandatory referrals (category A refers to very serious

TABLE 8.6. Distribution of Beds in Massachusetts DYS System in 1990, by Residential Type

Category type	No. of sites	No. of beds	Beds/site	% dist.
A. *Pretrial detention*				
Secure	7	128	18.3	51
Nonsecure	6	122	20.3	49
Subtotals	13	250	19.2	100
B. *Transitional management programs*				
Secure	NA	64	NA	38
Nonsecure	NA	103	NA	62
Subtotals	NA	167	NA	100
C. *Out-of-home care/treatment/custody programs*				
Secure	14	210	15.0	32
Group homes	36	360	9.7	53
Forestry camp	1	36	36.0	05
Foster care	7 (agencies)	65	NA	10
Subtotals	51 (+ sites)	661	11.7[a]	100
D. *Living at home*				
Outreach and tracking	NA	317	NA	100
E. *All types combined*				
Secure	21	402	19.1	29
Nonsecure residential[a]	43	676	14.2	48
Outreach tracking	NA	317	NA	23
Subtotals	64	1,395	15.8[a]	100

Note. See sources in Table 8.6. NA = not applicable.
[a]Excludes foster care.

violent offenses and category B to serious violent and property offenses) and one category of optional referrals. While awaiting classification, the 250 youth are placed in a secure transitional management program; there are 64 beds allocated to this function, with about 3.91 admissions per bed during the year, with an estimated average stay of 93 days (i.e., 365 days divided by 3.91).

The 580 remaining youth who are not presumptively eligible for secure treatment are sent to a nonsecure transitional management program for an evaluation. The DYS system allocates 103 beds for this function, with about 5.64 admissions per bed during the year, with an estimated average stay of 65 days (i.e., 365 days divided by 5.64).

Only 70% of the youth referred for classification to a secure unit are declared eligible for secure treatment (about 175 cases). Classifications are performed by a central panel composed of three persons appointed by the DYS commissioner. Begun in 1981, in order to reduce the interregional disparity in sentencing and to ensure that the decision-making process is "uniform and fair," the panel members use a "classification grid" to "determine the need for security, the length of stay, and the specific program placement" (Schwartz & Loughran, 1991, p. 10). The classification grid appears to be a combination of legislative and regulatory requirements; it is used to make decisions concerning the type and duration of restrictiveness for new, recommitted, or revocation cases. The major offense categories and the associated time assignments are as follows:

1. *Category A—Mandatory referrals.* This category refers to all types of murder and manslaughter charges, as well as homicide by vehicle. Youth 13 to 16 years old can be assigned a minimum of 12 months to a maximum indeterminate stay. Release is mandated at age 18, unless extension is granted by the court.

2. *Category B—Mandatory referrals.* This category refers to armed robbery, assaults with a dangerous weapon, arson, kidnapping, possession of a firearm, and sexual offenses involving a victim. Youth 13 to 16 years old can be assigned a minimum of 6 months to a maximum of 14 months. Case conferences can lead to early release or an extension of the maximum.

3. *Optional referrals.* This type refers to behaviors that present a "risk and danger to the community and/or to himself/herself or who exhibits a persistent and escalating pattern of delinquency." Youth 14 to 16 years old can be assigned a minimum of 4 months to a maximum of 12 months. Case conferences can lead to early release or an extension of the maximum.

4. *Revocation referrals.* This type refers to any juvenile deemed to have violated his/her "conditional liberty" as determined by a revocation hearing. Youth 14 to 17 years of age can be assigned a minimum of 4 months and a maximum of 12 months. Case conference can lead to early release or an extension of the maximum (Austin et al., 1991).

The bottom part of Figure 8.1 discloses that the total number of youth initially assigned to a secure treatment facility is calculated to be about 175 (i.e., 70% of 250). Using this figure, it is calculated that about 21% of all new commitments are initially assigned to a secure facility (i.e., 175 divided by 830). The remaining pool of youth are assigned to a variety of nonsecure DYS facilities and dispositions.

Table 8.6 summarizes the distribution of beds within the total DYS system for new, recommitted, and revoked youth. By arranging the information by out-of-home category, it is possible to describe the extent of restrictiveness of the system in 1990 by number of sites, beds, size, and the proportional allocation. Secure beds comprise 51% of the pretrial detention beds, 38% of the transitional management programs, and 32% of the out-of-home care/treatment/custody programs. If all types are combined, it is evident that 29% of the program "slots" (i.e., beds plus tracking assignments) were allocated to "secure" programs in 1990.

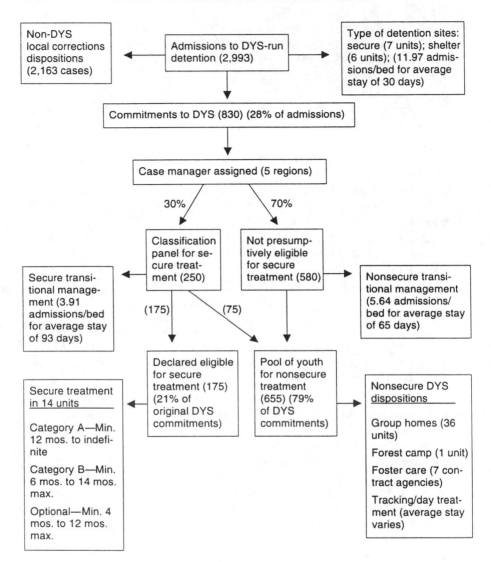

FIGURE 8.1. Flow of corrections cases in Massachusetts in 1990. Data from Schwartz and Loughran (1991, pp. 7–12) and Austin et al. (1991, pp. 2–5).

Whereas the proportion of DYS beds allocated to secure programs in 1990 is certainly smaller than the 1968 training school system, it is also much higher than occurred in the 1970s. This comparison holds whether we focus on initial youth assignments (21% to 10%), proportion of all out-of-home placement beds (32% to 18%), or a combination of all active nondetention slots (24% to 9%) (based on data contained in Table 8.6 and calculations of data in Coates et al., 1978, p. 22).

Besides responding to legislative mandates and political and civic critics in making initial assignments, DYS has also implemented extensive use of "intermittent and relatively short periods of secure confinement" as part of its operational practices for *all* cases (Austin et al., 1991, p. 5). According to the NCCD researchers, the tracking of a cohort of 819 youth disclosed that during a 24-month commitment period, the 696 nonviolent offenders experienced an average number of three distinct stays in a secure facility (of undisclosed type) while in the DYS system. This information is presented graphically in a comparison of the DYS's handling of nonviolent and violent chronic offenders versus a traditional youth corrections system over a 24-month period (Austin et al., 1991, p. 6). In this comparison, "traditional" youth are released from a training school after a stay of 9 to 12 months, but after release they are reconfined in a secure facility on a temporary basis an average of one time for an average stay of about 90 days. The DYS violent chronic offenders stay in a secure facility for about 8 to 12 months but after release are reconfined in a secure facility on an intermittent basis an average of two times for an average stay of about 30 days each time. These types of intermittent or temporary stays at a secure facility can occur without a revocation hearing. How this use of secure confinement during a commitment sentence is regulated by DYS is unknown, as the practice of intermittent confinement has not been the focus of a detailed study.

The use of temporary confinement is, however, not new in juvenile corrections. It was associated with the first community-based correctional projects attempted in California in the 1960s (see Lerman, 1975). In the California project of the 1960s, temporary detention was used as a means of avoiding bringing youth to a local juvenile court or avoiding revocation of parole, as well as a means of punishing deviant behaviors. If this occurs in the operational practices of the DYS system, then it is quite conceivable that the differences in the rates of court arraignments between the 1984–1985 and 1970 cohorts may be due to the Massachusetts rediscovery of the multiple uses of intermittent confinement.

Besides the varied uses of secure confinement and out-of-home placements, the DYS also makes certain that all residential programs provide 5 hours of academics daily, individual and group counseling, vocational training, medical and recreational services, and attention by a case manager. These and other services are either provided directly or purchased from private providers and other public agencies. On a statewide basis, about 45 private agencies account for a total of 90 contracts to provide residential and non-residential services to DYS youth. According to observers and officials, the DYS uses the following mechanisms to ensure the quality of its programs and humane treatment of DYS wards: (1) monitoring by program managers and case managers, (2) monitoring by the contracting departments, (3) soliciting youth grievances, and (4) programs of technical assistance (Coates et al., 1978; Schwartz & Loughran, 1991).

It is clear that creating and implementing a less restrictive system for youthful offenders is much more complex than redesigning the delivery of mental health or child welfare services. The need to balance accountability for past deeds, protection against future risk, and provision for competency development yields a blueprint sketch. But a detailed plan requires a specification of the type, degree, and duration of social controls, as well as the components of a treatment and service package that can be attached to very restrictive, moderately restrictive, and less restrictive residential facilities. The implementation of the correctional ideal in practice, by Massachusetts, disclosed that the blueprint can be operationalized but the DYS model contains elements of intermittent secure control that have not yet been incorporated into the ideal plan.

Besides offering doses of intermittent secure confinement to nonviolent, as well as dangerous and chronic, offenders, the DYS also offers pretrial detention to virtually all youth. As currently operated, the nonviolent offenders have a better than 50% chance of being detained in a secure facility *prior* to being assigned to a nonsecure transitional program (see Figure 8.1). The implementation of the correctional ideal in practice, by Massachusetts, discloses that the DYS model contains elements of secure confinement that have not yet been incorporated into the ideal blueprint.

A full comparison of the DYS model as an exemplar of the correctional blueprint would require that the total number of days for each secure confinement be tallied to include pretrial detention, as well as transitional program, initial placement, and intermittent confinements by number of days, in order to assess how differently the total number of secure confinement days of a 2-year commitment to the 1990 DYS system compares with a 2-year commitment to the 1968 training school system (or a current "traditional" system). In addition, a comparable calculation and comparison could be computed for nonsecure placements in pretrial, transitional, initial commitment, and intermittent doses of nonsecure residence. Until we engage in this important social arithmetic, as well as an assessment of the use of temporary confinement to avoid court arraignment, there will be an incomplete social accounting of the full, human implications of ideal and actual practices of this widely known model. In addition, the full fiscal implications of the ideal and actual practices cannot be fully calculated until all types of residential placements of short and long duration are counted and the costs added up.

Summary and Conclusions

The models of system reform chosen for discussion—decategorization and the DYS model of community-based corrections—share a number of similarities that may not be readily apparent but are worth noting. Both model systems share an interest in reducing out-of-home placements, including a reduction in the use of restrictive settings. However, the bottom-up approach to planning chosen by Iowa's state child welfare leaders displays a potential variability in how systematically local counties pursue these goals with specific reduction targets. While the correctional model delivers services at a local level, too, the decisions about out-of-home placements are primarily decided at a state level.

A reading of the system characteristics identified as an integral part of the correctional blueprint reveals that child welfare planning in Iowa also emphasizes the following features: (1) coordination of services, (2) provision of a broad array of services, and (3) flexible funding. Budget neutrality is also emphasized by the Iowa model, and this is matched by the correctional blueprint emphasis on cost efficiency. In practice, DYS officials are proud of the fact that the average correctional costs per committed youth are less than those of a traditional correctional model (even though their calculations may not have included all the monetary costs associated with confinement at the initial, transitional, and intermittent phases of a 24-month commitment period).

Both models are also interested in creating and maintaining information systems capable of providing evaluative feedback on programs and services to youth. However, both models, in practice, reveal an inability to identify all the unintended, as well as intended, social and fiscal costs associated with their reform efforts. Child welfare officials in Scott County reported only on the success of reducing state institutional placements for delinquents, without providing evidence that local detention and secure residential placements did not substitute for the state-level reduction in frequency or duration. Similarly, the DYS and even outside researchers have not systematically added up the social and fiscal costs associated with confinements at all the stages of a commitment career and the possible substitution of intermittent confinement for court arraignment in estimating rates of effectiveness.

The systems of child welfare and juvenile corrections have, as noted, an overlap in purpose and in the strategies of delivering programs. What is often overlooked is that they also have a distinct overlap in the target populations that are the focus of their respective goals and service strategies. An unknown portion of the target populations in the decategorization counties of Iowa are official and unofficial status offenders and juvenile delinquents. Iowa recognizes the importance of this population by insisting that one of the members of the local community presenting a plan must be a juvenile court judge. The overlap exists in funding out-of-home placements as well as in target populations and service delivery strategies and mechanisms. Given these facts about intersystem connections, it would be quite useful for child welfare reforms to take into account the correctional blueprint for juveniles by acknowledging that their overlap activities involve dealing with the issues of offender accountability and public safety. If they did so, there could be an open discussion and debate about the relative balance that the local community seeks in delivering competency development services within a social control package of out-of-home placements and restrictions on liberty. It is also conceivable, as in Ventura County, that the intersystem discussions could include the mental health and school systems.

Whether serious and frank intersystem discussions occur, it is critical that each system fully address the social control features of its community-based programs. These local programs combine varying degrees of restriction on liberty with an array of services. In evaluating these programs, it is critical to identify all the restrictions in terms of type, degree, and duration—as well as the types of services. This can be done routinely in any well-designed "tracking" system. It does not require an outside research evaluation team or a random experimental design. Instead, we are dealing with the issue of program accountability for all aspects of what is actually delivered to local youth. Communities should be concerned about ratios of detention to court appearances, lengths of detention stays without convictions, the extent of transitional programs of confinement, and the number and duration of intermittent detention—as well as the designated, long-term placement. If they were, then quarterly and annual reports could report on the frequency rates and duration of the types of out-of-home confinements and placements. Presumably, these reports could document whether secure confinement of all types, duration, and location were decreasing for local youth and to what extent alternate modes of social control were employed. By becoming aware of the relative changes in the utilization of *all* modes of offender accountability, communities could accurately determine whether the reforms (of child welfare and/or juvenile corrections systems) did, in fact, result in the use of less restrictive measures.

State officials responsible for allocating child welfare and correctional funds could also be held accountable to report on how funds were used, in practice, to deliver social control and service programs. Policymakers and officials, at a state level, should be able to acquire data on how the state is progressing toward the stated goal of reducing the restrictiveness of programs targeted to children and youth. Social audits of the disbursement of funds, as well as fiscal audits, are appropriate activities for state officials. In addition, state policymakers and officials might concern themselves with examining the fairness of how intermittent confinements, an integral part of community-based reforms in many localities, are actually decided and delivered for program and legal infractions.

The evaluation of the first nationally known correctional community-based project in California, in the 1960s, provided potent evidence that temporary confinement of supervised youth was associated with capricious decision making about breaking program rules and 20 days of solitary confinement for a majority of youth (Lerman, 1975, pp. 35–50). The questionable community-based practices of the 1960s, first identified in California, may have become an operational component of the Massachusetts DYS reform system in the 1980s and 1990s. Until we obtain the necessary evidence, it may be imprudent to assume that the DYS model, as practiced, is an appropriate exemplar to fully emulate. It is quite likely that a more detailed inquiry into all the social control practices and procedures of the DYS may reveal a greater use of restrictive measures than has been popularly disseminated. However, a comparison with existing training school models may still disclose that the DYS is a more humane model—even if its effectiveness in reducing illegal behaviors is comparable. Unfortunately, we do not now possess the data that would permit a balanced assessment of the total social control-treatment package of restrictions and services. Researchers identifying with the ideals of child protection have an obligation to learn more about the everyday social control practices, procedures, and consequences for youth before making an informed decision to unequivocally recommend the DYS model.

THE REGULATION OF OUT-OF-HOME PLACEMENT AS A CHILD PROTECTION STRATEGY

The discussions of system reforms, contained in the previous sections, were guided by a belief that preventing out-of-home placement or reducing the risk of living in a restrictive placement was a viable strategy for minimizing incidents of abuse and neglect. To enhance the likelihood that new system designs will yield minimal cases of maltreatment in any day or overnight program component, the discussion attempted to identify quality assurance mechanisms and procedures that promoted individual treatment plans and services of a high standard. For example, mental health system designs included scheduled case treatment reviews and case management, utilization and peer reviews, and program accountability measures. The DYS model relied on program and contract monitoring and solicitation of youth grievances, as well as case management. In addition to providing quality assurance mechanisms and procedures to prevent or reduce placements, states and communities can be expected also to improve their capabilities of learning about and responding to incidents of abuse and neglect when children are actually placed out of home. This section discusses some critical elements in a regulatory approach to enhancing a child protection policy.

The focus of the discussion centers primarily on the responsibility of the public sector and the way officials, parents, citizens, advocates, and children can use statutory language and enforcement mechanisms for preventing and minimizing maltreatment. There is, of course, also a place for voluntary organizations to participate in the regulation of out-of-home services. For example, the Child Welfare League of America, organized in the 1920s, has over the years published and disseminated to member organizations ideal "standards" for foster care, shelters, group homes, and residential treatment centers (Child Welfare League of America, 1963, 1988; Steiner, 1981).

Despite the availability of national standards and the continuing professionalization of all out-of-home services for children, the number of reported incidents occurring in out-of-home care facilities has risen by an appreciable amount. The state of New Jersey, considered to have one of the best records in keeping track of complaints of institutional abuse, investigations and substantiations, reported 481 complaints in 1980 and 2,110 in 1988 (excluding foster care in both years)—a rate of increase of about 339% (Rindleisch & Nunno, 1992). This rate of increase exceeds the growth of intra-familial cases of abuse and neglect for the nation (Besharov, 1983) for a comparable period, from 1.1 million incidents in 1979 to 2.3 million in 1988—a rate of increase of about 109%.

Although we lack comparable trend data for foster care, there is evidence that awareness of this out-of-home placement as an additional source of potential maltreatment is also growing. A Colorado study of 325 complaints of out-of-home maltreatment reported to a statewide review team for investigation revealed that foster care parents and foster siblings accounted for about 40% of the reports. About 38% of the foster home referrals were confirmed by the review team (using a standard of credible evidence), compared to 39% institutional referrals and 18–19% for group home and residential treatment referrals (Rosenthal, Motz, Edmonson, & Groze, 1991). Given the lack of substantiation in the facilities reporting the greatest number of incidents (residential treatment centers and group homes combined), foster care homes represented about one half of all substantiated cases identified by the Colorado review team (for the period 1983–1987). In New Jersey, substantiated foster reports accounted for about 43% of all out-of-home substantiated case in 1990 (New Jersey Bureau of Research, Evaluation, and Quality Assurance, 1991, Tables 12, 16).

The public sector has responded to these nonfamilial risks via a variety of statutory amendments to older child abuse laws, as well as by pursuing other regulatory mechanisms. This section discusses the following: (1) statutory protections for minors entering inappropriate care, (2) statutory definitions of abuse and neglect in out-of-home care, (3) upgrading licensing capabilities and responsibilities, (4) enforcement of statutory standards, (5) subsidizing and promoting child advocates, and (6) using research surveys to monitor placements.

Statutory Protection for Minors Entering Inappropriate Care

The legal regulation of admissions into out-of-home care varies by the statutory foundations associated with each of the three major systems of care, treatment, and custody. Since the advent of the *Gault* decision by the U.S. Supreme Court in 1967, the juvenile justice system has developed the most circumscribed definitions and procedures for committing delinquent youth into a correctional facility (*In re Gault*, 1967). As Linney (1984) notes, "due process protections have been offered for commitment proceedings in particular, but have not generally been extended to disposition decisions" (p. 225). If adjudications find youth guilty of serious offenses, then many states mandate secure confinement for an explicit period of time—as in Massachusetts "mandatory referrals" (see section "System Reform in Massachusetts"). However, the majority of American youth arrested for delinquency have committed offenses that are not serious; when these cases are referred to juvenile courts, the state statutes provide judges with a substantial amount of discretion (see Maguire & Flanagan, 1991, p. 433, for 1990 reports on arrests of youth under age 18). Judges, with the assistance of probation staff may or may not choose the least restrictive alternative.

The *Gault* case did not directly refer to child welfare cases, but since the 1960s, decisions concerning the placement of children have become more circumscribed by a greater attention to the standards and procedures for the removal of children from their families (see, e.g., Mnookin & Weisberg, 1988, pp. 349–453). Prior to 1962, most out-of-home placements occurred on a "voluntary" basis, with minimal judicial oversight. In 1962, federal AFDC (Aid to Families with Dependent Children) amendments required a "judicial determination" if any federal funds were to be used in foster home or foster institution placements (U.S. House of Representatives, 1962, Title IV-A). In 1967, the AFDC-Foster Care program was expanded and all states were required to offer foster care services to AFDC youth (if judicially determined). In 1980, Congress reversed the practice of providing foster care funds to states "without any strings attached" and attempted to provide incentives to "reunify the family or to prevent or eliminate the need for removal of the child from home" (Mnookin & Weisberg, 1988, p. 451). Federal law now requires an assessment of the out-of-home status of each child every 6 months and service programs to return youth to their families or help them become adopted. It could also be useful to obtain the opinions of child care staff because they have been found to have much stronger doubts about the placements in their facilities than the workers in child protection agencies (Rindfleisch & Rabb, 1984b).

Some states have tightened their laws to narrow the grounds for removal, thereby reducing the discretion of judges and child welfare official (Mnookin & Weisberg, 1988, p. 452). One state, New Jersey, in an effort to reduce the entry and length of residential placement, expanded the definition of neglect in 1987 as follows: "Neglect also means the continued inappropriate placement of a child in an institution as defined in section . . . with the knowledge that the placement has resulted and may continue to result in harm to the child's mental or physical well being" (N.J.A.S., chap. 6, §9:6–1).

The New Jersey definition of an abused child has also been broadened to include the following:

> A child who is in an institution as defined in section . . . and (1) has been so placed inappropriately for a continued period of time with the knowledge that the placement has resulted and may continue to result in harm to the child's mental or physical well-being or (2) has been willfully isolated from ordinary social contact under circumstances which indicate emotional or social deprivation. (N.J.A.S., chap. 6, §9:6–8:9)

For the purpose of the statute, "an institution includes, but is not limited to, a correctional facility, detention facility, day care center, residential school, shelter and hospital" (N.J.A.S., chap. 6, §9.6–8.21).

While the juvenile justice and child welfare systems have had their discretion to initiate and maintain placements circumscribed by legislation and the courts, the admissions policies for the psychiatric hospitalization of children have undergone the smallest amount of legal regulation (Melton, 1984; Weithorn, 1988). The rates of psychiatric hospitalization per 100,000 youth under age 18 have increased by over 170% between 1971 and the mid-1980s, while the rates for juvenile corrections actually decreased and the rates for child welfare increased less than 25% (Lerman, 1991). The increase in use of proprietary psychiatric hospitals has been so large that Weithorn referred to the increase as an example of "skyrocketing admission rates" (i.e., a gain of over 1,300% from 1971 to 1985). (Weithorn, 1988; Lerman, 1991).

Weithorn argues that psychiatric hospitalization for youth is minimally regulated by statute or administrative procedures by most states. A challenge to a civil commitment of a minor by parents, without a due process hearing, was struck down by the U.S. Supreme Court in 1979 (*Parham v. J.R.*). The Court held that all that was required was an informal review of the parent's request by a physician functioning as a "neutral fact finder." The decision has been sharply criticized as being based on dubious assumptions about the impartiality of medical opinions paid for by parents, the benign nature of mental hospitals, the consequences of hospitalization, and the utility of third-party review (Melton, 1984). Weithorn (1988) criticizes the decision as being unaware of the harmful impact on the physical and emotional well-being of children. She refers specifically to an array of risks linked to hospitalization that have been documented in the literature: feelings of powerlessness and helplessness, stigma, heavy doses of psychiatric medication, invasion of privacy, loss of self-control, and restrictions on normal activities and liberty. Besides the inherent risks and restrictiveness of psychiatric hospitalization,

Weithorn also summarizes several studies that question the efficacy of hospitalization in comparison to less restrictive alternatives.

Given the high risks and questionable efficacy associated with psychiatric hospitalization, Weithorn (1988) argues that a state juvenile commitment statute should be drawn up so that mental hospitals would be defined as an "option of last resort." Instead, there would be enacted a "statutory presumption against institutional alternatives." This standard would be worded to accomplish the following:

> Those seeking to hospitalize a minor should be required to demonstrate, with clear and convincing evidence, that less restrictive alternatives are inappropriate, and that hospitalization is likely to provide resources or approaches that are necessary to treat the problem and are available only in the hospital setting, or are essential in the present or immediate future, to protect the physical safety of the individual or others. Demonstration that less restrictive alternatives are not appropriate should include documentation of those alternatives that were tried and were shown to be unsuccessful. Only in a situation of imminent danger to the child or others should this requirement be waived, and then only until an imminent danger subsides. (p. 833)

It would be expected that a judicial or administrative panel hearing would use the statutory presumption and the facts of the case to assess all psychiatric hospitalization. Weithorn cites Connecticut and Virginia statutes as examples of states in which evidence must be presented that less restrictive alternatives to mental hospitalization are not appropriate.

The use of a statutory presumption standard could also be applied to civil removal of children and youth for 24 hours or more by child welfare authorities and judicial hearings of removal for juvenile status offenses. The use of such a standard could provide a balance of consideration in assessing the potential harm of a placement *prior to* a nonemergency removal and the potential harm to self or others by remaining in the current residence. If this standard were applied at entry and then coupled with the New Jersey statutory standard of defining inappropriate placements as instances of abuse and neglect, the policy of child protection could gain two potentially potent tools to promote a child protection policy.

Expanding the Definition of Abuse and Neglect to Institutions

The original definitions of child abuse and neglect were constructed to deal with intrafamilial incidents of maltreatment of minors. As interested persons, and even observers, became aware that abuse and neglect also occurred in the places designated as sites of protection, treatment, and safe custody, they also became aware that current definitions were inadequate. Critics claimed that statutory definitions were being "stretched" to accommodate the concern about behaviors in out-of-home placements (Rindfleisch & Rabb,

1984b; Nunno & Motz, 1988; U.S. Senate Subcommittee on Child and Human Development [Senate Hearings], 1979, pp. 250–275). The tolerance levels for permissible physical, social, and emotional behaviors in out-of-home placements were held to be much narrower than what might be the acceptable range for parents and relatives of children (Nunno & Motz, 1988).

One of the earliest staff guides for preventing child abuse and neglect in institutions, by Harrell and Orem (1980), argued that parental discretion in raising children and utilizing disciplinary measures was much broader then the discretion permitted under authority of the state in child placements. In addition, the responsibilities of government for meeting explicit standards of child care and adequacy concerning childrearing practices were greater than those applied to parents. For example, corporal punishment and deprivation of food as types of punishment by parents are not against the law in most states, but these techniques of discipline would be considered quite inappropriate if used in schools, day care facilities, or out-of-home placements. As of 1989, a survey of state child protection service liaisons to local agencies indicated that a majority of states had still not changed their statutes to clearly distinguish institutional child abuse and neglect as distinguishable from intrafamilial definitions (Rindfleisch & Nunno, 1992).

If states articulated precise statutory definitions of out-of-home abuse and neglect, as was done in North Dakota, Wyoming, New York, and Ohio, the task of dealing with instances of maltreatment could be made easier. Distinct statutory definitions could, according to knowledgeable observers, accomplish the following: (1) ease the task of enforcement for licensing and abuse/neglect investigative units, (2) provide clearer standards of behavior for residential administrators to educate and socialize child care staff regarding impermissible behaviors, and (3) also clearly notify foster parents that even though they are not members of a residential staff they, too, are obliged to refrain from using disciplinary measures that are permitted to be used by parents (Rindfleisch & Nunno, 1992).

In the absence of clear statutory distinctions, it is also unlikely that incidents will be reported and tabulated in a central registry. As of 1989, only 21 of 50 states were able to provide reports on out-of-home complaints of abuse or neglect. However, of the 21, only 15 were able to verify whether the complaints were substantiated (Rindfleisch & Nunno, 1992, Table 1). Until states are willing to identify the problem, maintain records, and publicly report their results, it would be difficult to ascertain whether progress was being made in dealing with the problem.

Upgrade Licensing Statutes to Include Quality Assurance Standards

A 1980–1981 survey of licensing statutes identified several areas that could improve the capabilities of state licensing organizations to regulate out-of-home residence. Three recommendations that may still be valid in the 1990s are as follows:

1. Eliminate exemptions, which exist in many states, from licensing of facilities and/or homes that house children;
2. Require each facility, as a condition of becoming licensed, that specific written policies and procedures exist pertaining to the identification, investigation, and reporting of suspected cases of abuse and neglect; and
3. Require written disciplinary policies, with precise prohibitions (with examples) of measures that are instances of abuse and neglect (Rindfleisch, 1984).

The case for improving public regulation and licensing of child care and treatment facilities has usually relied on more than a century of experience in investigating and monitoring institutional facilities (Bremner, Barnard, Hareven, & Mennel, 1971). A recent study, in the field of child day care, provides empirical support for the belief that stringent licensing standards and regulations, if backed up by enforcement or voluntary compliance, can influence the quality of a facility's environment. Local social environments in five states were positively influenced by regulations and standards compliance, so that children were much less likely to be treated harshly by day care providers (Phillips, Howes, & WhiteBook, 1992). The empirical findings that regulatory policies can influence the humane treatment of children indicates that a further specification of the nonphysical features of program standards can contribute to the humane quality of child care environments.

Besides incorporating the regulatory improvements suggested by Rindfleisch, a broad child protection prevention policy might want to emphasize the addition of standards of quality for health, education, nutrition, and other developmental needs of children. For example, Combs-Orme, Chernoff, and Kager (1991) recently reviewed studies of the health status of children in foster care and present an astonishing image of basic deficiencies. According to their assessment of the literature, the following facts can be documented:

1. At least 75% of America's foster children have significant health problems;
2. Foster children have high rates of developmental delay, dental problems, growth problems, and mental health difficulties;
3. Recommended schedules for well-child care are not followed for many foster children;
4. In many cases, health problems of foster children go unrecognized by case workers and foster parents;
5. When problems are detected, timely referrals may not be made for assessment or diagnosis; and

6. Timely compliance with treatment recommendations after diagnosis may also be a problem.

Until recent court decisions against state departments and individual caseworkers, there were few explicit policies pertaining to basic standards of health care for foster children. The first judicial recognition of foster child-health care issues emerged in *G.L. v. Zumwalt* (1983, discussed in Mnookin & Weisberg, 1988). Voluntary organizations have attempted to formulate standards (e.g., the American Academy of Pediatrics and the Child Welfare League), but public statutory policies "remain poorly defined and vary among communities in terms of the types of services that are mandated, how and when those services must be delivered, and the type of documentation that is required" (Combs-Orme et al., 1991, p. 166). In addition, the primary health care financing for foster care children, Medicaid, has been found to be "inadequate for promoting health care utilization" (Combs-Orme et al., 1991, p. 166).

Given these problems, the child welfare field can expect legal advocates to file additional class action suits at a state level or even in a federal court. One legal scholar has recently included the "woeful inadequacy" of medical care for foster children as part of a case for the "constitutional protection of foster children from abuse and neglect" from child welfare agencies that are derelict in meeting minimum professional standards (Mushlin, 1988). Rather than wait for court decrees, it would be appropriate to pass statutes requiring health care services to be available to out-of-home children who meet the standards of medical service set forth by the Academy of Pediatrics and the American Dental Association, and that they be available on a priority basis at all times. Quality assurance units within licensing organizations— independent of the placement units—could be mandated to operate utilization and peer reviews, using adequately kept records and observation, to monitor compliance. Combs-Orme et al. (1991) report that even the simple availability of 24–hour telephone consultations, continuity of medical providers, and reduced waiting times for appointments increased the utilization of health care in inner-city neighborhoods. Comparable progress might also be made for foster care children if policies and enforcement mechanisms monitored the implementation of basic standards of health care quality.

The expansion of licensing mandates and monitoring mechanisms would, of course, require increased staff if the quality standards were to be seriously enforced. The inclusion of community-based foster care placements would be expected, but the experience of the past decade has documented that the number of licensing staff positions has not kept pace with the expansion in the number and variety of placement types (Senate Hearings, 1979, pp. 551–558). To do a decent job in monitoring public standards of care requires a recognition of staffing ratios to the number of placement types and a concomitant flow of public funds. Although quality assurance of decent health care availability and utilization by out-of-home children may be costly, it is difficult to conceive of a preventive child protection policy that does not include health as an integral part of promoting the welfare of youth.

Enforcement of Institutional Abuse Standards

The enforcement of institutional abuse standards involves consideration of at least five issues: (1) scope of enforcement jurisdiction, (2) independence of the investigation, (3) protection of "whistleblowers," (4) making judgments about substantiation, and (5) assessing the results of investigation. Each is discussed here.

Scope of Enforcement Jurisdiction

Since the publication of federal regulations in 1987, out-of-home care has been defined as including family day care, group day care, and center-based day care, as well as 24-hour residential-type homes and facilities (*Federal Register*, 1987). States also have the option of including other child care settings, including public and private day schools, summer camps, after-school programs, and even transportation on school buses. One state's Institutional Abuse Investigation Unit (IAIU) (New Jersey), often cited as an exemplar of child protection enforcement, includes all these out-to-home settings as within the scope of a definition of institution and, therefore, receives complaints alleging abuse or neglect from all of these sources (Rindfleisch & Nunno, 1992; McCoy & Manon, 1989).

An expansive definition, when it occurs in a leading state such as New Jersey, can have an enormous impact on the workload of an investigative agency. For example, in 1990, New Jersey's IAIU received 1,984 allegations that required an official inquiry and determination of whether maltreatment actually occurred (using a "preponderance of evidence" standard) (Sec. 601). The 1990 reports of institutional abuse (McCoy & Manon, 1991) were distributed as follows:

	No.	%
Child day care/day camp	312	15.7
Day schools/public or private	857	43.2
Bus companies	119	6.0
Residential/group homes	329	16.6
All other resid. facilities	367	18.5
Total	1,984	100.0

If a jurisdiction such as New Jersey chooses to include day schools and bus companies as a type of institutional abuse, it must expect the possibility that over 49% of the reports will refer to day schools and the transportation to and from these sites. If these reports were excluded from the count, the count of institutional abuse in 1990 would be 1,008 reports rather than 1,984—a substantial reduction of 976 reports. Further, if our major concern were 24–hour residential facilities, then only 696 reports represented the universe of "institutional" allegations of maltreatment in 1990, and not 1,984. (These reports exclude foster home care.)

It is quite evident that the choice of an institutional definition can have an enormous impact on our image of the extent and location of the problem. Using New Jersey's records over the past decade, it is striking how the inclusion of nonresidential reports can shape our image, over time, of the growth of institutional abuse or neglect.

Table 8.7, Part A, discloses that the total reports of maltreatment increased almost 200% between 1980 and 1985 (from 481 to 1,428), and then increased at a much slower rate for the next 5 years (only 39%). However, the changes were not uniform when type of setting is considered. Day care and day schools recorded the sharpest increases between 1980 and 1985 (268% and 804%, respectively), while the 24–hour residential homes and facilities witnessed a much lower rate of increases from 1980 to 1989 (86% and 56%). As noted, between 1985 and 1990 the total number of reports increased at a more moderate rate than the previous 5 years (39% vs. 199%). However, during this time, day care reports remained virtually the same (a bare 2% increase) and all other residential facilities decreased 13%. Day schools continued to increase, albeit at a lower rate of increase (79%), and residential/group homes increased by 49%.

TABLE 8.7. Reports of Institutional Abuse or Neglect in New Jersey, by Type of Setting for 1980, 1985, 1990

Setting	1980	1985	1990	% change 1980–85	% change 1985–90
A. *Number of reports by setting*					
Day care/day camp	38	306	312	268%	2%
Day schools	53	479	857	804	79
Bus companies	NC	NC	119	NC	NA
Residential/group home	119	221	329	86	49
All other residential facilities	271	422	367	56	–13
Totals	481	1,428	1,984	196	39
B. *Distribution of reports by setting, in percentages for each year*					
Nonresidential (1–3)	19%	55%	65%	(see above)	
All residential (4–5)	81	45	35		
N	(481)	(1,428)	(1,984)		

Note. New Jersey Institutional Child Abuse Project, 1982a, 1982b, 1982c, 1985; New Jersey Bureau of Research, Evaluation and Quality Assurance, 1991. NC = not counted; NA = not applicable.

While we lack decent evidence, it appears improbable that the category "all other residential facilities" has improved its treatment to such an extent that reports have now decreased between 1985 and 1990. This category includes the most secure and restrictive settings in the state: detention centers and training schools, psychiatric units in general hospitals and mental hospitals, and crisis centers and shelters. Unlike the residential/group homes, they are not under contract to receive placements from the state child welfare agency, nor do they received routine visits from case workers. The trend data, by setting, raise the distinct possibility that reports are a function of public visibility, scrutiny, standards of conduct, and willingness to report, as well as the actual misbehavior of adults. The virtual explosion of day care and day school complaints from 1980 to 1985 and the continued rise in day school complaints, when coupled with the reduction in reports of maltreatment in the states most secure facilities, suggest that the changes in official reports are responsive to variables other than just adult misbehavior.

Part B of Table 8.7 provides cogent evidence that nonresidential complaints now comprise nearly two thirds of all the reports of institutional abuse in the state of New Jersey in 1990, compared to less than one fifth in 1980. This shift in the distribution of reports has implications beyond our assessment of the extent and location of the problem of institutional abuse within a state. If the state's IAIU were to deal with all complaints equally, then the acquisition and allocation of resources would influence the distribution of screening, investigating, recording, and remediating all allegations. Without further research, it would be difficult to determine whether fiscal and staff resources have shifted to deal with the preponderance of nonresidential cases. Given the widespread attention by the media to allegations of maltreatment in the most visible sites—day care and day schools—it is quite unlikely that the IAIU has failed to shift more resources toward these sources of complaints in 1990 than occurred in 1980 or 1985.

Understanding the operational scope of jurisdiction of an institutional enforcement unit is critical for interpreting trends and allocation of resources within a county or a state. But it is also important to understand that any inter-state comparisons of institutional abuse and neglect rates over time, or within a time period, is profoundly affected by the definitions employed by each reporting organization. If states follow the lead of New Jersey, and include foster care reports (as of June 17, 1991), as additional "institutional" sources of maltreatment, then the counting, interpretive, and enforcement problems will become even more complex (McCoy & Manon, 1991). In 1990, for example, New Jersey reported that 236 foster parent and 111 adoptive home allegations were substantiated, compared to 107 institutional staff allegations that were substantiated (McCoy & Manon, 1991, Table 2). If these new sources had been included in the 1990 total of institutional substantiated cases, the number would have increased from 107 to 454 affirmed cases—a rise of 324%.

The broad national definition of institutional abuse and neglect, and the discretion of states to enlarge the broad definition, presents advocates, officials, and interested citizens with an array of enforcement choices. Regardless of how a state chooses to define institutional abuse, it is incumbent upon reporters and users of statistical counts to disaggregate the data by setting, so our images of the problem can be congruent with reality, the extent and location of the problems can be identified accurately, and the unintended and intended consequences of our definitional policy choices openly addressed.

Independence of the Investigation

According to federal regulations, states are required to designate an independent agency to receive and investigate reports of the allegations that involve the acts, or failures to act, of an affected agency. However, the operational definitions of independent detachment, as employed by the 50 states, varies a great deal. Rindfleisch and Nunno (1992) found the following approaches used in dealing with this detachment issue:

1. Local child protection agencies are involved in foster care placements and supervision of cases, yet 34 states designate these types of organizations to investigate allegations of maltreatment by foster parents (28 do it alone and 6 do it in cooperation with other official agencies).

2. Local child protection agencies are also directly involved in making residential placements, yet 29 states designate them to investigate institutional abuse and neglect allegations (18 do to alone and 11 do it with other official agencies).

Two national standard-setting agencies, the American Bar Association and the American Public Welfare Association, with the cooperation of the American Enterprise Institute (1987), have recommended that local placement agencies handle only intrafamilial and foster family allegations. They recommended that all other out-of-home care complaints be handled by specialized units of professionals. Although this recommendation would affect the 29 states that have local protection agencies investigate complaints against residential facilities, it would leave untouched the potential conflicts of interest occurring in the 34 states where local agencies investigate their own foster care placement recommendations and supervision of cases. The projected consensus by the standard-setting agencies is, therefore, only a partial solution to the issue of independence of investigation in out-of-home cases. Perhaps the compromise solution was offered in deference to the local agency members interests represented by the American Public Welfare Association.

The 34 states can choose to abide by this recommendation or they can wait until a flagrant case of abuse or neglect in a foster care home is publicized on the front page of local newspapers and the nightly television news broadcasts. When the mass media can publicize the story that the agency investigates its own cases, then states might respond, as New Jersey did. On June 17, 1991, after a foster care case and a local public agency received extensive publicity in the mass media, New Jersey henceforth decided to refer all allegations of foster care maltreatment to the investigative staff under the direction of the statewide IAIU. Perhaps public and political pressure will help to overcome the resistance to impartiality offered by standard-setters who are not always independent of the local agencies.

Protection of "Whistleblowers"

In 1979, when the maltreatment of children in residential facilities surfaced as a national concern, a U.S. Senate subcommittee held hearings (Senate Hearing, 1979). At the hearings, references were made to the importance of encouraging the staff of institutions—who are closest to the everyday operations of residential facilities—to come forward with their direct observations of abuse and neglect. Policymakers recognized that in order to function as "whistleblowers" on maltreatment, employees had to be protected from losing their jobs, being demoted, or experiencing other retribution from the administrators of the offending facility. The hearing chairman, Senator Alan Cranston (D–Cal.), referred to the inclusion of a whistleblower provision in the draft of federal legislation on child protection (Senate Hearings, 1979, p. 163). Although the bill was supported at that time by the U.S. Attorney General's office, it failed to become law before the beginning of a new administration. Since that effort to include federal legal protection for whistleblowers, there has been no federal legislation on this subject (as of 1992).

    States, of course, have the option of enacting legal protection for whistleblowers. The importance of doing so, is supported by empirical research. Rindfleisch (1984) found, in a national survey of supervisors and direct care workers in residential facilities and a survey of local child welfare workers, that residential staff were significantly more likely to be able to recognize the seriousness of examples of child maltreatment than were local child protection staff. Further, they were also more likely to define "serious harms" as instances of potential abuse or neglect than local workers (Rindfleisch, 1984 p. 36). However, the study also found that "willingness to act" was strongly influenced by variables undermining a "commitment to act," defined as loss of job, loss of agency funding, and anger of fellow staff members (Rindfleisch, 1984, pp. 73–74). As Rindfleisch (1984) concluded: "One potentiating condition for translating knowledge that abuse or neglect has occurred is the presence of persons who are willing to take protective action in the face of incurring substantial risks to themselves" (p. 74).

    An example of a state's attempt to protect "whistleblowers" in their role of direct observers and reporters of child abuse or neglect is the enactment by New Jersey of a 1987 amendment to the legislative chapter on "Abandonment, Abuse, Cruelty, and Neglect." In the section on providing "immunity from liability" for making a report, the act was amended as follows:

> A person who reports or causes to report in good faith an allegation of child abuse or neglect pursuant to section 3 of P.L. 1971 c.437 (C.9.6–8.10) and as a result thereof is discharged from employment or in any manner discriminated against with respect to compensation, hire, tenure or terms, conditions or privileges of employment, may file a course of action for appropriate relief. . . .
>
> If the court finds that the person was discharged or discriminated against as a result of the person's reporting an allegation of child abuse or neglect, the court may grant reinstatement of employment with back pay or other legal or equitable relief. (N.J.S.A. Chap. 6, §9.6-8.13)

At this time there appears to be an absence of research on whether whistleblower statutes, comparable to the one enacted in New Jersey, have had an impact on the willingness to act of knowledgeable administrators, supervisors, or staff of residential facilities. Nor is it known whether they have had an impact on nonresidential programs (e.g., day care and day schools). Of course, even in the absence of empirical evidence of effectiveness, it might be considered good public policy to enact a whistleblower statute in order to symbolize a concern about the personal risks to employees, if they function as prosocial defenders of children's rights, and their right not to be subject to occupational maltreatment.

Making Judgments about Substantiation

There is an emerging consensus that out-of-home investigations of abuse and neglect—especially in residential settings—require specialized units of professionals with the "necessary expertise and authority" to make judgments about specific allegations of maltreatment (Rindfleisch & Nunno, 1992; Rindfleisch & Hicho, 1987; Rosenthal et al., 1991). The specific attributes of the expertise required to assess the allegation as substantiated or not is usually not discussed. However, one independent state unit, the IAIU of the Division of Family and Youth Services of New Jersey, has attempted to utilize the "best advice" offered by three sources: (1) The Ohio Department of Human Services, concerning the indicators of institutional abuse or neglect; (2) Cornell University's specification of interviewing techniques to examine potential witnesses; and (3) the American Bar Association's decision-making model for weighing the results of the investigation and making a judgment about the allegation. This "best advice" is integrated into a detailed manual (McCoy & Manon, 1989, revised 1991). Because this state's work is widely respected, the manual's guidelines for conducting and completing investigations is worth summarizing briefly.

Appendix A of the guide contains a reprint of the indicators of child abuse and neglect in institutions set forth by the Ohio Department of Human Services draft manual. The list and discussions of indicators cover the following topics: (1) how to identify a physically abused child, including marks or welts, cuts or scratches, broken bones or skull fractures, bite marks, internal injuries, or scars; (2) how to identify cases of "general abuse," including such disciplinary actions as placing in isolation without monitoring, denial of meals, denial of visiting permission, denial of clothing, and refusal to substitute soiled bedding; (3) how to identify sexual abuse, including instances of rape and sexual intercourse of all types, body manipulation, genital exposure, bestiality, and pornographic activities; (4) how to identify a neglected child, including inadequate or improper supervision that could jeopardize well-being, exposure to dangers by failure to provide basic necessities, and education and health services; (5) how to identify emotional abuse or emotional neglect, including ridicule and degrading words or acts, promoting a negative living environment, and using cruel modes of discipline and punishment; (6) factors that lead to child abuse and neglect by institutions, including inadequate policies and procedures, insufficient or inadequate training of staff, and programming practices; and (7) common situations that can lead to physical and sexual abuse and neglect, including inappropriate techniques used in handling instances of verbal or physical aggression, not breaking up fights, removal of angry staff for "cooling off," and redirecting children not following instructions.

Appendix I of the guide provides instructional tips on interviewing techniques provided by staff of the Family Life Development Center, Cornell University. The Cornell guide covers (1) the interviewing process, emphasizing the solicitation of statements from the victim and witnesses, so a matching of facts can occur and be credibly assessed; (2) guidelines and recommended questions for interviewing the victim, taking into account the victim's age, verbal ability, handicaps, and relationship to the alleged abuser; (3) interviewing the alleged perpetrator, taking into account that the allegation can bear serious consequences; and (4) interviewing appropriate institutional staff, including supervisors, medical staff, and other professionals.

The IAIU manual incorporates a decision-making "matrix" for weighing the evidence secured in the investigation of an allegation of abuse or neglect (authored by Wells, 1985, for the American Bar Association National Legal Resources Center for Child Advocacy and Protection). The IAIU's introductory discussion of decision making and the sections on assessing findings (sections 500 and 600) rely primarily on the work of Wells. The Wells model is based on the assumption that decisions about complex events are influenced by observations, knowledge, and values, and these are "inextricably linked with one's habits of information processing" (McCoy & Manon, 1989, p. 5). Besides acquiring the difficult skills of making accurate descriptions, investigators need to be knowledgeable about facility operations, personnel practices, and child development in order to screen and process information. Investigators are warned to continually test theories with evidence and not be afraid to let go if evidence does not sustain provisional judgments. Supervisors can help train investigators to break down decisions into separate tasks of observation, processing of information for detection of relationships, employing causal inference to determine whether one event actually causes or explains another event, predicting the probability of an event occurring again, and testing whether the accumulated facts support a theory about the allegation (McCoy & Manon, 1989).

It is unknown at this time whether the New Jersey staff, or other units using the Wells/ABA Model of decision making, are more reliable (i.e., consistent) in their judgments about allegations than investigators that are not trained to utilize this method of collecting, processing, and judging information. This suggested model of decision making is ripe for investigation. Efforts to fund research studies of units utilizing these types of aids to decision making could assist the entire field of child protection by actually demonstrating the relative reliability of deploying a systematic method for reaching judgments of maltreatment. The professionalization of investigative work could thereby be enhanced by being supported by a body of verified knowledge.

Assessing the Results of Investigative Decisions

Most reports issued by states that refer to the outcomes of investigations provide only two types of decisions: substantiated or unsubstantiated (e.g., U.S. Advisory Board on Child Abuse and Neglect, 1990, p. 15, referring to the substantiation figures obtained from a 50-state survey analyzed by Daro & Mitchell, 1990). However, in practice, agencies may find that the four-fold classification of decisions, used by the New Jersey IAIU unit, captures the actual judgments of complex legal and social events more precisely:

1. *Substantiated cases.* The allegation is sustained using the legal standard of preponderance of evidence.
2. *Unsubstantiated with concern.* Concern exists that an incident of abuse neglect actually occurred, but the allocation of blame cannot meet the legal standard of preponderance of evidence.
3. *Unsubstantiated without concern.* An incident occurred, as alleged, but the facts do not support the categorization of abuse of neglect.
4. *Unfounded.* The alleged incident did not actually occur as reported, or the allegation was found to be inherently improbable or false (McCoy & Manon, 1989).

If we use only the first decision category, "substantiated," then New Jersey's IAIU work resulted in only 10.1% of the 1,984 allegations classified as "reports substantiated" (MCoy & Manon, 1991, Table 16). However, if we inquire whether any more cases raised "concern" about institutional abuse or neglect, the 1990 data reveal that an additional 40.6% of the cases are legally unsubstantiated but are indicative of concern. In other words, readers of the report can be concerned about 50.7% of the reports, not 10.1%. We know that the state takes the second category, "unsubstantiated with concern," seriously because it often makes recommendations for corrective actions in such cases (and expects compliance). Recommendations for "unsubstantiated with concern" cases included better in-service training on the use of proper restraint techniques, disciplinary actions against staff, changes in policy or procedures to reduce or eliminate the recurrence of the "inappropriate or unjustifiable intervention and/or behavior" (McCoy & Manon, 1989, p. 2). A 1985 study that studied whether facilities actually complied with the recommended "corrective actions" reported a compliance rate of 90% (New Jersey Institutional Child Abuse Project, 1985). Even if this self-report is on the high side, there is cogent evidence that all parties treat the "unsubstantiated with concern" cases quite seriously.

In effect, investigators of institutional abuse or neglect are forced to make three distinct types of critical decisions: (1) Is the allegation baseless or is there merit to the complaint? (2) If there is merit, do the facts support the legal definition of preponderance of evidence? (3) If the legal standard cannot be met, do the total facts warrant social concern by responsible state authorities? It is apparent that just paying attention to a legal concern can mask a reasonable cause for social concern (in a ratio of about 4 to 1, using 1990 New Jersey data). If we pursue this reasonable line of inference, it is also useful to be aware that the rates of legal and social concern can vary by the source of complaint—whether it stems from a nonresidential or residential setting. Legal concern, in New Jersey, is most likely to be associated with the most secure facilities (16.9%) and least likely to be associated with day care programs (7.1%). Social concern without a legal basis (i.e., "unsubstantiated with concern") is highest for bus companies and day schools (48.7% and 48.2%, respectively), whereas it is lowest for day care (28.2%). If we add up the legal concern and the nonlegal social concern to assess the rates of total legal social concern, then New Jersey's official investigation of out-of-home complaints (excluding foster care) reveals the following rank order:

Bus companies	59.6%
Day schools	56.5
Residential/group	48.9
All other residential	48.8
Day care	35.3

The results indicate that schools are associated with the largest amount of concern, whether it be on a bus or inside a school. Conversely, day care facilities rank appreciably lower. The residential facilities generate a total social concern in between schools and day care. While these insights are undoubtedly useful in understanding the extent and location of reports that are of broad concern, it is important to remember that these rates are related to whether incidents are even reported. If out-of-home youth, as well as residential staff, are reluctant to blow the whistle by "snitching," complaints cannot be referred for investigation and decision making.

The Contribution of Advocacy Efforts

In 1984, Rindfleisch completed a 3-year study of "the state of the art of child protection in child welfare institutions and children's protective agencies in the 48 contiguous states" (p. 1). It was the first comprehensive national study of a problem that had existed since the opening of the New York House of Refuge in 1824 but had never been systematically studied on a national level (Pickett, 1969; Bremner et al., 1971). One of the major conclusions of the national study concerned the best case-finding techniques for identifying and ensuring harm-free care. Rindfleisch (1984) concluded the following:

> Providers of care (CPS staff also) are not supportive of the introduction of third parties (advocates) or resident dependent techniques (telephone hotlines or complaint boxes). Providers perceive that residents have needs; they are less likely to affirm residents rights. Harmful acts or omissions are defined as organizational lapses (training/selection problem) rather than as abridgements of residents' rights. A substantial number of respondents in our survey of residential facilities and child protection agencies mistook our request for information about institutional abuse and neglect complaints for complaints about residents' parents. They view themselves as part of the solution, not part of a problem.
>
> The results of the "Willingness to take Protective Action" clearly support the introduction of an advocate as one method to increase the likelihood that harmful events will be recognized and reported. "Administrative Support for Reporting" had negligible effect on the willingness to take protective action. (p. 78)

If a similar survey were conducted in 1994, there is a strong likelihood that a similar conclusion would be written about the introduction of an advocate as a third-party defender of children's rights. Actually, advocacy has occurred throughout our history, albeit on a limited scale and in a sporadic manner, via citizens groups and public exposure in mass media outlets (Bremner et al., 1971). Since the 1960s, the practices of out-of-home residences have come under the scrutiny of the courts and publicly subsidized, full-time advocates attached to specific human service systems. The potential contributions of each new advocacy "method"—legal class action suits and public subsidization of advocates—are worth noting and discussing briefly. In addition, the importance of utilizing research surveys of placed-out children as an advocacy method are discussed.

Class Action Suits as a Method of Advocacy

Ever since the ground-breaking cases of *In re Gault* (1967) in the field of juvenile justice and corrections and *Wyatt v. Stickney* (1971) in the fields of mental illness and developmental disabilities, federal courts have begun to accept the arguments of advocates that the state, functioning *in loco parentis*, or as a guardian, could not be presumed always to be acting in the interests of children or adults experiencing or faced with institutional confinement (Cohen, 1980). Since the early 1970s, federal and state courts have become increasingly receptive to class action suits complaining of the following state-sponsored, or -subsidized, actions in children's residential facilities: solitary confinement and the use of tranquilizing drugs in New York; supervised beatings, indiscriminate use of drugs, and mail censorship in Indiana; use of tear gas, physical abuse, solitary confinement, denial of contact with family and friends, and contacts with case workers and psychologists in Texas; dirty and unsanitary rooms in Oregon; beatings and kicking of children while shackled and hog-tied in Florida; and verbal, physical, and sexual abuse in Oklahoma (Schwartz, 1989, pp. 1–21).

Recently, class action lawsuits on behalf of foster children and against state and local agencies have been successful in gaining enforcement of federal and state statutes promoting the best interests of the child. In 1982, Massachusetts was forced to comply with the foster care requirements of the Child Welfare Act of 1980, by specifically doing the following: (1) reducing case loads to no more than 20 per worker, so that workers could carry out their child protection responsibilities; (2) providing each child with a specific case plan; (3) reviewing a child's foster care status at least every 6 months; and (4) assigning cases to a caseworker within 24 hours (Mnookin & Weisberg, 1988, pp. 452–453). A year later, in Missouri, advocates obtained a legal consent decree that has been described as a "model of this type of decree" (Mushlin, 1988, p. 273). In *G.L. v. Zumwalt* (1983), the decree dealt with 15 distinct aspects of foster care, including the following: caseworker case loads, foster care compensation, medical and dental examinations, selection and supervision of foster homes, and investigation of suspected instances of foster parent abuse and neglect (summarized by Mushlin, 1988, p. 273). For each topic covered by the decree there are specific standards for assessing the performance of the child protective agency. Agency staff must maintain accurate medical records, including a complete medical history, records of dental and eye examinations, and details of the types of inoculations and medications, and have a specific schedule for frequent agency visits of the home (Mushlin, 1988). Mushlin argues that these types of decrees can provide "structural injunctions" for improving services and enforcing standards of care outside the home. Active involvement, over time, of legal counsel (representing the child) in the monitoring of the performance indicators of the decree is deemed imperative.

If citizens groups were able to fund a coordinated legal strategy in order to obtain a series of structural injunctions, as promoted by Mushlin, the foster care systems of the affected states could make progress in reducing the incidence of abuse and neglect and promoting the normal development and rights of children in all types of out-of-home care funded by public subsidies. The pace of the progress would depend not only on the availability of funds and legal resources and talent and the receptivity of the courts, but also on the responsiveness of the defendants of the class action suits, namely states and local human service agencies. In each of the cases discussed in this section, officials complied with the judgments of the court without appealing to the U.S. Supreme Court. If appeals were made in the 1990s, however, the current majority might be receptive to arguments on behalf of the child welfare agencies functioning *in loco parentis*, with restricted state and local budgets. Until that counterstrategy is used and tested at the highest judicial level, the willingness of state and local officials to be "forced" to comply with standards and practices they accept may be an important hidden ingredient of a legal class action strategy.

Subsidizing Child Advocates with Public Funds

In 1975, the federal government enacted the Developmental Disabilities Assistance and Bill of Rights Act, which mandated that each state and territory establish a Protection and Advocacy System for Persons with Developmental Disabilities (PADD) by October 1977 as a condition for receiving a basic state grant allotment. The governor of each state is free to designate one or more programs to serve as part of PADD, but he/she must ensure that the system is independent of the state planning council or "any agency which provides treatment, services, or habilitation to person with developmental disabilities." Agencies designated to provide PADD services must have the ability to pursue legal, administrative, and other remedies to protect the rights of individuals under federal and state statutes. According to the National Association of Protection and Advocacy Systems, a voluntary national organization created by the state and local agencies, PADD activities include the following: (1) investigating, negotiating, or mediating solutions to problems identified by clients, families, or agency representatives; (2) providing technical assistance to attorneys, government agencies, and service providers; (3) providing legal counsel and litigation services to persons or groups unable to obtain legal services; and (4) training advocates, consumers, volunteers, professionals, and other parties (National Association of Protection and Advocacy Systems [National Association], 1991, p. 2).

In 1976, the U.S. Congress appropriated about $1.5 million to fund the activities of PADD, but by 1991 its budget had grown to about $21 million. A federally subsidized PADD now exists in every state, U.S. territory, the District of Columbia, and Puerto Rico. In 1989, PADD investigated 3,947 distinct abuse and neglect cases, and in 1990 a total of 3,320 (National Association, 1991, p. 3). However, a number of these cases involved class action suits, so the numbers affected by the allegations are substantially larger than the annual case counts of maltreatment investigations. For example, in 1990, the Wyoming PADD filed a class action suit against the state alleging abuse and neglect at the state's only institution for persons with mental retardation; Wyoming lists 8 abuse and neglect cases (National Association, 1991, pp. 7, 38), but there are 97 residents in the state school (National Association, 1991, p. 29). The New York PADD investigated 279 reports of abuse/neglect involving children, but it is unknown how many other persons were affected. In 1990, a total of 2,280 cases went to full litigation on behalf of PADD clients throughout the nation.

In 1986, the federal government mandated (Protection and Advocacy for Mentally Ill Individuals Act of 1986 [PAMII Act]) a comparable system for the field of mental health—Protection and Advocacy for Persons with Mental Illness (PAMII). PAMII engages in activities comparable to PADD. Federal funds for PAMII grew from $9.5 million in 1986 to $15.6 million in 1989 (PAMII Act, p. 3). In 1989, PAMII investigated 6,692 abuses cases and 11,575 neglect cases—a total of 18,267 reports; in 1991, the figures were 8,342 for abuse and 12,897 for neglect—a total of 21,342 (PAMII Act, p. 4). Investigations involved physical and sexual assaults, guardianship complaints, overmedication, neglect in treatment and care, inappropriate restraints and seclusion, and other allegations—including client deaths.

Given the precedents of the federal authorization and funding of PADD and PAMII activities for two vulnerable populations (of all ages), it appears reasonable to propose that similar programs with federal subsidies could be authorized for child and youth. If the legislation were targeted to address children and youth at risk of out-of-home placements and residences, the programs could remain focused on 1–1.4 million children on an annual basis (see section on Estimates of Youth at High Risk). While the proposed Protection and Advocacy System for Children and Youth (PACHY) could have specific targets, it could have a mandate to cover *all* systems dealing with children, with a primary focus on child welfare, juvenile corrections, and mental health.

Prior to promoting specific legislation and implementing mechanisms for PACHY activities, it be would useful to be aware of the strengths and limitations of PADD and PAMII. One recent study of PADD efforts to deal with the investigations of abuse and neglect can provide initial insight into issues that might need to be addressed if a comparable protection and advocacy system were inaugurated on a national scale for children and youth. Zuckerman, Abrams, and Nuehring (1986) found that PADD offices vary in the statutory authority undergirding their activities. For some state the federal statute is the sole authority; in other states, a specific state law was also passed; in still others an administrative rule or executive order was issued to define the PADD goals, powers, and position within the formal structure of the state government. Some PADD organizations are located in the governor's office; others contract with private, nonprofit, legal rights organizations; and still others have established offices in autonomous state agencies (Zuckerman et al., 1986, p. 197).

In a questionnaire to which 43 states responded, Zuckerman et al. (1986) found that the size of the budgets varied by a wide margin, because some states supplemented federal funds. Federal funds are allocated on the basis of population, extent of need by the PADD population, and financial need of the state (Developmental Disabilities Assistance Act, 1986). The average annual budget was about $254,000, but the range was from less than $100,000 for 13 states to $1.2 million for one state and an average annual budget of about $739,000 for 5 states. About 86% of the directors surveyed rated their current budgets as very inadequate (54%) or not adequate (32%). Given these restrictive resources, the majority of agencies allocated less than one full-time equivalent to assessing abuse and neglect problems in residential facilities (Zuckerman et al., 1986, pp. 198–199).

The major barrier to PADD activities was identified as a lack of legal authority to gain access to clients or to records located in residential facilities unless help was requested by a resident or interested party seeking assistance for the resident. Twenty-four of the 43 states participating in the survey (56%) cited this impediment; they were forced to undertake "joint investigations with agencies vested with investigative privileges" (Zuckerman et al., 1986, p. 199). They also cited other barriers: (1) fears of staff or parents, (2) organizational opposition, (3) prejudicial attitudes toward the rights of the disabled, and (4) inadequate staff and resources.

Additional studies of PADD and PAMII agencies—with different organizational locations, budget sizes, and legal authority—could enhance our knowledge of this federally subsidized mechanism as a prototype for a PACHY effort. Meanwhile, citizen advocacy groups might begin to consider how $15.6 million to $21 million of federal funds might be captured for proactive efforts on behalf of children and youth at risk of out-of-home placement or living in substitute-care residences.

Using Research Surveys in the Service of Advocacy

Many studies of abuse and neglect in out-of-home settings have reported on the difficulty of obtaining the cooperation of staff. But another large group that is reluctant to penetrate the "conspiracy of silence" are the youthful victims and witnesses of abuse and neglect (Harrell & Orem, 1980, pp. 36–47). Besides the fear of retribution by threatening or powerful adults, many youth are loathe to "snitch" or "squeal," even if it is on their own behalf, because of threats from peers (New Jersey Institutional Child Abuse Project, 1985, p. 10). While continual efforts to gain the trust and confidence of children and youth are worthwhile, there are distinct services that researchers can perform to identify and document settings and/or persons who are perceived to permit, condone, or practice abuse and neglect.

A recent survey by Fanshel, Finch, and Grundy (1989a, 1989b), of 106 former foster care children followed up in their adult years (for the Casey Foundation in Washington State) revealed some startling data: Of 45 girls interviewed in the follow-up, 11 girls (24%) said they had been "sexually molested in their Casey foster homes or reported being aware of another Casey child in the same home being molested" (Fanshel et al., 1989a, 1989b, p. 474). The foster father was identified as the source of abuse in most cases. Of the 61 boys followed up, 5 boys were molested. These figures are a prevalence figure over the "career" of the 106 foster children, so we do not know the proportion of new cases (i.e., the incidence) that occurs each year, or how many separate incidents occurred over the career. In addition to sexual abuse, Fanshel et al. (1989b) learned about even more incidents of physical abuse. They concluded that "children need access to a private and available source to make complaints of abusive conditions in the home" (p. 474). They supported their recommendation with the following information gained from the 106 interviews:

> While constituting a minority of the subjects, those who did not fare well in foster care placements in the program were quite vocal and often biting in their criticisms. In addition to molestation, their complaints about their foster families were varied and included physical abuse, harsh discipline, favored treatment of their own children, unrealistic expectations of what the subject could accomplish, and sheer incapacity to understand troubled children . . . Some subjects commented that meetings with the social worker in the presence of a foster parent did not allow them to speak freely, with fear of removal from the home being a matter of deep concern. Criticism was also presented that their social workers did not deal with core issues in their lives, such as their feelings about loss of their parents, their difficulty in getting over a disrupted adoption, and their dealing with expectations of their foster parents. (p. 474)

Fanshel et al. recommend that children in foster care be available for an interview with a "children's representative." They did not discuss who the representative might work for, and report to, but it seems quite reasonable to integrate this role into the proposed PACHY. However, because children would still be residing in a foster home or residential facility, they might be wary of being forthcoming with a PACHY representative. An additional method for securing the views of those in placement is to rely on a retrospective approach. Fanshel et al. (1989b) suggest that "all agencies should make efforts to provide feedback" (p. 475). This suggestion is also worth following up and incorporating into the ongoing capabilities of PACHY—both for quality assurance and for potential investigative purposes.

In order to capture the feedback of children and youth, it would be imperative that the work not be performed by amateurs but rather by competent survey researchers functioning with autonomy from any service organization. Rather than set up the unrealistic goal of expecting all agencies to conduct follow-ups, it would probably be more realistic to undertake this research function as a legitimate responsibility of the public sector, to make sure that subsidies are not promoting adverse experiences for children and youth. This responsibility could be accomplished by stratified random sampling of youth leaving specific types of out-of-home placements. Because turnover in placements is quite high, the respondents would still be youthful.

The retrospective follow-ups would involve little or no threat to the youthful respondents, but they could be asked to provide consent for the information to be used for the purposes of remedying an abusive or neglectful setting. Policies and procedures governing the request of consent from youthful respondents could be guided by the extensive thought and effort that the field of psychology has already devoted to issues of competency to understand issues of custody, testimony, voluntary treatment, and informed consent (Repucci, Weithorn, Mulvey, & Monahan, 1984).

The use of survey research to provide information for the purposes of quality assurance and child protection would constitute new activities for most researchers. Pilot projects might be funded in order to determine how best to obtain relevant information in an understandable and efficient format, and also how best to report and utilize negative reports that pass the threshold of credible allegations. From an ethical perspective, if the potential use of confidential material is openly discussed with the respondents and permission is obtained to pursue their reports, researchers should be able to create a valuable role within a protection and advocacy system.

Summary and Conclusions

Earlier sections of this chapter focused on describing and critically assessing system reforms that indicated that out-of-home placements could be reduced, particularly in the most secure types of facilities. These system reforms were viewed as part of a broader prevention effort for reducing abuse and neglect in out-of-home placements. A summary and conclusions for promising system reforms in the fields of mental health, child welfare, and juvenile corrections can be found at the end of these sections.

This final section focused on improving existing efforts to regulate the out-of-home residences that are used when prevention efforts are perceived to have failed in dealing with individual or family problems. A major issue is the statutory standards that mandate the use of the most restrictive facilities only as a last resort, when all other efforts have been thoroughly exhausted. Borrowing from the work of Weithorn (1988), this last section discussed a "statutory presumption" against restrictive placements in psychiatric hospitals, residential treatment centers, and locked correctional facilities. This statutory presumption standard is based on the reasonable assumption that the potential risk of abuse and neglect increases with the restrictiveness of the residence. Further, there is an absence of an empirical basis, using an effectiveness criterion, for using these types of residences over less restrictive alternatives.

A second area of regulatory improvement can occur if states legislatively recognize that standards of behavior by foster parents and residential staff and administrators are much narrower than those permitted to parents and close relatives. The public sector cannot tolerate slaps, restrictions, and ridicule that may be allowed to parents by current concepts of childrearing and legal standards of familial abuse. Therefore, there has been a consistent effort by knowledgeable persons to have states give up "stretching" traditional definitions of abuse and neglect and to provide amendments that specify the narrower boundaries that are impermissible in out-of-home residences.

A third area focused on upgrading licensing practices regarding out-of-home placements. Besides the usual focus on physical standards of varied residences, licensing statutes and regulations could be expanded to include health standards and practices as significant requirements to meet in order to gain or renew a license. The national data on the poor health of children in foster care highlight the necessity of taking much stronger action in this area than is currently occurring in many communities throughout the country.

A fourth area focused on enhancing protection by improvements in enforcement. The need to create and maintain an independent unit to investigate allegations of out-of-home abuse and neglect is now widely recognized, but the practices of many states indicate that the separation of placement and investigatory powers is still not sufficiently distinct in practice. In states in which independence between services and enforcement of allegations has been established, the possibility exists that the scope of jurisdiction of the investigative units has been broadened far beyond the original definitions of institutional abuse to include public and private day schools, day care, camps, and bus companies. While these nonhome organizations may require scrutiny, there is evidence that they receive much more attention than the more restrictive, 24-hour out-of-home facilities that were the original targets of public concern. In an exemplary state, like New Jersey, two thirds of the complaints received by the state's institutional abuse investigation units are devoted to nonresidential types of child care organizations (i.e., schools, day care, and bus companies). Instead of the problem of stretching family definitions of abuse and neglect, we are witnessing a stretch of institutional definitions to cover nonresidential facilities—and, thereby, minimizing the allocation of resources to the primary targets of abuse and neglect.

Improvement of enforcement also requires a greater amount of statutory protection on a national and state level to protect the employment benefits, rights, and privileges of persons functioning as whistleblowers of unacceptable practices and behaviors. A national statute could symbolize that America is as concerned about child maltreatment occurring with federal welfare funds as we are about military contract malfeasance occurring with defense department funds.

Experience with more than a decade of separate institutional abuse investigation units has highlighted the unique types of expertise required to perform the complex tasks of data gathering and decision making. Studies are needed to assess the reliability and usefulness of training investigators to use specific indicators of institutional abuse and neglect, interviewing techniques to assembl_ facts, and a decision-making model for making judgments about the facts that could substantiate the allegations.

The experience of an exemplary investigative unit discloses that the enforcement field needs to address two types of substantiation of allegations: legal and social. Legal substantiation refers to an allegation being supported by facts that can meet a statutory standard of preponderance of evidence (or a comparable legal standard). However, there are many allegations that do not meet a technical legal standard, but the facts are sufficient to evoke a social concern that remedial action should be recommended (with implicit threats of subsidy withdrawals or licensing citations). Actions that are legally unsubstantiated but trigger a social concern can occur at a ratio of about 4 to 1. It would be prudent to openly address the distinction between a legal and social concern about institutional forms of abuse and neglect and articulate the evidentiary standards that distinguish the two types of concerns. This conceptual and regulatory distinction will become even more important as independent institutional abuse units assume the responsibility for assessing the allegations against foster parents. Unlike residential facilities, foster parents lack the resources to contest a legal definition of concern. To be fair to foster parents, the standards using both legal and social concerns for their residence should be similar to those used in assessing the more powerful residential organizations.

The final area of regulatory improvement pertains to the expansion of advocacy efforts on behalf of children by supporting the following: (1) class action suits that can monitor and enforce national and state legislative standards pertaining to out-of-home placements, (2) federal subsidization of protection and advocacy systems for children and youth that are comparable to what has already been done for the developmentally disabled and mentally ill, and (3) survey research efforts that systematically interview random samples of youth leaving all types of out-of-home placements used by a community. All three protection and advocacy efforts could prove useful in overcoming the documented resistance of placement organizations and service providers to monitor and enforce public standards pertaining to out-of-home care, treatment, and custody. The threat of legal action has proven useful in all of the fields associated with children and youth services. The subsidized support of these efforts, as well as negotiations, by third-party, independent protection and advocacy systems has also been documented.

Survey research efforts would be a new departure for monitoring the quality and regulatory standards of all types of out-of-home placements. Besides proving useful for upgrading practices and identifying persons and settings associated with maltreatment, these survey efforts could provide baselines for measuring improvement in our efforts to protect children and youth. Competent social science researchers added to the array of experts necessary to protect children and youth could only realize their potential if they are employed by independent advocacy organizations. Given the potential for researchers to contribute to quality assurance, child protection, and the evaluation of our regulatory efforts, a good case can be made for including these activities as a national requirement for obtaining child welfare, mental health, and juvenile justice funds from the federal government. An effort to generate improvements in child protection by obtaining information from the primary sources—youth experiencing the benign intentions of public authorities—could prove to be the most strategic recommendation contained in this chapter.

REFERENCES

American Bar Association, American Enterprise Institute, & American Public Welfare Association. (1987). *Child abuse and neglect reporting and investigation: Policy guidelines for decision making* (J. Besharov, Rapporteur). Washington, DC: Authors.

American Psychiatric Association. (1987). *Diagnostic and statistical manual of mental disorders* (3rd ed., rev.). Washington, DC: Author.

Attkisson, C., Dresser, K., & Rosenblatt, A. (1991). *Service systems for yough with severe emotional disorders: System of care in research in California.* San Francisco: University of California, Institute for Mental Health Services Research, San Francisco.

Au Claire, P., & Schwartz, I. (1986). *An evaluation of the effectiveness of intensive home-based services as an alternative to placement for adolescents and their families.* Minneapolis: University of Minnesota, Hubert Humphrey Institute of Public Affairs.

Austin, J., Elms, W., Krisberg, B., & Steele, P. (1991). *Unlocking juvenile corrections: Evaluating the Massachusetts Department of Youth Services.* San Francisco: National Council on Crime and Delinquency.

Barton, W., Streit, S., & Schwartz, I. (1991). *A blueprint for corrections.* Ann Arbor, MI: Center for the Study of Youth Policy.

Behar, L. 1985. Changing patterns of state responsibility: A case study of North Carolina. *Journal of Clinical Child Psychology, 14,* 188–195.

Behar, L. (1986). A model for child mental health services: The North Carolina experience. *Children Today, 15,* 16–21.

Behar, L. (1991). *Close to home: Community based mental health for children.* Raleigh, NC: North Carolina Division of Mental Health/Developmental Disabilities.

Besharov, D. (1983). Child protection: Past progress, present problems, and future directions. *Family Law Quarterly,* (2), 151–172.

Bremner, R., Barnard, J., Hareven, T., & Mennel, R. (Eds.). (1971). *Children and youth in America: Documentary history* (3 vols.). Cambridge, MA: Harvard University Press.

Bruner, C. (1989). *Is change from above possible? State-level strategies for supporting street-level services.* Paper presented to the Association for Public Policy Analysis and Management Eleventh Annual Research Conference, Des Moines, Iowa.

Burchard, J., & Clarke, R. (1990). The role of individualized care in a service delivery system for children and adolescents with severely maladjusted behavior. *Journal of Mental Health Administration, 17*(1), 48–60.

Burns, B., & Friedman, R. (1990). Examining the research base for child mental health services and policy. *Journal of Mental Health Administration, 17*(1), 87–98.

Butts, J., & Streit, S. (1988). *Youth correction research: The Maryland and Florida experience.* Ann Arbor University of Michigan School of Social Work, Center for the Study of Youth Policy.

Child Welfare Act, 42 U.S.C. §675 (1980).

Child Welfare League of America. (1963). *Standards for services of child welfare institutions* (Report of the Committee on Standards for Residential Group Care). New York: Author.

Child Welfare League of America. (1988). *Standards for services to abused and neglected children and their families.* Washington, DC: Author.

Coates, R., Miller, A., & Ohlin, L. (1978). *Diversity in a youth correctional system: Handling delinquents in Massachusetts.* Cambridge, MA: Ballinger.

Cohen, F. (1987). *The law of deprivation of liberty: A study in social control—Cases and materials.* St. Paul, MN: West.

Combs-Orme, T., Chernoff, R., & Kager, V. (1991). Utilization of health care by foster children: Application of a theoretical model. *Child and Youth Services Review, 13,* 113–129.

Cornsweet, C., Rosenblatt, A., Harris, L., & Attkisson, C. (1991). *Use of mental health services among severely emotionally disturbed children and adolescents in San Francisco.* San Francisco: University of California, Institute for Mental Health Services Research, San Francisco.

Dembo, R., Williams, L., LaVoie, L., Berry, L., Getreu, A., Wish, E., Schmeidler, J., & Washburn, M. (1989). Physical abuse, sexual victimization and illicit drug use: Replication of a structural analysis. *Violence and Victims, 4,* 121–138.

Developmental Disabilities Assistance and Bill of Rights Act, 42 U.S.C. §6010 (1984).

Elmore, R. (1978). Organizational models of social program implementation. *Public Policy, 26,* 185–228.

Elmore R. (1979). Backward mapping; Implementation research and policy decisions. *Political Science Quarterly, 94*(4), 601–616.

Fanshel, D., Finch, S., & Grundy, J. (1989a). Modes of exit from foster family care and adjustment at time of departure of children with unstable life histories. *Child Welfare, 68*(4), 391–402.

Fanshel, D., Finch, S., & Grundy, J. (1989b). *Foster children in life-course perspective: The Casey Family Program experience. Child Welfare, 68*(5), 467–478.

Federal Register. (1987). Final rules Part 1340—Child abuse and neglect prevention. 45 C.F.R. ch. XIII.

Feldman, L. H. (1991). Evaluating the impact of intensive family preservation services in New Jersey. In K. Wells & D. Biegel (Eds.), *Family preservation services: Research and evaluation* (pp. 47–71). Newbury Park, CA: Sage.

Friedman, R. (1987). *Service capacity in a balanced system of services for seriously emotionally disturbed children.* Unpublished manuscript. University of South Florida, Florida Mental Health Institute, Tampa.

Gault, In re, 387 U.S. 1 (1967).

G. L. v. Zumwalt, 564 F. Supp. 1030 (W. D. Mo. 1983).

Harrell, S., & Orem, R. (1980). *Preventing child abuse and neglect: A guide for staff in residential institutions* (DHHS Publication No. OHDS 80-30255). Washington, DC: U.S. Government Printing Office.

Institute of Medicine. (1989). Research on children and adolescents with mental, behavioral, and development disorders. Washington, DC: National Academy of Sciences.

Joint Commission on Mental Health of Children. (1969). *Crisis in child mental health: Challenge for the 1970s.* New York: Harper & Row.

Jordan, D., & Hernandez, M. (1990). The Ventura Planning Model: A proposal for mental health reform. *Journal of Mental Health Administration, 17*(1), 26–47.

Kassar, D. (1991). *Iowa Child Welfare Decategorization Project.* Des Moines, Iowa: Iowa Department of Human Services/Adult, Children, and Family Services. (Application submitted to Harvard University Innovations in State and Local Government 1991 Awards Program, JFK School of Government)

Lengyel, M. (1990). Foster child abuse in Pennsylvania: Pursuing actions against the county placement agency. *Dickinson Law Review, 94,* 501–526.

Lerman, P. (1968). Evaluating institutions for delinquents. *Social Work, 13,* 55–64.

Lerman, P. (1975). *Community treatment and social control.* Chicago: University of Chicago Press.

Lerman, P. (1982). *Deinstitutionalization and the welfare state.* New Brunswick, NJ; Rutgers University Press.

Lerman, P. (1990). *Counting youth in trouble living away from home* [mimeograph]. Ann Arbor, MI: Center for the Study of Youth Policy, School of Social Work.

Lerman, P. (1991). Counting youth in trouble in institutions: Bringing the United States up to date. *Crime and Delinquency, 37*(4), 465–480.

Linney, A. (1984). Deinstitutionalization in the juvenile justice system. In N. Repucci, E. Mulvey, & J. Monahan (Eds.), *Children, mental health, and the law* (pp. 211–282). Beverly Hills, CA: Sage.

Maguire, K., & Flanagan, T. (Eds.). (1991). *Sourcebook of criminal justice statistics, 1990.* Washington, DC: U.S. Department of Justice, Bureau of Justice Statistics.

Maluccio, A., & Marlow, W. (1972). Residential treatment of emotionally disturbed children: A review of the literature. *Social Service Review, 46,* 230–251.

Milazzo-Sayre, L., Benson, P., Rosenstein, M., & Manderscheid, R. (1986, April).

Use of inpatient psychiatric services by children and youth under age 18, United States, 1980. *Mental Health Statistical Note No. 175*. Washington, DC: Department of Health and Human Services.

McCoy, P. J., & Manon, S. M. (1989, April). *The management and investigation of institutional abuse cases*. Trenton, NJ: New Jersey Institutional Child Abuse Project, Division of Youth and Family Services.

McCoy, P. J., & Manon, S. M. (1991, June 17). *The management and investigation of institutional abuse cases* (rev. for foster care). Trenton, NJ: New Jersey Institutional Child Abuse Project, Division of Youth and Family Services.

McDonald & Associates, Inc. (1990). *Evaluation of AB 1562 in home care demonstration project: Vol. 1. Final report*. Sacramento, CA: Author.

Melton, G. (1984). Family and mental hospital as myths: Civil commitment of minors. In N. Repucci, L. Weithorn, E. Mulvey, & J. Monahan (Eds.), *Children, mental health, and the law*. Beverly Hills, CA: Sage.

Mnookin, R., & Weisberg, D. (1988). *Child, family and state: Problems and materials on children and the law* (2nd ed.). Boston: Little, Brown.

Moran, M. (1991, March 1). Initiatives throughout country bring child MH care home. *Psychiatric News*, pp. 9–17.

Mushlin, M. B. (1988). Unsafe havens: The case for constitutional protection of foster children from abuse and neglect. *Harvard Civil Rights—Civil Liberties Law Review, 23*, 200–280.

National Association of Protection and Advocacy Systems. (1991). *1990 Annual Report on State Programs*. Washington, DC: Author.

National Institute of Mental Health. (1967–1980). *Statistical notes*. Washington, DC: Public Health Service.

New Jersey Bureau of Research, Evaluation and Quality Assurance. (1991, April). *Child abuse and neglect in New Jersey 1990 Annual Report*. Trenton, NJ: Division of Youth and Family Services.

New Jersey Institutional Child Abuse Project. (1982a, June). *Institutional child abuse and neglect: A training guide for child care staff in residential institutions*. Trenton, NJ: Division of Youth and Family Services.

New Jersey Institutional Child Abuse Project. (1982b, July). *Institutional abuse and neglect: A guide for investigators*. Trenton, NJ: Division of Youth and Family Services.

New Jersey Institutional Child Abuse Project. (1982c, September). *Institutional child abuse and neglect in New Jersey: 1978 to 1980*. Trenton, NJ: Division of Youth and Family Services.

New Jersey Institutional Child Abuse Project. (1985). *Contributory factors to child abuse and/or neglect in residential facilities and in other out-of-home child care settings*. Trenton, NJ: Division of Youth and Family Services.

Nunno, M., & Motz, J. (1988). The development of an effective response to the abuse of children in out-of-home care. *Child Abuse and Neglect, 12*, 521–528.

Ohlin, L., Coates, R., & Miller, A. (1977). *Reforming juvenile corrections: The Massachusetts experience*. Cambridge, MA: Ballinger.

Parham v. J. R. 442 U.S. 584 (1979).

Phillips, D., Howes, C., & WhiteBook, M. (1992). The social policy context of child care: Effects on quality. *American Journal of Community Psychology, 20*, 25–51.

Pickett, R. (1969). *House of refuge: Origins of juvenile reform in New York State, 1815–1857.* Syracuse, NY: Syracuse University Press.

President's Commission on Mental Health. (1978). *Task panel reports subcommittee to the President's Commission on Mental Health* (Vols. 1–4). Washington, DC: U.S. Government Printing Office.

Protection and Advocacy for Mentally Ill Individuals Act, 42 U.S.C. § 10801 (1986).

Rabb, J., & Rindfleisch, N. (1985). A study to define and assess severity of institutional abuse/neglect. *Child Abuse and Neglect, 9,* 285–294.

Repucci, N., Weithorn, L., Mulvey, E., & Monahan, J. (1984). *Children, mental health, and the law.* Beverly Hills, CA: Sage.

Rindfleisch, N. (1984). *Identification, management and prevention of child abuse and neglect in residential facilities* (Vol. 1). Columbus, Ohio: Ohio State University Research Foundation.

Rindfleisch, N., & Hicho, D. (1987). Institutional child protection: Issues in program development and implementation. *Child Welfare, 66*(4), 329–342.

Rindfleisch, N., & Nunno, M. (1992). Progress and issues in the implementation of the 1984 Out-Of-Home Care Protection Amendment. *Child Abuse and Neglect, 16,* 693–700.

Rindfleisch, N., & Rabb, J. (1984a). How much of a problem is resident mistreatment in child welfare institutions? *Child Abuse and Neglect, 8,* 33–40.

Rindfleisch, N., & Rabb, J. (1984b). Dilemmas in planning for the protection of children and youth in residential facilities. *Child Welfare, 63*(3), 205–215.

Rosenblatt, A., & Attkisson, C. (1992). Integrating systems of care in California for youth with severe emotional disturbance: A descriptive overview of the California AB 377 Evaluation Project. *Journal of Child and Family Studies, 1,* 93–113.

Rosenthal, J., Motz, J., Edmonson, D., & Groze, V. (1991). A descriptive study of abuse and neglect in out-of-home placement. *Child Abuse and Neglect, 15,* 249–260.

Rutherford, A. (1974). The dissolution of the training schools in Massachusetts. In B. Krisberg, & J. Austin (Eds.), *The children of Ishmael: Critical perspectives on juvenile justice* (pp. 515–534). Palo Alto, CA: Mayfield.

Schlenger, W., Etheridge, R., Hansen, D., & Fairbank, D. (1990). *Alaska CASSP case study report* (Final Report of the CASSP Initial Cohort Study, Vol. II: Individual Case Study Reports). Rockville, MD: National Institute of Mental Health.

Schwartz, I. (1989). *Justice for juveniles: Rethinking the best interests of the child.* Lexington, MA: Heath.

Schwartz, I., & Loughran, E. (1991). *Restructuring youth corrections systems.* Ann Arbor, MI: Center for the Study of Youth Policy, School of Social Work.

Sewall, R. (1990). *Answers from AYI.* Juneau, Alaska: Individualized Services Consulting.

Silver, S. (1990). A comparison of children with serious emotional disturbances served in residential and school settings. *Proceedings of Second Annual Research Conference on Children's Mental Health: Building a Research Base.* Tampa Mental Health Institute.

Stroul, B., & Friedman, R. (1986). A system of care for severely emotionally disturbed youth. Washington, DC: Georgetown University, NIMH Child and Adolescent Service System Program Technical Assistance Center.

Stroul, B., & Goldman, S. (1990). Study of community-based services for children and adolescents who are severely emotionally disturbed. *Journal of the Mental Health Administration, 17*(1), 61–77.

Sunshine, J., Witkin, M., Atay, J., & Manderscheid, R. (1991, January). Psychiatric outpatient care services in mental health organizations, United States, 1986. Mental Health Statistical Note No. 194. Washington, DC: Department of Health and Human Services.

Thomas, G. (1975). *A community oriented evaluation of the effectiveness of child caring institutions* (Final Report to the Office of Child Development of the Department of Health, Education and Welfare). Athens, GA: University of Georgia, Regional Institute of Social Welfare Research.

U.S. Advisory Board on Child Abuse and Neglect. (1990). *Child abuse and neglect: Critical first steps in response to a national emergency.* Washington, DC: U.S. Government Printing Office.

U.S. Advisory Board on Child Abuse and Neglect. (1991). *Creating caring communities.* Washington, DC: U.S. Government Printing Office.

U.S. Bureau of Census. (1988). United States population estimates, by age, sex, and race: 1950 to 1987. *Current Population Reports* (Series P-25, No. 1022). Washington, DC: U.S. Department of Commerce.

U.S. House of Representatives. (1962). *Compilation of the Social Security Laws.* Washington, DC: U.S. Government Printing Office.

U.S. Senate Subcommittee on Child and Human Development. (1979). *Abuse and neglect of children in institutions, 1979* (Hearings before the Subcommittee of the Committee on Labor and Human Resources, United States Senate). Washington, DC: U.S. Government Printing Office.

Van Den Berg, J. (1989). *The Alaska Youth Initiative: Program background.* Juneau, Alaska: Alaska Division of Mental Health and Developmental Disabilities.

Van Den Berg, J., Sewell, R., & Kubley, K. (1991, January). *Executive summary: Annual report on the Alaska Youth Initiative* [mimeograph]. Juneau, AK: Division of Mental Health and Developmental Disabilities, Child and Adolescent Mental Health Services.

Weithorn, L. (1984). Children's capacities in legal contexts. In N. Repucci, L. Weithorn, E. Mulvey, & J. Monahan (Eds.), *Children, mental health and the law* (pp. 25–58). Beverly Hills, CA: Sage.

Weithorn, L. (1988). Mental hospitalization of troublesome youth: An analysis of skyrocketing admission rates. *Stanford Law Review, 40*(3), 773–838.

Wells, K., & Biegel, D. (1992). Intensive family preservation services research: Current status and future agenda. *Social Work Research and Abstracts, 28*(1), 21–27.

Wells, S. (1985). *How we make decisions in Child Protective Services intake and investigation.* Chicago: American Bar Association National Resource Center for Child Advocacy and Protection.

Whittaker, J., & Maluccio, A. (1989). Changing paradigms in residential services for disturbed/disturbing children: Retrospect and prospect. In R. Hawkins & J. Breiling (Eds.), *Therapeutic foster care: Critical issues* (pp. 81–102). Washington, DC: Child Welfare League of America.

Wyatt v. Stickney, 325 F. Supp. 781 (M.D. Ala. 1971).

Young, T., Pappenfort, D., & Marlow, C. (1983). *Residential group care, 1966 and 1981* (Mimeo Preliminary Report). Chicago: University of Chicago School of Social Service Administration.

Zuckerman, M., Abrams, H., & Nuehring, E. (1986). Protection and advocacy agencies: National survey of efforts to prevent residential abuse and neglect. *Mental Retardation, 24*(4), 197–201.

Index

439